3RD EDITION

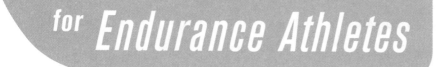

SPORTS NUTRITION

for Endurance Athletes

MONIQUE RYAN, MS, RD, CSSD, LDN

VELO press

BOULDER, COLORADO

Disclaimer

The information in this book is intended for educational and instructional purposes, and is not meant to substitute for the advice provided by your own physician or dietitian.

velopress®

3002 Sterling Circle, Suite 100
Boulder, Colorado 80301-2338 USA
(303) 440-0601 · Fax (303) 444-6788 · E-mail velopress@competitorgroup.com

Distributed in the United States and Canada by Ingram Publisher Services

Library of Congress Cataloging-in-Publication Data
Ryan, Monique, 1962–
Sports nutrition for endurance athletes / Monique Ryan.—3rd ed.
  p. cm.
Includes biographical references and index.
ISBN 978-1-934030-82-0 (pbk.: alk. paper)
1. Athletes—Nutrition. 2. Exercise—Physiological aspects. I. Title.
TX361.A8R95 2011
613.2'024796—dc23

         2011041273

For information on purchasing VeloPress books, please call (800) 811-4210 ext. 2138 or visit www.velopress.com.

This paper meets the requirements of ANSI/NISO Z39.48-1992 (Permanence of Paper).

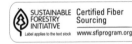
SUSTAINABLE Certified Fiber
FORESTRY Sourcing
INITIATIVE
Label applies to the text stock www.sfiprogram.org

Cover design by *the*BookDesigners
Cover photo by Justin Bastien
Interior design and tables by Erin Johnson
Sweat Calculator design by Charlie Layton
Composition by Chris Davis

Text set in Warnock Pro Light.

12 13 14 / 10 9 8 7 6 5 4 3 2 1

CONTENTS

Preface   vii

Acknowledgments   ix

PART I
YOUR DAILY PERFORMANCE DIET

Optimal Nutrition for Training and Health   I

1   Daily Hydration Essentials: Drinking It In   3

2   Energy Nutrients for Optimal Health and Performance:
Building a Solid Nutrition Base   17

3   Vitamins, Minerals, and Electrolytes:
The Nuts, Bolts, and Spark Plugs of Your Diet   49

PART II
YOUR TRAINING DIET

Fine-Tuning Your Diet for Top Performance   75

4   Your Daily Training Diet: Eating for Optimal Recovery   77

5   Food and Fluid Intake for Training and Competition:
Timing Is Everything   127

6   Weight Loss, Muscle Building, and Changing Body Composition:
Boosting Your Strength-to-Weight Ratio   175

7   Ergogenic Aids: Separating Fact from Fiction   201

PART III
SPORT-SPECIFIC NUTRITIONAL GUIDELINES

Putting Your Sports Nutrition Plan into Action   231

8   Nutrition for Triathlon (and Other Multisport Events)   233

9   Nutrition for Cycling (Road Cycling, Mountain Biking,
Track Cycling, and Cyclocross)   263

10   Nutrition for Distance Running   285

11   Nutrition for Swimming   303

PART IV
SPECIAL NUTRITIONAL CONSIDERATIONS

Meeting and Managing the Challenges   315

12	The Athlete with Unique Nutrition Considerations	317
13	Performance Boosts and Problem-Solving with Nutrition	353
14	Nutritional Strategies for Extreme Environments	365

APPENDIXES

Appendix A	Glycemic Index of Foods	377
Appendix B	Glossary of Vitamins and Minerals	381
Appendix C	Comparison of Sports Nutrition Products	384
Appendix D	Creating the Optimal Training Diet	387
Appendix E	Sample Menus	396
Appendix F	Estimating Sweat Loss—Worksheet	403

Selected Bibliography	405
Index	413
About the Author	421

PREFACE

When the first edition of *Sports Nutrition for Endurance Athletes* was published in 2002, and then the second edition in 2007, triathletes, cyclists, runners, swimmers, and adventure racers devoured the wealth of practical, sport-specific nutritional advice found within its covers. Over the years, it has been rewarding and gratifying to hear from readers, clients, and coaches across North America that the book has been an indispensable tool and resource for their training and race programs. With the burgeoning participation in endurance sports, it seemed not only logical but imperative to write the third edition that you are now holding in your hands. As a dedicated endurance athlete, you take your nutrition plans very seriously, and whether this book has found you at the start, peak, or post-event phase of your training season, you need to have the latest and best cutting-edge nutrition strategies.

Of course, cutting-edge sports nutrition research continues to develop, expand, and flourish. This book provides you with a practical working guide to that research. The third edition of *Sports Nutrition for Endurance Athletes* provides updated guidelines that are scientifically sound and practical for athletes participating in endurance and ultra-endurance sports, particularly in the areas of fueling before, during, and after training, and strategies for training and competition or event day.

Navigating the current tide of popular nutrition information can be confusing for the endurance athlete. Many popular diet plans extol the dangers and evils of carbohydrates. Of course, carbohydrate intake has played a key role in the development of sports nutrition and continues to play an important role in exercise performance and recovery. The key to carbohydrates for the endurance athlete is how much, what type, and when to consume carbohydrates. High-quality carbohydrate foods support both health and performance, and the nutritional impact of your training also requires the appropriate use of sports nutrition products when training and racing.

This book is ultimately about improving the quality of your training and performance in events and competition, but endurance athletes know that good health also enables lasting participation in their chosen sport. Part I is filled with updated information on the links among your daily food choices, optimal health, and disease prevention, with a perspective that supports your daily hours of dedicated training and longevity in your endurance career.

Part II contains the greatest amount of updated material, with the well-researched principles that truly distinguish your diet as an endurance athlete. From your perspective, nutritional timing and portioning are everything. The section on immediate post-training nutritional recovery has been expanded, the information about hydration and electrolyte strategies for training and competition has been fine-tuned, and the nutritional guidelines for muscle building have been updated. Most important, Part II outlines how to adjust and periodize your nutritional intake for the various training cycles so that your daily training diet can be tailored more specifically to each training block and to each exercise session within these blocks. More specifics are given on estimating your energy needs and nutritional requirements for specific training days, and how to adjust these estimates for weight and body fat loss. It is best if you employ weight management strategies that suit an endurance athlete, without compromising energy and recovery, rather than the latest fad weight-loss diet or extreme measures. Use the sample menus in Appendix E, vegetarian included, to help you get started on your latest sports nutrition plan.

Current recommendations on the proper use of the ever-expanding offering of sports nutrition ergogenic aids as outlined in Chapter 7 will help you use these products wisely and safely.

Part III explains how to apply sports nutrition principles to training and competition in a particular endurance sport. These chapters contain detailed practical guidelines for various racing distances and disciplines. The race nutritional strategies of an Ironman® competitor differ from those of a short-course triathlete, and fueling strategies for a mountain bike race differ from those of a cycling road race. This part of the book specifies how to adapt the general principles to your specific sport.

Part IV is dedicated to specific health concerns for endurance athletes, providing guidance as to how diet and nutrition are related to these conditions. Throughout the book, guidelines and food choices that fit a vegetarian diet are also highlighted.

As before, this book addresses nutritional strategies relevant to recreational athletes, serious age-groupers, and elite endurance athletes. Whatever your goals and level of participation, an optimal sports nutrition plan is ultimately about making your participation in your sport more effective, more rewarding, and just plain fun.

ACKNOWLEDGMENTS

Thanks to all the endurance athletes out there who have embraced this book over the past decade. It has been gratifying to reach enthusiastic cyclists, triathletes, runners, and swimmers who digest and absorb the contents of the book as they train, recover, and compete. Staying on top of all the latest research in sports nutrition is just plain fun for me, and having this great finished product to share with you is my pleasure. I promise that there will always be more sports nutrition advice to support you in your quest to be the best endurance athlete you can be.

While the polished, finished product makes it all look so easy, much work goes into bringing this book to your table. One of the best parts of updating and revising this book every few years is working with the great team at VeloPress. Many thanks to Renee Jardine for embracing the new workings of the third edition, to Casey Blaine for guiding those ideas to fruition, to Kara Mannix for her attention to detail, to Michelle Asakawa for making things clean and clear, and to Dave Trendler for spreading the word for several years to come.

PART I

YOUR DAILY PERFORMANCE DIET

Optimal Nutrition for Training and Health

Proper nutrition is essential for any athlete, but it plays a particularly important role for endurance athletes because of the special demands and stresses of their sport. Whether you are an enthusiastic recreational participant or a serious competitor, the subject of nutrition—part art and part science—is well worth mastering. It involves choosing the proper foods, but knowing how much to eat—and when to eat it—is just as important as knowing what to eat. Eating right for your training regimen and competition schedule allows you to replace fuel burned during training and supplies the ingredients required to build strength and muscle. If you focus on optimal nutritional recovery from day to day, and from workout to workout, your efforts will be rewarded. You will derive the maximum benefit from your exercise program, and you will arrive at the start of an event or race in top nutritional shape. The bottom line is that when your diet meets the nutritional demands placed upon your body, you will perform at your best.

Bodies trained and primed for endurance sports require premium fuel for staying healthy throughout the season. If you suffer from lackluster training days, injuries, and more than a fair share of colds and bouts of flu, you may not be making the highest-quality fuel choices. When it comes to daily diet, endurance sport athletes need to obtain each of more than forty-five different nutrients required for optimal functioning of the human body.

Part I of *Sports Nutrition for Endurance Athletes* provides guidelines for building a training diet that will promote optimal health and a strong immune system. This section also identifies the most nutritious sources of carbohydrates, proteins, and fats; how to balance them for optimal training and health; and how to meet the fluid, vitamin, and mineral intakes necessary to build the foundation of a cutting-edge sports diet and good health.

Like any good diet, an endurance training diet emphasizes high-quality foods, variety, and balance among the food groups. But this wide-angle view of the endurance training diet is not enough—one needs to take a closer look to truly learn how to use nutrition to enhance performance. Many categories of foods are complex and provide several nutrients that work in tandem to keep an athlete's body well-nourished and healthy. Which foods complement each other, and how can one best approach meals and snack times throughout the day? How can an athlete make sure there is enough variety in his or her diet? Within each food group are nutrient-packed choices that are minimally processed, fresh, and wholesome. It is best for your lasting good health that you avoid the highly processed foods so prevalent in the North American diet. But how can this best be achieved? Chapters 1 to 3 focus on the details of applying solid nutritional principles to sports nutrition for the endurance athlete.

Quality eating for training and good health takes knowledge and planning, and having a working knowledge of food groups is a key first step. Foods can be categorized in different ways. We often think of basic outlines, such as the government food pyramid, the newer plate model, or even systems used by a variety of commercial diet programs. But these food group systems simply do not work for the endurance athlete. Foods are more often grouped according to carbohydrate, protein, and fat content, as the proper balance of these nutrients is required for optimal training

and recovery in endurance sports. However you look at it, there is an optimal combination of food groups that produce a cutting-edge diet for each endurance sport and for every individual athlete.

While grouping and categorizing foods can be useful in planning a healthy endurance sports diet, it can also lead to oversimplification. The next step in planning a healthy training diet is to look at some of the choices available within each of the main food groups to see what nutrients they provide. For example, some oils can be highly processed and are a very poor nutritional choice, while others are relatively healthy and can be beneficial. Animal proteins can contain varying levels of fat, and some meats are much too high in fat to be a regular part of any serious athlete's diet. Skim milk and yogurt, in contrast, contribute carbohydrates in addition to high-quality protein. Grains can be wholesome, high in fiber, and even provide small amounts of protein, or they can be highly processed and nutritionally very poor.

Ultimately, the goal is to come to appreciate which choices are the most nutritious and to design a diet plan that works for you. How you portion and time these healthy foods is what distinguishes your endurance training diet from an everyday diet geared toward good health. More information on how to determine food portions and how to time meals and snacks to complement your training program is provided in Part II.

DAILY HYDRATION ESSENTIALS

Drinking It In

Water is one of the most essential nutrients for the endurance athlete. Some two-thirds of your total body weight is water, and this remarkable substance plays an important role in every major organ and system keeping you alive. We've all seen the need for hydration in a sweat-logged athlete. But for the athlete, the distraction of daily life can make it easy to forget to keep drinking water regularly. Many athletes also have not taken the time to learn and practice valuable daily hydration strategies. While much research and emphasis has been placed upon an endurance athlete's fluid intake directly before, during, and after training or racing, emptying your bottles of fluid during a swim, bike ride, or run is only one of many hydration strategies essential for top performance. Paying attention to daily fluid intake during nonactive hours is also important. Nevertheless, daily water and fluid intake is often a secondary nutritional consideration, and many athletes frequently fall short on the everyday consumption of this life-sustaining nutrient.

Years of hydration research indicate that athletes should try to prevent even mild levels of dehydration. Although an athlete may not always be aware of how much he or she is sweating, even relatively small fluid losses during training and competition can be significant

Daily fluid requirements average 2.5 to 3 quarts daily (2.5 to 3 L).

Even slight dehydration impairs athletic performance.

Hydrate throughout the day at regular intervals.

Sweat losses during training often exceed daily fluid requirements.

Monitor urine color to check hydration status.

enough to hinder performance. And sweating doesn't take place only during hot weather; it takes place in the gym, in cool weather, and during outdoor winter workouts as well. Studies demonstrate that even in thirst-inspiring hot weather, athletes usually fail to replace all the fluid that is lost through sweat during training and competition. To prevent any adverse performance effects, every athlete should arrive for training sessions optimally hydrated, and to do so means staying on top of your daily fluid intake.

WATER: THE FIRST NUTRIENT

Much marketing fuss has been made about the optimal ingredients for the fluids that athletes require. But before the plethora of sports-related drinks and designer fluids flooded the market, there was simply water. Clear and calorie-free, water is basic and unpretentious and flows naturally into an active sport life with no packaging or gimmicks attached. Don't take basic H_2O for granted. Carbohydrates may be the premium fuel for your energy tank, but when you are about to train or compete in your sport, your fluid stores should be topped off as well. You can go a few weeks without food but will only survive a few days without water.

Water plays an integral role in the optimal functioning of your body both during training and during rest and recovery. Well-hydrated muscles are high in fluid content—in fact, water makes up 70 to 75 percent of an athlete's muscle tissue. Fat tissue is relatively low in water content, at about 10 percent. Even bones, though seemingly solid, are about 32 percent water. Consequently, muscular athletes will have high water content when adequately hydrated. Water is stored in many body compartments, and it moves freely among these various spaces.

As the predominant component in our body, water performs many important functions:

- About two-thirds of your body's water is stored inside your cells, giving them their shape and form. The rest of the water in your body surrounds these cells and flows within your blood vessels.
- Water is the main component of your blood. Blood carries oxygen, hormones, and nutrients such as glucose to your cells.
- Water provides structure to body parts, protecting important tissues such as your brain and spinal cord and lubricating your joints. When fluids become depleted through sweating, both your cells and blood decrease in water content and volume.

- Muscle glycogen holds a considerable amount of water, and water removes lactic acid from exercising muscles, which can be an advantage to well-hydrated athletes.
- Water aids digestion through saliva and stomach secretions and eliminates waste products through urine and sweat.
- Water is essential for the proper functioning of all your senses, particularly hearing and sight.
- As the primary component of sweat, water plays a major role in body temperature regulation. It enables you to maintain a constant body temperature under various environmental conditions because it allows you to continually make adjustments to either gain or lose heat.

Clearly the role water plays in maintaining your overall health is extremely important. That's why you can't live without water for more than a few days. But the role that water plays in your performance is equally vital. Being even slightly underhydrated dramatically impedes top athletic performance.

Your fluid balance is simply the result of your intake of fluids versus your output of fluids. Intake is the net result of the water and other hydrating fluids we consume, the water in some of the foods we eat, and the metabolic water produced by our bodies. When you are not training, urine output represents your greatest fluid loss, or output, but sweating during exercise can result in significant fluid losses. Fluid is also lost in feces and in the air you exhale; through exposure to warm or humid weather, living in a dry climate, or living and training at altitude all increase fluid losses; and when traveling, especially by plane.

How much water do you need? Most people have heard the oft-quoted recommendation to consume eight 8-ounce cups of fluid (4 quarts, or about 1.9 L) daily, mainly in the form of water. In 2004, when much public attention was focused on dietary water requirements, the Food and Nutrition Board of the Institute of Medicine (IOM) released Dietary Reference Intakes (DRIs) for water and various electrolytes. Because of the large variations in water needs among individuals, the IOM panel established Adequate Intake (AI) levels of 130 ounces, or about 16 cups (3.8 L), daily for men and 95 ounces, or about 12 cups (2.9 L), for women.

But of course daily fluid losses can vary greatly depending on your level of training, whether you are male or female, and your individual sweat rate. The daily fluid needs of active males can increase to 4.75 quarts (4.5 L), but requirements for male endurance athletes can often be in excess of 10.5 quarts (10 L) daily, depending on sweat losses during training, and perhaps slightly lower for women. Estimating fluid requirements beyond the basic AI recommendations is really about replacing fluid at a rate close or equal to your own individual sweat rate and total sweat losses for a particular day of training. Further guidelines for replacing training sweat losses are provided in Chapter 5.

At rest, the fluids your body needs can be slowly replenished throughout the day as you make a conscious effort to drink enough water every one to two hours to replace these fluid losses. You should be aware, however, that climate, clothing, and other factors can affect daily water requirements. While thirst is often thought of as the primary human drive that pushes us to drink, it is important for athletes not to rely on thirst alone but to develop regular drinking habits and behaviors to maintain a good level of daily hydration and monitor their own hydration status. By the time someone becomes thirsty, his or her body has already sensed a decrease in the level of fluids or an increase in sodium concentration. So in reality, you get thirsty only when you have already experienced some fluid loss or alterations in your sodium status, both of which are affected by the prolonged periods of sweating that endurance athletes regularly experience. By then, an athlete's performance level would already have decreased. So for an endurance athlete in training, one of the most important concepts to learn is that it is unwise to rely on thirst only for daily hydration needs. Doing so may result in falling short of both optimal fluid intake and optimal performance or recovery.

CAFFEINE: IS IT TRULY DEHYDRATING?

In North America, about 90 percent of adults regularly consume caffeine, mainly in liquid form, whether from cola, tea, coffee, or other caffeine-laced beverages. Caffeine is also present in cocoa and chocolate. Given this statistic, it is safe to assume that most endurance athletes ingest caffeine on a daily basis and perhaps even during training and competition. While the proper use of caffeine can enhance physical performance (see Chapter 7), it has long been labeled as a diuretic, or a substance that actually increases fluid losses by increasing urine production. Athletes have often been cautioned to limit their daily caffeine and not to count caffeine-containing beverages toward total daily fluid intake.

Is caffeine truly dehydrating? For almost a decade scientists have challenged this assumption about caffeine. Reassessments of existing data and new studies of the effects of caffeine on the hydration status of athletes show that, while caffeine often does act as a mild diuretic, stimulating urine production from the kidneys, it does not produce a greater increase in urine volume when compared with the same volume of water or caffeine-free fluid consumption. One study compared the effects of caffeinated and noncaffeinated beverages (both caloric and calorie-free) on the daily hydration status of healthy males. Over a twenty-four-hour period, there were no significant hydration differences among the various beverages. Another study had athletes rehydrate with a caffeinated beverage between exercise periods. The researchers found little evidence to support that caffeine can slow down an athlete's efforts to rehydrate. Bottom line: Caffeine is not the powerful diuretic it was once thought to be.

Endurance athletes can rest assured that a moderate daily intake of caffeine of about 1.4 to 2.7 milligrams per pound (3–6 mg/kg) of body weight should not compromise their daily hydration status when consumed within the context of a well-balanced diet. Caffeine intakes safely falling into this range would be 230 to 460 milligrams of caffeine for a 170-pound (77 kg) man, or 190 to 380 milligrams for a 140-pound (64 kg) woman. A can of soda contains about 40 to 45 mil-

TABLE 1.1 CAFFEINE CONTENT OF FLUIDS

PRODUCT	SERVING SIZE (OZ.)	(ML)	CAFFEINE CONTENT (MG)
COFFEE			
Coffee, grande, Starbucks	16	470	550
Coffee, tall, Starbucks	8	240	250
Coffee, brewed, drip	8	240	185 (95–290)
Coffee, brewed, percolated	8	240	130 (65–270)
Coffee, instant	8	240	105 (50–190)
Mocha Frappuccino®, Starbucks	16	470	95
Espresso, double, Starbucks	2	60	70
Espresso, Starbucks	1	30	40 (30–50)
Coffee, decaffeinated	8	240	5 (3–8)
Espresso, decaffeinated, Starbucks	1	30	6
TEA			
Tea, black, loose leaf	8	240	25–110
Tea, oolong, loose leaf	8	240	12–55
Iced tea, sweetened	12	350	70
Tea, green, loose leaf	8	240	30
SODA			
Movie theater soda, large	44	1,300	500
Soda, large	20	590	220
Mountain Dew®	12	350	54
Coca-Cola®	12	350	46
Diet Coke®	12	350	46
Dr. Pepper®	12	350	46
Pepsi-Cola®	12	350	38
DAIRY DRINKS			
Hot chocolate, nonfat, no whip, grande, Starbucks	16	470	25
Hot cocoa, homemade	12	350	5–12
Milk, chocolate, fat-free	8	240	5–8
Cocoa, Swiss Miss®	1 env. (15 g)		3
Cocoa, Nestlé® Rich Chocolate	1 env. (20 g)		0
White hot chocolate, whole milk, whip, venti, Starbucks	20	590	0
Milk, fat-free	8	240	0

ligrams of caffeine, but the amount of caffeine in a cup of coffee varies widely depending on how the coffee is brewed (for the caffeine content of some beverages, see Table 1.1). Certainly, caffeine-containing drinks should not compromise the majority of your fluid intake.

Avoid excessive doses of caffeine, however, as high amounts are associated with side effects such as nervousness, gastrointestinal upset, irritability, and insomnia. Higher doses can also negatively affect your hydration status and do not result in performance improvements much beyond the moderate doses. Heavy coffee drinkers may find that the acidic nature of the drink can cause reflux.

ALCOHOL: THE NONNUTRITIVE NUTRIENT

One might expect that endurance athletes would be among those inclined not to drink alcohol, given their greater awareness of health issues and their desire to perform well in training and competition. Still, many who do drink may not be aware of how it can affect their athletic performance. It is important for an athlete to use alcohol sensibly, as it does not play any role in physical recovery and could have mild to serious detrimental effects upon performance. Abuse of alcohol can impair health by contributing to cirrhosis of the liver and other diseases, and drunk driving is always dangerous and irresponsible. Alcohol abuse can lead to many kinds of health and social problems. But let's take a look at the implications of alcohol specifically for endurance sports enthusiasts.

Although alcohol is considered a drug, it provides calories just as foods do. But as far as your body is concerned, alcohol is merely an onslaught of empty calories. These calories are not used for energy in the same way as carbohydrates, proteins, and fats. Beer and wine contain only small amounts of carbohydrates and only trace amounts of protein, vitamins, and minerals. In fact, alcohol can interfere with how your body uses vitamins and minerals. Half an ounce of pure ethanol is the equivalent of one drink—that is, 12 ounces (360 ml) of beer (150 calories), 4 ounces (120 ml) of wine (100 calories), or 1.25 ounces (38 ml) of liquor (100 calories). Despite originating from fermented carbohydrates, alcohol is metabolized in your body as fat. Alcohol by-products are converted into fatty acids, which are stored in your liver and sent to your bloodstream. For this reason, alcohol is not the best nutrient choice if your goal is to be a lean athlete. Consuming four or more drinks daily raises your odds of developing obesity by 46 percent.

In the media much has been made of alcohol's protective effects against heart disease. Like fruit and vegetables, red wine and dark beer contain antioxidants called polyphenols, which are believed to protect against cancer. But while moderate amounts may raise the desirable and protective high-density lipoprotein cholesterol (HDL), too much alcohol may actually increase your risk of heart disease. Three or more alcoholic drinks daily can raise your blood pressure as well as the level of harmful blood fats in your body called triglycerides, which, when combined with a low amount of the good cholesterol, HDL, make for a health profile associated with an increased risk of heart disease. Consumed in excess over a long period, alcohol may not only elevate blood pressure but also increase the risk of stroke and, of course, liver damage. Excessive intake of alcohol also increases risk of mouth, esophageal, stomach, liver, breast, and colon cancer. Even one drink a day can slightly raise breast cancer risk in women. Chronic alcohol abuse also increases the risk of developing osteoporosis and can accelerate aging of the brain.

Consuming too much alcohol too soon after training or racing can impede recovery. Alcohol is a diuretic that causes your body to lose more fluid than it takes in. That's why you need to replace losses even after drinking moderate amounts of alcohol. Alcohol may also interfere with glycogen or carbohydrate fuel synthesis in the muscles and liver. Athletes with soft tissue damage or bruising may also want to consider that alcohol is a blood vessel dilator. Consuming alcohol after exercise may aggravate swelling or bleeding and impair healing.

Excessive alcohol consumed shortly before training, or even the night before, can impair fine motor ability and coordination, increase risk of dehydration, and weaken fuel stores. Alcohol adversely affects your brain's ability to process information and therefore delays your reaction times. Know your limits, and be aware of how they change with your training and fitness level. Keep in mind that people metabolize alcohol at different rates depending on their body size. Average-sized men metabolize slightly less than one drink per hour, whereas smaller men and women take longer to metabolize this same amount.

If you do choose to indulge once in a while, have a large glass of water with each alcoholic drink. Consider that when you are resting from your sport, your top priority as an athlete is recovery. Too much alcohol can compromise how effectively you recovery. Table 1.2 provides an outline of the calorie and alcohol content of various alcoholic beverages.

TABLE 1.2 ALCOHOL AND CALORIE CONTENT				
ALCOHOL	SERVING SIZE (OZ.)	(ML)	CALORIES	ALCOHOL CONTENT (G)
Gin, distilled, 90 proof	1.5	45	110	15.9
Wine, table, red	5.0	150	125	15.6
Wine, table, white	5.0	150	121	15.1
Whiskey, distilled, 86 proof	1.5	45	105	15.0
Beer, regular	12.0	350	156	14.4
Vodka, distilled, 80 proof	1.5	45	97	14.0
Liqueur, 63 proof	1.5	45	160	13.5
Beer, light	12.0	350	103	11.0

HOW TO HYDRATE PROPERLY

It is essential that you stay on top of your fluid needs by drinking a minimum of 11 to 16 cups (2.7–3.8 L) of fluid daily for basic hydration requirements when not training. Try to drink on a schedule of 8 ounces (240 ml) every hour on average. Water should make up about half of your daily fluid intake, but you can also receive hydration benefits from other fluids. Juice, dairy milk, soy milk, soup, and various sports nutrition supplements can be good choices. Some foods—especially fruits and vegetables—contain a high percentage of water and can also contribute fluid to your daily diet. Endurance athletes with very high energy requirements can consume high-calorie drinks such as juices and smoothies to assist them in meeting their fluid, carbohydrate, and energy needs. Caffeinated beverages can be incorporated into your diet in reasonable amounts, but they should not be your first choice prior to and after training. Overdoing your caffeine intake can also interfere with your sleep patterns and make you nervous and jittery.

ALCOHOL AND YOU

If you drink alcohol, drink sensibly:

- Avoid alcohol within at least 24 hours of competition or a demanding training session.
- After training or competition, refuel and rehydrate with nonalcoholic drinks.
- Consume alcohol in moderation during heavy training cycles.
- Remember that soft drinks, fruit juices, energy drinks, and other mixers add calories to the alcohol mix.
- Alcohol tends to increase your appetite and food intake.
- Avoid alcohol if you have a soft tissue injury or bruising.
- Consume 8 ounces (240 ml) nonalcoholic fluid for every alcohol drink consumed.

CHECK YOUR HYDRATION STATUS

You can monitor your hydration status by checking the color and quantity of your urine. Clear or lemonade-colored urine reflects adequate fluid intake, while darker or apple juice–colored urine, or a smaller volume of urine, indicates that you need to step up your fluid intake. Urine tends to be more concentrated when you first wake up, but it should become clearer throughout the day. You should urinate at least four full bladders every day. Certain vitamin supplements can darken or add a neon-glow quality to your urine, so volume rather than color may be a better indicator of hydration status if you take them. Regular monitoring of your weight during heavy training periods can also be helpful in judging fluid balance. If you notice significant weight losses at morning weigh-ins, this may be an indicator of chronic dehydration.

It is definitely worthwhile to focus on your daily fluid intake and make the effort to improve in this area. Athletes who have developed techniques for increasing their fluid intake have consistently found that improved hydration results in enhanced recovery and higher energy levels. Improving your hydration levels is really very simple. Just plan ahead and make sure that water and other hydrating fluids are available for consumption throughout the day. This will ensure that you begin your training sessions with a well-hydrated body.

DESIGNER WATERS AND COVERT CALORIES

Today you can choose from a number of "designer" waters, often called "enhanced waters," offering everything from vitamins, minerals, and antioxidants to herbs and caffeine in the mix. Some are flavored with no added sweeteners, while many are flavored and sweetened with a sugar substitute, or flavored and sweetened with a sugar (or a combination of sugar and sugar substitute). The choices can be confusing, and in their advertising these drinks are often confused with sports drinks or the carbohydrate-electrolyte beverages with specific scientific formulations that endurance athletes consume during exercise to replace fluid, carbohydrate, and electrolyte losses.

Read the labels to know just what you are buying. Perhaps your plan is to obtain your vitamins and minerals from a variety of foods and one multivitamin mineral supplement, and you would prefer not to consume too many sugary calories. Check on serving sizes; many bottles contain multiple servings. Waters with added sugar typically

DAILY HYDRATION STRATEGIES

- Start your day with hydration in mind. Consume liquids such as juice, dairy milk, soy milk, or any other milk substitute at breakfast. Liquid hot cereals and juicy fruits, such as melons, also contribute to your fluid intake. A moderate dose of a caffeinated beverage is fine in the morning.
- Don't rely on caffeinated beverages for your hydration needs. After a moderate intake of caffeine, switch to decaffeinated coffee, decaffeinated tea, herbal tea, and other caffeine-free beverages.
- Carry water with you at all times—for example, when you commute and while you are at work or school.
- Incorporate 100 percent real fruit juices, soy or cow's milk, yogurt, and water into meals or snacks.
- Spruce up your water with lemon, lime, or a small amount of juice for flavor.
- Consume 24 ounces (720 ml) of fluid 2 hours before exercising, and 8 to 16 ounces (240–480 ml) additional fluid 30 minutes before exercising to ensure that you start training well hydrated.

provide 70 to 125 calories per 20-ounce bottle (check the serving size on the label), making them close in calories to a soft drink, but minus the carbonation. Some waters clock in at zero calories, but keep an eye on their use of artificial sweeteners. With zero calories and no artificial sweeteners, some of these waters simply provide flavor for individuals who do not like to drink plain water, and for this reason they do encourage good fluid intake.

Herbal and vitamin-enhanced waters may not provide significant amounts of these nutrients per serving; however, if you drink them frequently you could potentially consume enough to take in too much of some of these substances. Currently there is no scientific backing for the idea that consuming oxygen-enriched water can boost energy by increasing the oxygen content of red blood cells, as the advertisements for these products claim.

If one of your goals as an endurance athlete is to decrease weight and body fat, you may be rethinking what you put on your plate, but what you consume from a cup may have as great an impact on your body composition.

Sugar-sweetened drinks contribute the most calories in many American diets, not only soft drinks, but also fruit-flavored drinks and sweetened iced teas. These beverages may also be edging out healthier drinks that provide vitamins and minerals. Sweetened drinks are often available in large or super-sized amounts. And liquid calories may not have the same satisfying effect as solid foods, as slurping replaces chewing, not giving your brain as much to register that you have eaten. While there may be timing intervals during a demanding training period when liquid recovery drinks and the additional calories are needed and welcome, those products also provide specific nutrients for the recovery process, rather than empty calories. So be aware of liquid choices, their calories, and their nutrient contribution, and use them appropriately. Table 1.3 outlines some of the designer waters on the market today.

TABLE 1.3 DESIGNER WATERS

WATERS	SERVING SIZE (OZ.)	(ML)	CALORIES	PRODUCT CONTENT
Aquafina FlavorSplash, Citrus Blend	20	590	0	Sucralose
Clearly Canadian, Wild Raspberry	20	590	63	High-fructose corn syrup, sucralose, natural flavors
Dasani Flavored Water, Lemon	20	590	0	Sucralose
Fruit$_2$O, Natural Grape	20	590	0	Sucralose
Glaceau Endurance Vitamin Water	20	590	125	Fructose, added vitamins and minerals
Hint Water	20	590	0	Natural flavors, unsweetened
Sport Owater, Peach Mango	20	590	87	Pure cane sugar, natural flavors
Propel Fitness Water, Berry	20	590	25	Sucralose, vitamin- and mineral-fortified

WATER: BOTTLED OR TAP?

Americans currently consume more than 9 billion gallons of bottled water per year. In recent years the bottled water industry has taken a hit for the landfill problem that plastic bottles generate. Recent reports indicate that bottled water is not necessarily safer than tap water.

Tap water does contain substances other than water. Depending on where you live, it can provide varying levels of minerals such as fluoride, calcium, sodium, magnesium, iron, zinc, lead, and mercury. While calcium and fluoride may be beneficial, lead and mercury are not. As a health-minded athlete and consumer, you may also be concerned about microbial contamination and pesticide residues in water.

Unlike bottled water, tap water is regulated under the strict standards of the Environmental Protection Agency (EPA), but there are some contaminants that the EPA does not regulate. Your local water municipality is required to supply you with an annual "Right to Know Report" every July. This report lists contaminants detected in your drinking water and notes any violations that have occurred in the past year. Your water provider is also required to test for microbes several times daily. You can contact your local water municipality to obtain the names and numbers of certified testing labs to have the water from your tap checked. Levels of lead and copper in your water may be higher than official reports indicate because of deterioration of household plumbing and faucets.

For healthy adults, tap water in the United States is a very safe option, but that doesn't mean that you can't make your water safer. If you discover that your water is not of the best quality, filtered water may be a viable option. Many filters attach right to the tap and can filter out lead and other contaminants. Another convenient filtering method is a pour-through filter that can be placed in a special pitcher and kept in your refrigerator. More expensive filters include an under-the-sink model that requires a permanent connection to your water pipe. Reverse osmosis filters are considered the best of this type and can filter out lead, mercury, minerals, some pesticides, and microorganisms. Whole-house filters are the most expensive and are installed where the water meets the main water pipe. The benefit is that this type covers all the water used in the house.

An independent organization called NSF International sets standards for and certifies water filtration systems. Its website, www.nsf.org, lists filters and the contaminants that each is certified to reduce in your water. Look for a filter with a pore size of less than 1 micron in diameter. Be sure to follow the manufacturer's directions for replacement of the filter cartridge.

continues

WATER: BOTTLED OR TAP? *continued*

Because it is convenient to have a portable water supply when commuting and working, carrying a reusable bottle filled with tap water is a great solution. You won't have to pay for bottled water or toss the bottle when finished. Just make sure that you wash your bottle daily with hot, soapy water to keep it safe from bacteria. You can even purchase stainless-steel bottles that do not contain unsafe components found in plastic bottles.

Should you determine that bottled water is a more convenient option for you, understand there is no guarantee that it is microbe-free or safer than tap water. About one-quarter of all bottled water comes from municipal water supplies. Bottled water can also be spring water, mineral water, well water, or distilled water. Unlike EPA-regulated tap water, bottled water is regulated by the Food and Drug Administration (FDA). It is not tested for the parasites cryptosporidium and giardia, and it is tested only once weekly for microbes. It is convenient, however, and many consumers like the taste of certain brands.

Look for brands of bottled water that maintain the NSF International certification. To do so, water bottlers must send daily samples for microbial testing to an independent lab and maintain records of filter changes and other quality checks. You can also determine if your brand of water is NSF-certified by visiting the NSF's website.

Think before you drink:

- Drink only 100 percent fruit juice, and know your limits. One 4-ounce serving supplies 60 calories for most juices. Look for vitamin C sources and even calcium-fortified drinks.
- Use low-fat milk whenever possible.
- Order coffee drinks with fat-free milk and skip the whipped cream.
- Request sugar-free syrup for coffee drinks or ask for fewer pumps of regular syrup.
- Beware of frozen coffee drinks and other choices that resemble milk shakes. Aim for the "skinny lattes."
- Smoothies can range from 200 to 800 calories per serving. Choose the lower-calorie versions and smaller portions.

ATHLETE PROFILE

Daily Hydration Strategies: Nora

Nora is a collegiate cyclist who complained of daily fatigue as well as poor recovery from training and frequent upper respiratory infections. She indicated that she was having particular difficulty with hydration during early-morning training sessions. A recent check at the student health center indicated that she was in fact dehydrated.

During her 2-hour morning workouts, Nora consumed carbohydrate gels and blocks, but less than 8 ounces of water. Her daily hydration intake was also limited, with less than 1 quart of water consumed daily. Nora reported that her urine became darker in color throughout the day.

Based on her initial assessment, Nora was first advised to improve her daily hydration strategies. She was experiencing significant dehydration during her morning training session and was not sufficiently rehydrating post-workout and throughout the day. For every pound of weight lost during her morning training session, Nora was advised to consume 24 ounces of fluid over the 3 hours after training. To enhance the rehydration process, this fluid should be consumed with food and other fluids that naturally contain sodium. Daily hydration should continue in the 3 hours post-training, with about 8 to 10 ounces of fluid obtained from water, milk, and juice. Hydration status should be verified by checking urine color throughout the day.

To minimize the dehydration incurred during these early-morning training sessions, Nora was also instructed to check her sweat loss rate and increase her fluid intake to 24 ounces (720 ml) per hour. She continues to refine her hydration strategies both on and off the bike.

ENERGY NUTRIENTS FOR OPTIMAL HEALTH AND PERFORMANCE

Building a Solid Nutrition Base

2

**AT A GLANCE
KEY POINTS**

Carbohydrates are an athlete's main fuel.

Carb requirements vary with training intensity and duration.

Emphasize wholesome, unprocessed carbs from whole grains, fruits, and vegetables.

The glycemic index is a more accurate carbohydrate classification than *simple* and *complex*.

Protein requirements are easily met in a well-planned diet. Avoid overdoing it.

Every diet needs some healthy fat.

Being an endurance athlete comes with a number of perks: You get to spend many hours outdoors doing a sport that you love, you enjoy the health benefits of being in top physical shape, and, not least, you can consume modest to generous portions of a variety of delicious and healthy foods. The endurance athlete's diet is definitely not one of zealous restriction and self-sacrifice. Because these athletes participate in vigorous physical activity year-round, they have many days and training cycles that demand a high energy intake. The training hours they put in on a weekly basis require them to take in adequate amounts of carbohydrates, proteins, and fats. Consuming enough of these nutrients allows them to replace fuel stores used in training, make the most of recovery time between training sessions, and, ultimately, arrive for competition in the best form possible with fuel to burn.

But this doesn't mean that endurance athletes can eat anything they feel like eating. Training bodies rely on premium, high-quality fuel for staying healthy. This chapter focuses on the foods that provide the foundation of your daily training diet and discusses how your food choices impact your health, immune system, and well-being. Popular diets often promote a specific balance of carbohydrates, proteins, and fats—low-carb, high-protein, Mediterranean, gluten-free, and no sugar, among them; the list is long, and there is always a new addition. But some of these, such as the recently popular low-carb diets, raise serious concerns for endurance athletes, not least because of their recommendation to eliminate many of the healthy grains and fruits that are key to optimal nutrition. Clinical studies have repeatedly demonstrated that as the duration and intensity of an endurance athlete's training increase, so too does his or her need for carbohydrates. Exactly how much of this fuel an athlete requires for various training days is outlined in Chapter 4. The current chapter focuses on the best food choices for endurance athletes rather than on portion sizes, total calories, and gram counts.

It is important to keep in mind whom the newest popular diet is intended for: probably not an endurance athlete. Even if one of your goals this season is to lose weight and decrease body fat, you still need to consume an adequate training diet, with just the right amount of carbohydrates at the right time. One advantage that popular low-carbohydrate diets have provided is an opportunity for sports dietitians to highlight the importance of consuming nutritious carbohydrates rather than sugar-loaded sweets and empty calories, and appropriate portions of nutrient-dense carbohydrate choices.

CARBOHYDRATES: THE ATHLETE'S FUEL

Carbohydrates are a major source of fuel for endurance athletes during training. While nutrition plans should always be personalized to an athlete's training program, medical history, and genetics, if your carbohydrate intake does not provide a sufficient amount of fuel for your training and recovery, you will not perform at your best. As an endurance athlete, one of your top priorities is to target your carbohydrate intake to match the intensity and duration of your training. Of course, to stay healthy during the training and competition season your carbohydrate choices should be of the highest quality possible, for the various nutrients they provide will keep your immune system strong and your body functioning optimally.

SIMPLE CARBOHYDRATES

Many athletes are familiar with the traditional classification of carbohydrates. Simple carbohydrates, often called "sugars," consist of one or two molecules. One-molecule carbohydrates, or monosaccharides, include glucose, fructose (found in fruit), and galactose and are the easiest to digest. Two-molecule carbohydrates, or disaccharides, include:

• Sucrose = 50% glucose + 50% fructose: Often referred to as table sugar, sucrose is also found in cane sugar, brown sugar, high-fructose corn syrup, maple syrup, molasses, and many fruits, and is added to many foods.
• Lactose = 50% glucose + 50% galactose: Found in milk and dairy products.
• Maltose = glucose + glucose: Does not contribute large amount of carbohydrate to the diet, but can be added to foods. It is found in sprouted grains, malted cereals, malted milk, and beer.
• High-fructose corn syrup: 45% glucose + 55% fructose: a manufactured disaccharide that can vary in fructose content. It is often added to processed foods.

COMPLEX CARBOHYDRATES

Carbohydrates that contain three to twenty molecules are oligosaccharides. This category includes many manufactured carbohydrates, such as maltodextrins (found in some sports drinks). Oligosaccharides also include healthy carbohydrates such as raffinose and stachyose, which are found in legumes.

Other complex carbohydrates, or polysaccharides, are composed of more than twenty and sometimes up to thousands of carbohydrate, or glucose, molecules joined together. This group includes amylose and amylopectin. The vast majority of carbohydrates in the plant world, such as those found in cereals, rice, corn, potatoes, and wheat, are polysaccharides, and most of them are broken down into glucose for absorption. Complex carbohydrates should be a main source of carbohydrate energy for an athlete. Glucose polymers, a string of glucose molecules, are also complex carbohydrates and can be found in sports drinks and carbohydrate gels. Complex carbohydrates provide indigestible fiber, such as cellulose, hemicellulose, gums, and pectins, and are very important for gastrointestinal health and disease prevention.

SIMPLE OR COMPLEX—HOW DO CARBS FIT INTO AN ATHLETE'S DIET?

All of this may sound overly complicated at first. In fact, the terms "simple" and "complex" are often used incorrectly to describe carbohydrates and have created a lot of confusion—

particularly for athletes who consume many carbohydrate-containing sports nutrition products.

Is it necessary to know how to classify carbohydrates and to understand the scientific terminology in order to simply frame a healthy training diet? The short answer is yes. The reason is that it is important for endurance athletes to appreciate that they may incorporate different types of carbohydrates into their diet at different times for specific performance-related reasons.

For example, a wide variety of sports drinks, gels, and recovery drinks now contain various types of simple or manufactured complex carbohydrates. Are these products healthy or useful, and if so, at what points in your training day or cycle should you use them? When choosing among them, what should you look for? Some of these manufactured carbohydrates may be marketed as "complex" because they are made of chains of molecules that are seemingly superior to the simple sugars found in similar products. They are designed to quickly deliver energy to your working muscles during exercise because they are easily tolerated in the gut and easily digested. These carbohydrates are not necessarily more nutritious than others or superior in terms of providing health benefits or boosting athletic performance, however. There is no particular reason to consume them when you are not in the midst of vigorous physical exercise. They can, however, do the job they were designed to do—fuel your body during exercise. If you like the taste and your digestive system tolerates them well, they may be worthwhile and right for you.

QUALITY IS KEY

Keeping up-to-date on the science of carbohydrates also allows the endurance athlete to distinguish fact from fiction when it comes to dietary advice. For years nutrition experts said that simple carbohydrates such as fructose and other sugars cause a rapid rise and subsequent fall in blood sugar levels that results in fatigue, and that these sugars are therefore less nutritious. Conversely, it was maintained that complex carbohydrates resulted in a more gentle blood glucose rise and occurred in more nutritious foods. In the world of black-and-white thinking, simple carbohydrates were considered "bad" and complex carbohydrates "good." Although this classification might seem logical, scientific data from the past decade indicate that the advice is outdated. What endurance sport athletes should be concerned about is the quality of the carbohydrates they are consuming on a daily basis, emphasizing nutritious and wholesome sources while decreasing nutrient-poor, refined sources. Complex carbohydrates can be wholesome carbohydrates that provide vitamins, minerals, and fiber, but they can also be refined carbohydrates mainly from processed foods that provide little other than calories. Wholesome carbohydrates are not always of the complex variety, and refined carbohydrates are not always simple sugars. Fruit contains simple carbohydrates but is packed with nutrients, whereas products made from white flour, such as white bread, contain complex carbs but often have a much lower vitamin and mineral content. Refined products have the fiber and nutrients stripped away, and while some vitamins are added back, it may not be as much as was originally present; in addition, the fiber is still absent.

Grain sources are much more nutritious in their natural state. For optimal training and good health, choose wholesome carbohydrates. They are a very important component of your diet because they are high in nutritional value.

In addition to being wholesome or refined, carbohydrates can be categorized according to how they affect blood sugar (or blood glucose) levels. The belief that simple carbohydrates cause a rapid rise in blood glucose and that complex carbohydrates cause a slower rise is outdated. Research has demonstrated that each carbohydrate food produces its own unique blood glucose or blood sugar profile, which does not correlate with the simple-versus-complex classification.

THE GLYCEMIC INDEX: EFFECT ON BLOOD GLUCOSE

The ranking system that describes the blood glucose profile of a food is referred to as the glycemic index (GI), and it represents how quickly a particular food increases blood glucose. In this system, a blood glucose profile of 50 grams of pure glucose is given a glycemic index of 100. Other carbohydrates are tested in 50-gram doses and compared with glucose. The glycemic index of a food is classified as follows:

- High-glycemic or quick carbohydrates have a GI greater than 70.
- Moderate-GI carbohydrates are in the 55 to 70 range.
- Low-GI carbohydrates are less than 55.

Table 2.1 provides an abbreviated list of the glycemic index ranking of high-carbohydrate foods, while a more extensive listing is provided in Appendix A and at www .glycemicindex.com. Interestingly, fruits generally have a low glycemic index, despite containing simple carbohydrates, whereas white potatoes and white rice, which contain

TABLE 2.1 GLYCEMIC INDEX AND GLYCEMIC LOAD OF FOODS

FOOD	SERVING SIZE (OZ.)	(G/ML)	CARBOHYDRATES PER SERVING (G)	GLYCEMIC LOAD PER SERVING	GLYCEMIC INDEX (50 G)
HIGH-GLYCEMIC FOODS (GI >70)					
Potato, white without skin, baked	5	150	27	26	98
Rice, instant, white	5	150	42	37	87
Rice Krispies™ cereal	1	30	26	22	82
Cornflakes™ cereal	1	30	26	21	80
Total™ cereal	1	30	22	17	76
Waffles	1.1	35	13	10	76
Cheerios™ cereal	1	30	20	15	74
Watermelon	4	120	6	4	72
Bagel, white, frozen	2.3	70	35	25	72
Millet, boiled	5	150	36	26	71
Bread, white	1	30	14	10	71
MODERATE-GLYCEMIC FOODS (GI 55–70)					
Shredded Wheat cereal	1	30	20	13	67
Pineapple	4	120	10	6	66
Oat kernel bread	1	30	19	13	65
Muffin, banana oat and honey	1.7	50	26	17	65
Raisins	2	60	44	28	64
Couscous, boiled	5	150	35	21	61
Oat bran, raw	0.3	10	5	3	59
Spaghetti, white, durum wheat	6	180	44	26	58
Muesli	1	30	19	11	55
All-Bran™ cereal	1	30	21	12	55
LOW-GLYCEMIC FOODS (GI <55)					
Buckwheat	5	150	30	15	51
Bread, whole-grain	1	30	13	7	51
Banana, ripe	4	120	25	13	51
Rice, brown	5	150	33	16	50
Porridge oatmeal	8.5	250 ml	23	11	49
Grapefruit juice	8.5	250 ml	20	9	48
Sweet potato	5	150	25	11	44
Pear, Bartlett	4	120	8	3	41
Apple	4	120	16	5	34
Yogurt, fruited	6.7	200 ml	105	35	33
Milk, skim	8.5	250 ml	13	4	32
Spaghetti, whole-grain	6	180	44	14	32
Peach	4	120	13	4	28
Lentils	5	150	18	5	28
Kidney beans	5	150	25	5	19

SOURCE: WWW.GLYCEMICINDEX.COM. ACCESSED 2011.

Note: Values can vary depending on form of food, how food is prepared, and type of study conducted.

complex carbohydrates, have a high glycemic index. Many factors influence the glycemic index of a food, including:

- Soluble fiber, which slows digestion, producing a lower blood glucose rise. Beans, lentils, peas, and oats are high in soluble fiber.
- Amylose and amylopectin, which are two types of starch. Amylose slows digestion and results in lower GI. Beans, lentils, peas, and basmati rice have a high amylose content.
- Wheat flour products, which have a high amylopectin content and consequently higher GI level.
- Processing, which reduces particle size and results in a higher GI. Breakfast cereals like Rice Krispies® have a higher GI than muesli.
- When a starch is swollen with water, which makes digestion faster and GI higher. Cooked potatoes have a high GI.
- Fat and protein, which slow stomach emptying and result in a lower GI. Potato chips have a lower GI than plain boiled potatoes. Eating chicken with rice or potatoes lowers the GI.
- Sugar content: Sugar is broken down into glucose and fructose, and fructose causes a slower rise in blood glucose, resulting in a lower GI.

So why should we pay attention to the glycemic index? Individuals with specific health concerns (such as diabetes) need to control blood glucose and elevated blood lipids by manipulating their carbohydrate intake based on the glycemic index of the foods. The glycemic index can also play a role in treating individuals diagnosed with metabolic syndrome, characterized by insulin resistance, or problems with the ability to use insulin appropriately. Ongoing research utilizes the glycemic index to help fine-tune dietary recommendations for individuals with these health concerns.

But athletes may also be able to use the glycemic index to their performance advantage by developing specific recommendations for manipulating carbohydrate intake before, during, and after training and competition. The performance and recovery applications of the glycemic index are reviewed in Chapters 4 and 5. For their daily diet, endurance athletes should experiment with various unprocessed, nutrient-dense, whole-grain carbohydrate foods to determine what works best for them, taking their individual food preferences and schedules into account.

CONSIDER THE GLYCEMIC LOAD

The glycemic index (GI) is a ranking of carbohydrates based on their immediate blood glucose effects. The glycemic load (GL) builds on the GI of a food to provide a more meaningful measure of how your body responds to the carbohydrates you consume. That's because the GL takes portion sizes into consideration. Not all carbohydrate food portions supply the 50-gram dose used in glycemic index testing; an individual may in fact consume a much smaller amount.

Glycemic load is the glycemic index of a food multiplied by the total grams of carbohydrates in the portion used, which is then divided by 100. One GL unit is about equal to the glycemic effect of 1 gram of glucose. You can add up the total GL of all carbohydrate foods eaten throughout the day and determine whether you are eating high or low on the GI/GL scale. The total daily GL in the typical American diet ranges from 60 to 180. On a low-GL day the GL units will add up to less than 80, whereas on a high-GL day the total will be greater than 120.

The general equation is:

$$GL = GI \times grams\ of\ carbohydrates\ per\ serving \div 100$$

Let's compare the GLs of carrots and corn. Carrots have a GI of 92, which is high, whereas corn has a more moderate glycemic index of 60. We'll assume that our hypothetical diner eats one-half cup of each, and that both are cooked. The math for carrots works out as follows:

$$92 \times 6 = 552,\ and\ 552 \div 100 = 5.52$$

Carrots have a GI of 92. One-half cup of cooked carrots has 6 grams of carbohydrates. The carrots have a GL of 5.52. The math for corn works out as follows:

$$60 \times 20 = 1,200,\ and\ 1,200 \div 100 = 12$$

Corn has a GI of 60. One-half cup of cooked corn has 20 grams of carbohydrates. The corn has a GL of 12.

Although carrots have a higher glycemic index than corn, the GL of carrots is lower than that of a similar portion of corn. Many moderate- to high-GI foods may not be consumed in the 50-gram portion test dose and could have a low GL. Alternately, a typical portion of a food that seems to rank low on the GI scale may actually have a high GL ranking.

A low GL for a carbohydrate serving is 10 or less. Moderate GL ranges from 11 to 19. High GL is 20 or more.

In order to achieve a lower-GI diet, consider the following carbohydrate choices:

- Plenty of fresh fruits, such as apples and oranges
- Low-GI starchy vegetables, such as sweet potatoes and yams
- Low-GI cereals, such as oatmeal and muesli
- Low-GI breads, such as those containing barley, rye, oats, sunflower seeds, and pumpernickel
- Low-GI grains like whole-grain pasta, oats, buckwheat, quinoa, and basmati rice

GO FOR THE GRAINS—THE WHOLESOME ONES

With the advent of carbohydrate-restricted diets, the group of carbohydrates most often eliminated and heavily restricted is grains. This is unfortunate because wholesome grains are good sources of carbohydrates, fiber, and B vitamins. Because they are so concentrated in carbohydrates, they are excellent choices for replenishing your body's carbohydrate stores—namely, muscle and liver glycogen, which becomes depleted from intense and demanding training sessions. Grains are easily obtained in the North American diet, but unfortunately many of the most accessible ones are refined grains rather than whole grains. Just as there are "good fats" and "bad fats" (a topic explored later in this chapter), in the typical North American diet there are good carbohydrates and bad carbohydrates.

For both optimal health and top performance (especially during the winter months), choose whole grains whenever possible. Whole grains literally come from the entire grain, which includes the endosperm, germ, and bran portion of the grain, thereby retaining all the desirable nutrients. In contrast, when refined grains are produced, the bran and germ are separated from the starchy endosperm. The endosperm is then ground into flour.

Whole grains are packed with vitamins, minerals, and phytochemicals, which have powerful antioxidant and disease-fighting properties that cannot be obtained from white bread, processed cereals, white rice, and even many "enriched" multigrain breads. Some of the phytochemicals found in whole grains are oligosaccharides, flavonoids, lignans, phytates, and saponins, many of which have powerful antioxidant properties. Whole grains also provide vitamin E and selenium. Studies have shown that regular consumption of whole grains can help to prevent heart disease, diabetes, and certain cancers, yet surveys indicate that most Americans consume less than one serving of whole grains daily. Consuming grains such as whole oats, barley, and bran can reduce the glycemic load of your diet. High-fiber, whole-grain breads that contain whole seeds have an even lower glycemic index.

Include a variety of whole grains in your diet. Even making simple changes, such as using brown rice instead of white rice and whole-wheat pasta instead of semolina pasta, will be beneficial. Buy 100 percent whole-grain breads and look for "whole grain" on the package, which indicates that more than half of the weight of the product comes from whole grains.

Athletes who are tired of the same wheat- and rice-based grain choices have a few more adventuresome options to choose from. There are many whole-grain alternatives, including amaranth, kasha (buckwheat), quinoa, spelt, and teff (see Table 2.2). They take a bit more cooking time than do pasta, rice, and potatoes, but they are nutritious and add variety to the diet. You can experiment with various seasonings to flavor these wholesome grains.

FRUITS AND VEGETABLES: THE HARVEST OF CHAMPIONS

You should place a strong emphasis on fruits and vegetables, not only for their carbohydrate content but also for the great health benefits that they offer. In fact, some health organizations and health researchers believe that fruits and vegetables should constitute the majority of our carbohydrate intake. Studies have shown that eating more fruits and vegetables can reduce your risk of heart disease, stroke, and some types of cancer. Because

TABLE 2.2 WHOLE-GRAIN ALTERNATIVES

GRAIN	DESCRIPTION	PREPARATION
Amaranth	• High in protein and fiber • Good source of vitamin E	Boil and eat as a cereal. Cook 1 c. grain in 3 c. water (or liquid) for 30 min.
Barley	• High in soluble fiber	Cook 1 c. grain in 3 c. water (or liquid) for 45 min.
Bulgur	• High in fiber, folate, magnesium, and iron	Cook 1 c. grain in 1.5 c. water (or liquid) for 10–12 min.
Kasha (buckwheat groats)	• High in fiber • Excellent source of magnesium	Serve as a cereal, as pilaf, or in pancakes. Cook 1 part groats in 2 parts water (or liquid) for 15 min.
Millet	• High in minerals • A staple in Africa	Serve with meat or cook as a cereal. Cook 1 c. grain in 2¼ c. water (or liquid) for 25–30 min.
Oats	• High in protein • Source of cholesterol-lowering fiber	Avoid instant varieties; steel-cut are more nutritious. Cook 1 c. oats in 4 c. water (or liquid) for 20 min.
Quinoa	• Oatmeal-like cereal • Excellent source of B vitamins, copper, iron, and magnesium	Rinse before cooking to remove bitter coating. Cook 1 c. grain in 2 c. water (or liquid) for 20 min.
Spelt	• High in fiber and B vitamins • A distant cousin to wheat	Use to make breads and pastas or in pilafs. Cook 1 c. grain in 4 c. water (or liquid) for 30–40 min.
Teff	• High in protein • Good source of iron and calcium	Cook 1 c. grain in 3 c. water (or liquid) for 15–20 min.

HOW TO EAT ENOUGH WHOLE GRAINS

Current whole-grain consumption in the U.S. is only 11 percent of the *total* U.S. grain consumption. The U.S. Department of Agriculture (USDA) 2010 Dietary Guidelines recommend that at least half of an adult's grain consumption consist of whole grains. One slice or 1 ounce (30 g) of bread or cereal equals one serving. The high level of fiber, vitamins, minerals, and antioxidants in whole grains can reduce risk factors for heart disease, cancer, and diabetes.

Cereals

Find whole-grain cereals that you enjoy for breakfast. Good choices include oatmeal, Fiber One®, Kashi Go Lean®, Heart to Heart®, All-Bran®, and Raisin Bran®. Read labels to make sure the first ingredient is wheat bran, whole wheat, whole-grain wheat, cornmeal, or whole oat flour. Choose cereal primarily for its fiber content. Aim for 5–8 grams per serving. Added sugars listed on the label, such as cane sugar, evaporated cane juice, and high-fructose corn syrup, have no real nutritive value and add empty calories. Also look out for hydrogenated oils.

Breads

Choose whole-grain breads, and don't rely on color, texture, or fiber content to judge true whole-grain content. Bread that is 100 percent "whole grain" is best; "enriched" wheat flour is not whole-grain. The terms "multi-grain" and "7-grain" do not guarantee a whole-grain product, nor does "made from whole grain." Look for the stamp of approval from the Whole Grains Council. It depicts shafts of wheat and the words "whole grain" followed by: "100%" if all grain ingredients are whole-grain, "Excellent Source" for at least 16 grams of whole-grain ingredients per serving, and "Good Source" for 8 grams of whole-grain ingredients per serving.

Select a whole-grain bread with a short ingredients list and without high-fructose corn syrup. Some breads labeled as "soft," "light," or "double fiber" may have added fiber or improved texture, but they may not contain the healthy phytonutrients found in true whole-grain products. For a lighter texture, try bread made from "white whole wheat," though many of these breads are not 100 percent whole-grain.

Other Grains

Start by making whole substitutions for the grains you eat the most, such as rice and pasta. Just using brown rice instead of white rice will add fiber to your diet. One-quarter cup of dry brown rice contains 2 grams of fiber. A 2-ounce serving of whole-grain pasta can provide up to 6 grams of fiber.

fruits and vegetables are so packed with disease-fighting nutrients, the American Heart Association and the American Cancer Society both recommend five or more servings daily. How you put together your sport diet will ultimately depend on your food preferences and tolerances, need for convenience, personal health considerations, and carbohydrate training requirements. But chances are that boosting fruit and vegetable intake would be a step in the right direction for any athlete interested in optimal performance when cycling, running, or swimming.

Fruits and vegetables are distinguished by the thousands of substances they provide that protect our bodies from disease. These phytonutrients act as antioxidants and counteract the cellular damage that we encounter every day. Fruits and vegetables are also great sources of the immune-boosting vitamin A and the antioxidant beta-carotene, as well as other health-enhancing carotenoids. They also supply ample amounts of vitamin C, another important antioxidant and vitamin that performs many essential functions in your body, and the mineral potassium. In this section we will review not only some nutrient-packed fruit and vegetable choices for your training diet but also excellent sources of specific vitamins, minerals, and antioxidants.

Filling Up on Fruit

Fresh fruits, dried fruit, and fruit juice provide the endurance athlete with a significant and concentrated source of carbohydrates that deliver energy for training and fuel for recovery.

All fruits are nutritious, but some choices are extremely nutritious. Tropical fruits such as papaya, mango, kiwifruit, and guava have wonderfully high levels of vitamin C and carotenoids, which are potent antioxidants. Carotenoids are also found in significant amounts in deep yellow or orange fruits such as apricots, cantaloupe, and nectarines. Citrus fruits such as oranges and grapefruits are known for being great sources of vitamin C. Also found in fruits are phytonutrients such as catechins, flavonols, stilbenes, allicin, quercetin, ellagic acid, anthocyanins, limonin, zeaxanthin, and lutein, which appear to be increasingly important for maintaining good health.

The best way to obtain a variety of phytonutrients is to consume a variety of fruits. Dried fruits and real fruit juices will provide the most concentrated sources of carbohydrates for athletes with higher energy needs. Dried fruit, however, will not be as great a source of vitamin C, though it may provide more minerals and fiber than fresh fruit because it is so concentrated. Try to avoid dried fruits prepared with sulfites if you are sulfite-sensitive. (Sulfites are preservatives that trigger allergic reactions in some individuals.) Fresh fruits are also great sources of fiber and the highest in nutrients. See Table 2.3 for a list of optimal choices.

While the warm summer months are associated with a wide variety of fresh fruits, fresh produce is often not as abundant or reasonable in cost during the winter months. Choose fresh and eat fresh whenever possible, but don't disregard frozen and canned choices to keep a healthy supply of fruit in your diet year-round. The nutritional value of fresh fruits is too high to ignore, but any source of fruit is better than none. Flash freezing and other new technologies trap vitamins, minerals, and phytochemicals in fruit immediately after they are harvested, when produce is at its peak. When you peruse the supermarket aisles, purchase enough fresh fruits and vegetables to last three to four days, the amount of time it takes fresh fruit to lose its nutritive value when sitting in your refrigerator. If you shop twice weekly, pick up another fresh fruit stash later in the week. If you shop once a week (and it can be challenging to keep up a healthy sport diet if you shop any less frequently), buy a variety of frozen or canned fruit.

Choose frozen and canned fruits carefully. Avoid frozen brands that add extra sugar or syrup and canned varieties that are packed in heavy syrup, as this adds nonnutritive calories. Opt for fruit canned and packed in light juice and frozen fruit where the fruit is the sole ingredient on the package label. If you miss those delicious summer raspberries and blueberries at certain times of the year, don't forget the frozen version. Check for organic fruit in the frozen food aisle as well; it is increasingly available in mainstream stores. Frozen fruits should move about freely in the package; when they have fused into a solid block of ice, some nutrient loss has already occurred. Also avoid packages that are

TABLE 2.3 TOP FRUIT AND VEGETABLE CHOICES

GOOD SOURCES OF VITAMIN C	GOOD SOURCES OF CAROTENOIDS AND VITAMIN A	GOOD SOURCES OF PHYTONUTRIENTS
Artichokes	Apricots	100% real fruit juices
Blackberries	Broccoli	Apples
Broccoli	Canteloupe	Asparagus
Brussels sprouts	Carrots	Beets
Cauliflower	Guava	Blackberries
Kiwifruit	Kale	Blueberries
Mangoes	Mangoes	Cabbage
Okra	Nectarines	Cherries
Oranges	Peaches	Citrus fruits
Papayas	Red peppers	Cruciferous vegetables
Peas	Romaine lettuce	Grapes
Pineapples	Spinach	Kale
Potatoes	Sweet peppers	Leeks
Strawberries	Sweet potatoes	Onions
Tangerines	Swiss chard	Tomatoes
Tomatoes	Winter squash	Watermelons

sweating or stained with the color of the fruit that is inside; this indicates that the package was partially thawed and refrozen before reaching the supermarket. Once-thawed frozen fruit can be a bit more waterlogged than its fresh counterparts. Frozen fruits work well on top of hot cereals, pancakes, and waffles, and they are perfect for smoothies, which are great recovery drinks for endurance athletes.

Finding Veggie Heaven

Like fruits, vegetables provide a wide variety of vitamins, minerals, phytonutrients, and fiber to enhance your health. While a wide variety of vegetables are available in the spring and summer months at supermarkets and farmers' markets, great winter vegetable choices include broccoli, bok choy, Brussels sprouts, potatoes, sweet potatoes, and winter squash.

All vegetables are good, healthy choices, but some stand out, nutritionally speaking, and are even more concentrated in nutrients than fruit. Color is often a good indicator of a higher nutrient content in vegetables. Some stellar options are carrots, sweet potatoes, and red peppers, which are high in carotenoids. Spinach and romaine lettuce are good leafy choices for their vitamin C, folate, and phytonutrient content. Another group of vegetables that contain not only beta-carotene and vitamin C but also the cancer-fighting phytonutrients called "indoles" is broccoli, cauliflower, bok choy, collards, Brussels sprouts, and kale. See Table 2.3 for a useful list of nutrient-filled vegetables.

Each day, try to consume a variety of colorful vegetables that are yellow, orange, red, and deep green. Choose large servings of vegetables when you eat at home, as it can be challenging to obtain quality vegetable choices when eating out. Buy fresh vegetables when you know you will consume them within a few days, and store them in the refrigerator crisper drawer. When buying fresh, remember that carrots tend to retain their nutritive value a bit longer, whereas kale, broccoli, and green beans lose nutrients quickly. If your crisper drawers have humidity settings, set the level to high humidity for leafy green vegetables to extend freshness. Most other vegetables do best at a lower humidity setting, and some, such as tomatoes and onions, are best stored at room temperature.

Frozen vegetables are a good second choice. Frozen produce may even provide more beta-carotene because it is protected from light by packaging. Fresh tomatoes contain lycopene, a powerful antioxidant; canned and jarred tomatoes and tomato sauces contain even higher levels of available lycopene. Frozen and canned vegetables are preferable to fresh choices that have been sitting in your crisper too long, and they are a good winter alternative to your summer farmers' market produce. Frozen vegetables, like frozen fruits, should also move freely about in the package, indicating they have retained the full force of their nutritional value.

Avoid overcooking your vegetables in order to preserve all the wonderful nutrients they contain. Steaming above water level is the best choice for preserving nutrients in cooked vegetables, whereas boiling or allowing any contact with water during the cooking process results in the highest nutrient losses. When microwaving vegetables, use as little water as possible to preserve nutrient content, and check for doneness frequently to avoid overcooking them.

FITTING IN FIBER

Besides their many other benefits, wholesome and unprocessed foods provide the fiber that is such an important component of your diet. Despite the wide selection of high-fiber food choices at the supermarket, Americans obtain only about half of the recommended daily intake of 25 to 38 grams. This typical amount is not enough to obtain all of the known health benefits of fiber. Diets high in fiber can help:

- Increase feeling of fullness and assist in weight management
- Reduce the risk of colon cancer
- Improve gastrointestinal health
- Improve glucose tolerance and reduce risk of diabetes
- Reduce risk of high blood pressure, high blood lipids, and heart disease
- Stimulate the production of healthy bacteria in the gut

If you need more fiber in your diet, increase your intake slowly and drink plenty of water. Your gut can adapt and your body can secrete more of the enzymes and healthy bacteria that break down fiber, resulting in better tolerance. Most fruits and vegetables average 2 to 3 grams of fiber per serving. Dried peas and beans are loaded with fiber, providing 6 to 8 grams per one-half cup. Whole grains can provide 2 to 3 grams of fiber per serving. Check labels to make the best choices. Nuts and seeds are also great sources.

As an endurance athlete, you want to be strategic about the timing of your fiber intake. Consuming fiber at meals is important, but you may also want to modify your fiber intake in the meals and snacks consumed before training and in the days leading to competition. Endurance athletes may experience unwanted gastrointestinal symptoms during training and competition that could be aggravated by the wrong types of fiber consumed at the wrong times. It is important to know your own tolerances. On training days when your energy needs are especially high, too much fiber can be too filling and prevent adequate calorie intake.

SIFTING THROUGH THE SUGARS

Sugar is contained in foods that many of us view as treats or even comfort foods. According to the USDA, the United States has the highest consumption of sugars and caloric sweeteners in the world, with the average intake at 22 teaspoons per day. The American Heart Association recommends no more than 6 teaspoons daily for women, and 9 daily for men.

What Is Sugar?

The term *sugar* is commonly used to refer to simple carbohydrates composed of single and double carbohydrate molecules. Glucose, fructose, and galactose are the monosaccharides, or single-molecule carbohydrates, that serve as the carbohydrate building blocks of our diet. Disaccharides are composed of two molecules and include sucrose (table sugar) and lactose (milk sugar).

Depending on the food choices you make, the sugar in your diet is either *added sugar*, which is simply sugar added to food, or *naturally occurring sugar*, which is a natural component of foods and therefore not added in processing, preparation, or at the table. The key to smart sugar consumption is choosing the healthy natural sugars and downplaying the non-nutritive added sugars. Naturally occurring sugars include the fructose found in fruits and the lactose found in milk and yogurt. The food sources of these sugars are highly nutritious and contain a wide range of vitamins and minerals.

Risks of Added Sugars—the Facts on High-Fructose Corn Syrup and Juice

Added sugars are often found in foods low in nutritional value. Sucrose, commonly referred to as table sugar, is found mainly in desserts and snack foods with very limited nutritional value. Particularly prevalent is high-fructose corn syrup (HFCS), an added sugar produced by chemically altering cornstarch that is cheaper and sweeter than sucrose. HFCS is made up of about 55 percent fructose and 45 percent glucose. Some HFCS has higher fructose levels, at 90 percent, for an even sweeter flavor. HFCS is added to a variety of food products, including baked goods, breads, cereals, ketchup, and soft drinks, so read labels carefully. For over a decade there have been concerns regarding HFCS. Some experts contend that increased intake of HFCS is directly linked to the growing rate of obesity and type 2 diabetes in the United States. Other experts counter that it is simply the empty calories consumed from HFCS-containing products that contribute to obesity, and that weight gain is not inherent to the sweetener itself. Of course, all experts agree that this sugar is found in foods with very little nutritional value that are high in refined carbohydrates.

Fruit juice also requires careful consideration before consuming. In many cases, it is an excellent example of a natural sugar product gone bad. Any fruit juice you consume should be 100 percent juice, and not a juice drink or blend that provides some HFCS. But even real fruit juice is higher in simple sugar than whole-fruit counterparts. Look for "100 percent fruit juice" on labels and try to avoid the cheap fillers of apple juice and white grape juice. Read the ingredient list carefully. The juices that appear at the beginning of the list are present in the greatest quantity. Juices with color tend to have more antioxidants and phytonutrients, so purple grape juice, for example, is better than white grape juice.

How Much Is Too Much?

Sugars can make foods more palatable and need not be completely eliminated from your diet. But how much added sugar is too much? Nutritional surveys and logic indicate that as added sugar intake increases, intake of several vitamins and minerals decreases. Processed sugar calories should not replace appropriate servings of fruits, vegetables, whole grains, and low-fat dairy products, or the quality of your diet will suffer.

You do not have to eliminate sugar in your diet completely. The occasional dessert or piece of candy after a meal is fine as part of a well-balanced diet. If your active lifestyle demands an intake of 2,400 calories daily, your sugar intake should not exceed 240 calories, or 10 percent of total calories as recommended by the World Health Organization (WHO). This leaves room for some treats in a daily diet filled with wholesome choices.

Check Labels

Nutrition labels do not distinguish between added sugars and natural sugars in a food. Only the "total sugars" are listed, and this total can include both types. You can determine if added sugars are a major ingredient by referring to the ingredient list. Some added sugars to look for on the label are beet juice, brown rice syrup, cane syrup, corn syrup, corn sweetener, crystalline fructose, dextrose, evaporated cane juice, fructose, high-fructose corn syrup, invert sugar, malt syrup, maltodextrin, sucrose, fruit juice concentrates, molasses, honey, sorghum, and cane sugar. The closer the terms are to the beginning of the ingredients list, the greater the amount of added sugar in the product.

Fiber is also available in supplement form, but it is best to obtain most of your fiber from food so that it can work its wonders in conjunction with other nutrients. Fiber supplements may be promoted for treatment of various gastrointestinal disorders and may be effective as part of an overall dietary plan designed by a dietitian.

TYPES OF FIBER

Fiber is made up of a group of indigestible carbohydrates found in plant foods. It is calorie-free, as it is not absorbed by the body. Fiber in food products may be natural dietary fiber or manufactured functional fiber, with the total sum of these two fibers being the fiber amount listed on food labels. For decades, dietary fiber has been divided into two main categories, water-soluble and water-insoluble fiber. Both types are found in every fiber-rich food, though one usually predominates, and it is important to obtain fiber from a variety of sources.

Total Fiber = Dietary Fiber + Functional Fiber

Dietary Fiber

Insoluble fiber: The most familiar form of dietary fiber, insoluble fiber is found in wheat bran, whole-grain cereals, vegetables such as green beans and cauliflower, potato skins, flaxseed, other seeds, and nuts. This type of fiber aids digestion, moves potentially cancerous substances through the colon, and keeps colon function regular.

Water-soluble fiber: Less common in foods than insoluble fiber, water-soluble fiber acts like a sponge and can help control blood glucose and blood cholesterol levels. Good sources of water-soluble fiber include whole oats, oat bran, barley, psyllium seed husks, some fruits, and dried peas and beans.

Functional Fiber

This is nondigestible carbohydrates that are fermented in the colon to produce beneficial substances that enhance health, such as producing healthy bacteria in the gut, and discouraging the development of unhealthy bacteria.

PROTEIN POWER

Endurance athletes interested in maximizing power and strength as well as building endurance need adequate amounts of protein foods for top performance. Power athletes especially gravitate toward high protein intakes, but endurance athletes need high amounts of protein as well. This is because you burn some level of protein during training, you have a higher level of muscle mass than your sedentary counterpart, and you need to recover from the muscle damage that can occur during training.

Protein plays many important roles:

- Supports the growth, repair, and maintenance of muscles and other tissues in your body, such as tendons, ligaments, skin, hair, and nails
- Required to form hormones, enzymes, and neurotransmitters, all of which perform essential functions in your body such as the usage and storage of carbohydrates, proteins, and fat
- Functions as a key component of your immune system by creating antibodies
- Needed for the formation of hemoglobin, the substance that carries oxygen to the exercising muscles
- Serves as a fuel source during endurance exercise if your body's carbohydrate stores run low
- Crucial to controlling fluid volume in the body and maintaining water balance

Clearly, protein plays an important role for both optimal health and performance. Let's take a look at how our body creates proteins from the dietary protein that we consume from food.

ESSENTIAL AND NONESSENTIAL PROTEIN

There are different types of proteins, some of which we need to obtain from food in our daily diet, and others that we can make in our bodies. All are important for health and performance. Because many sports nutrition products contain manufactured sources of protein, it is important to understand the components of protein.

Proteins are composed of amino acids, which are the building units that create protein-based tissues. We obtain amino acids from the protein-containing foods we consume and from the breakdown of our muscle tissue. Amino acids that can be manufactured by our body are considered nonessential to our diet, as it is not required that we consume them in food. Conversely, amino acids that we cannot manufacture in our body are considered essential to our diet and must be obtained in adequate amounts for good health and optimal performance. Both essential and nonessential proteins perform all the important functions required of proteins. The terms can be misleading: In reality, "nonessential" amino acids are just as essential as "essential" ones to the proper functioning of the human body—we just do not need to obtain them from the foods we eat.

Proteins that we consume are digested into smaller protein molecules called polypeptides and eventually into the individual amino acids, which then go to the amino acid pool in your body. These amino acids can be drawn upon to synthesize protein-based tissues or can be used as energy if carbohydrate stores run low. The best way to ensure that your body can manufacture all the needed proteins is to consume a wide array of amino acids from a variety of foods and consume an adequate number of calories. With these ingredients, your body can synthesize proteins as needed.

PROTEIN REQUIREMENTS

Our bodies require about 0.6 to 0.9 gram of protein per pound of body weight (1.4–2.0 g/kg) depending on one's training program and body composition goals, or about 89 to 127 grams daily for a 140-pound (64 kg) female endurance athlete. Aim for the higher end of the range when there has been greater muscle damage from hard training. More protein is burned for fuel when your body's stores of carbohydrate or glycogen run low. Burning protein for energy creates some metabolic waste, however, and it is not the most efficient or cleanest way for an endurance athlete to burn fuel. This use of protein for training fuel is best prevented by eating a diet adequate in carbohydrates and by consuming carbohydrates during training.

EXCESS PROTEIN

For many athletes, daily protein intake actually exceeds protein requirements. Our culture encourages large protein portions, so generally our athletes get plenty of protein to meet their body's needs. Our bodies cannot use higher amounts efficiently—your body is better at processing amounts of 20 to 35 grams at one meal or snack. Excess protein will increase production of a waste product called ammonia, which is eliminated in urine and sweat (often giving sweat a pungent odor). Excess protein requires adequate fluid intake for processing of waste products.

Some athletes, however, may restrict certain foods in an attempt to limit or avoid fat intake, possibly placing themselves at risk. Consuming inadequate protein can interfere with regulation of metabolism in the formation of hormones and enzymes. Insufficient protein can also hinder muscle recovery in the hours after training because of protein's essential role in the building and repair of muscle tissue. Your protein requirements can change depending on your current training cycle and day-to-day variations in your training program, but on even the most demanding training days it should not be difficult to obtain an adequate amount of protein in your diet. If you consume too much protein, your body can either store the excess as fat or burn it for energy—which, again, is to be avoided.

PROTEIN SOURCES

Animal foods such as lean meats, poultry, fish, and eggs are the foods most concentrated in protein. Many of these animal proteins are also good sources of iron and zinc. High-quality plant sources of protein include soy products such as tofu and tempeh, dried peas and beans, and lentils. Low-fat dairy products are also an excellent source of protein as well as of the mineral calcium. What is important for optimal health is to choose lean protein sources, as this will reduce your intake of saturated fat. Too high an intake of

TABLE 2.4 PROTEIN CONTENT OF FOODS

FOOD	SERVING SIZE (OZ./C./TBSP.)	(G/ML)	PROTEIN (G)
ANIMAL FOODS			
Chicken, white	3 oz.	100 g	25
Pork, lean	3 oz.	100 g	23
Beef, lean	3 oz.	100 g	21
Fish, white	3 oz.	100 g	20
Eggs	2 whole		13
LEGUMES AND SOY PRODUCTS			
Tofu, firm	4 oz.	120 g	20
Lentils, cooked	1 c.	240 ml	18
Kidney beans, cooked	1 c.	240 ml	17
Tempeh	½ c.	120 ml	16
Black beans, cooked	1 c.	240 ml	15
Soy milk	1 c.	240 ml	10
Peanut butter	2 tbsp.	40 ml	8
DAIRY PRODUCTS			
Milk	8 oz.	240 ml	8
Yogurt	6 oz.	180 ml	8
Cheese	1 oz.	30 g	7
NUTS AND SEEDS			
Sunflower seeds	1 oz.	30 g	6.5
Almonds	1 oz.	30 g	6
Cashews	1 oz.	30 g	4.5
VEGETABLES			
Potato	5 oz.	150 g	5
Broccoli	1 c.	240 ml	5
Carrots	1 c.	240 ml	2

saturated fat is a risk factor for developing heart disease. Table 2.4 lists the protein content of certain foods per specified portion. Try to emphasize leaner choices of beef, lamb, and pork to limit your intake of saturated fat. Cheese is also high in saturated fat. Plant foods can also contribute to your total daily protein intake, although they do not always provide the same quality or amount of protein as animal sources do. More discussion of protein choices, protein requirements, and timing for specific types of training is provided in Chapters 5 and 6.

FAT: FACTS AND FIGURES

Fat is an important part of anyone's diet, but the role it plays for an endurance athlete is somewhat different from the role it plays for the typical sedentary person. Although fat is well-known as a concentrated source of calories, and often shunned for that very reason, it does play several key roles in keeping you healthy:

* Fat is a source of nutrients known as essential fatty acids. The two essential fatty acids, linoleic acid and alpha-linolenic acid, must also come from the foods you eat.
* Essential fatty acids help maintain the integrity of cell membranes and play a role in the growth, reproduction, and maintenance of skin tissue as well as general body functioning.
* Fat has an important role in the transport and absorption of the fat-soluble vitamins A, D, E, and K as well as the carotenoids.
* Fat can add a wonderful flavor to our meals and make them more filling and satisfying.

HOW MUCH FAT?

Much has been made of the quantity of fat consumed in the North American diet. A high fat content often characterizes convenience foods, restaurant meals, and especially fast foods. Fats are a concentrated source of calories, and excess fat beyond your requirement does not provide optimal fuel for your body and can crowd out valuable complex carbohydrates and proteins. Generally, endurance athletes may need anywhere from 20 to 25 percent of their dietary calories to be derived from fat. Consuming excess fat, or "fat loading," does not appear to improve performance. But it is important that endurance athletes consume adequate fat to replace the fat stored in the muscle for fuel, especially

BEING A VEGETARIAN ATHLETE

In recent years, many nutritionally aware athletes have decreased their intake of specific proteins, such as meats high in saturated fats. Some have gone a step further and replaced animal proteins with plant proteins. Vegetarians are individuals who have consciously made the choice to completely exclude animal foods from their diet, or to include only specific animal foods, such as dairy products, eggs, or fish, and obtain a significant portion or all of their protein from plant foods. Whether these dietary modifications are for health, environmental, ideological, or taste-related reasons, vegetarians need to pay close attention to their nutrition program to ensure adequate protein consumption and sufficient intake of specific vitamins and minerals. Vegetarian athletes must design a well-balanced diet suited to their training program.

"Vegetarianism" is a term that actually incorporates a range of dietary exclusions. A plant-based vegetarian diet may refer to one of the following descriptions:

Semi- or Near-Vegetarians: Eat small amounts of fish, poultry, eggs, and dairy products and avoid red meat.

Pesco-Vegetarians: Eat fish, dairy products, and eggs.

Ovo-Lacto Vegetarians: Eat dairy products and eggs.

Ovo-Vegetarians: Eat eggs.

Vegans: Eat no animal foods whatsoever.

If you are a vegetarian, you need to carefully choose foods that provide specific nutrients in your diet. These nutrients include protein, of course, but also iron and zinc, and—particularly if you exclude dairy products—vitamin B12, calcium, and vitamin D.

Throughout this book, the unique considerations of vegetarian athletes will be addressed in regard to specific nutrients. Of course, any athlete can choose to include more plant sources of specific nutrients—including high-quality plant proteins—in his or her diet. Plant foods are filled with health-promoting minerals and other nutrients. Vegetarians appear to have a lower risk of developing hypertension, certain cancers, heart disease, and diabetes. A plant-based diet also supplies plenty of carbohydrates for replenishing body fuel stores after training. Filling up on whole grains, fruits, and vegetables benefits any endurance sport athlete. Milk and yogurt, though sources of high-quality protein, add nice amounts of carbohydrate to your diet as well.

Like a diet containing meat and other animal protein, a vegetarian diet can be well planned and support your training efforts, or it can be overly restrictive, poorly planned, and counterproductive.

on days that include 4 or more hours of training. It is fairly easy to consume plenty of fat in the typical North American diet, and lowering your fat intake to the right balance for optimal training takes planning and knowledge. Another important consideration is that many North Americans don't consume the best types of fat and may need to increase their intake of specific essential fatty acids. Oils, butter, and margarine are all fats, also referred to as lipids, but they differ in some of their characteristics. Lipids that are solid at room temperature are called fats, while lipids that are liquid at room temperature are called oils.

WHAT TYPE OF FAT?

Fat comes in several chemical forms, some of which are healthier than others. Depending on their composition, fats are categorized as saturated or unsaturated. Unsaturated fats include both polyunsaturated and monounsaturated fats. Currently the American Heart Association sets the recommended range of total fat intake at 15 to 30 percent of total calories. Exceeding this range, particularly if you consume the wrong types of fat, such as saturated and trans fats, may increase the risk of heart disease, while going below it could result in essential fatty acid insufficiency in some individuals.

Saturated and Trans Fat

The most important general rule is to limit the amount of saturated and hydrogenated fats, or trans fats, you consume to 10 percent or less of your total caloric intake in order to prevent heart disease. Saturated fats and the trans fat produced from hydrogenation of liquid oils raise the harmful low-density lipoprotein (LDL) cholesterol, and trans fat can also lower the beneficial high-density lipoprotein (HDL) cholesterol. Undesirable saturated fat is found mainly in fatty animal foods such as cheese and whole-milk products, fatty cuts of meat, highly processed lunch meats, butter, lard, and shortening. Palm, palm kernel, and coconut oil are three highly saturated plant oils sometimes found in processed foods and commercial baked goods. More research is needed to determine if coconut oil supplies a more "neutral" saturated fat that does not contribute to heart disease.

Trans-fatty acids are created from liquid oils that are "partially hydrogenated." Hydrogenation turns liquid corn oil into margarine sticks and increases the shelf life of commercial products that contain the altered oils. Some common sources of trans fat are cookies, crackers, and snack chips. Check labels to limit hydrogenated oils as much as possible, particularly if they are listed as one of the first ingredients. If you consume margarine, choose products that list "liquid oil" as the first ingredient and that are marked as being "trans-fat free" per serving. Labels now list the trans fat content of a serving and can be marked as containing zero grams of trans fat if they have less than 0.5 gram of trans fat per serving.

Unsaturated Fats

Unsaturated fats can help lower LDL cholesterol when they replace saturated fats in your diet. Corn oil, safflower oil, sunflower oil, and walnut oil are all polyunsaturated. These oils should make up no more than one-third of your total fat intake and should be consumed in liquid form. Most health-care professionals advocate that monounsaturated fats constitute the majority of your fat intake. Many cultures that consume ample amounts of olive oil seem to have a decreased risk of heart disease, and monounsaturated fat seems to be the fat of choice for other health concerns as well. Good monounsaturated oils include olive oil, canola oil, avocado oil, almond oil, and hazelnut oil. Table 2.5 outlines oil, food, nut, and seed sources of the various types of dietary fats.

TABLE 2.5 SOURCES OF DIETARY FATS

| SOURCE | SATURATED | POLYUNSATURATED | | MONOUNSATURATED |
		OMEGA 6 (LINOLEIC ACID)	OMEGA-3 (ALPHA-LINOLENIC ACID)	
Foods	Bacon Butter, cream, cream cheese, lard, sour cream, shortening Coconut, coconut milk	Margarine (trans fat free) Mayonnaise Salad dressing with oils listed below Tahini or sesame paste Wheat germ	Fish (listed from highest to lowest EPA and DHA content): farmed Atlantic salmon, herring, wild Atlantic salmon, bluefin tuna, sockeye salmon, sardines, swordfish, mussels, sole, tuna, Atlantic cod Soy milk Tofu	Avocado Olives
Nuts, Nut Butters, and Seeds		Nuts: Brazil, English, pine nuts, soy nuts, walnuts Seeds: hemp, pumpkin, sesame, sunflower	Ground flaxseed Soy nuts	Nuts: almonds, brazil nuts, cashews, hazelnuts, macadamia, peanuts, pecans, pistachios Nut butters (trans fat free): almond butter, cashew butter, peanut butter
Oils	Coconut, fractionated palm kernel, lard, palm, palm kernel	Corn, cottonseed, grapeseed, hemp, pumpkin seed, safflower, sesame, soybean, sunflower, walnut	Canola, flaxseed, soybean, walnut	Almond, avocado, canola, hazelnut, olive, peanut
	Trans fat: Choose foods that are labeled "trans fat free." Avoid foods that include partially hydrogenated oil on the ingredients list and choose liquid, tub, or spray form margarines.			

Note: Some foods may be a good source of more than one type of fat.

ESSENTIAL FATTY ACIDS ARE IMPORTANT!

Unfortunately, what has gotten lost in some of this heart-healthy advice about mono-unsaturated oils is that some polyunsaturated fats should also be included in your diet. Here are some important facts about polyunsaturated fat:

- Linoleic and alpha-linolenic essential fatty acids are both essential fats and polyun-saturated fats.
- Linoleic acid is from a family of fats known as "omega-6" fats; alpha-linolenic acid is from the "omega-3" family of fats.
- Two other omega-3 fats, and two of the most potent, are docosahexaenoic acid (DHA) and eicosapentaenoic acid (EPA), both of which are abundant in fish such as salmon and tuna.

DHA and EPA are of great interest to health experts and to endurance athletes. Consuming these fats, as well as alpha-linolenic acid, is necessary to produce hormone-like compounds that can reduce unnecessary blood clotting, boost immune function, and reduce inflammation. High intakes of DHA and EPA may help to prevent heart disease and stroke and may improve conditions such as rheumatoid arthritis and depression.

Conversely, excess linoleic acid can produce hormones that lead to inflammation, promote blood clotting, and constrict arteries. Linoleic acid competes with alpha-linolenic acid, DHA, and EPA for use by the body; it is best not to consume an excess of linoleic acid and to make sure that you consume enough of the healthy omega-3 fatty acids.

Keep in mind that all of these essential fats are good for you. But what is desirable is to obtain the proper balance of essential fatty acids in your diet. Most North Americans consume an excess of linoleic fat (omega-6) and need to increase their intake of alpha-linolenic acid, EPA, and DHA (omega-3). Table 2.6 will guide you in choosing food sources of these fats. Try to emphasize fatty fish, and use soy and canola oils. Although olive oil is an excellent source of the healthy monounsaturated fat, it supplies very little of the essential fatty acids. Other good plant sources of alpha-linolenic acid are leafy green vegetables, walnuts, and flaxseed. Several foods are listed under both essential fatty acid headings, as they are rich in both.

TABLE 2.6 FOOD SOURCES OF ESSENTIAL FATTY ACIDS

FOOD	SERVING SIZE (OZ./C./TBSP.)	(G/ML)	ALPHA-LINOLENIC ACID CONTENT (G)
FOODS RICH IN ALPHA-LINOLENIC OMEGA-3 FATTY ACIDS			
Flaxseed oil	1 tbsp.	20 ml	6.6
Flaxseed, ground	1 tbsp.	20 ml	1.8
Soy nuts, roasted	½ c.	120 ml	1.8
Canola oil	1 tbsp.	20 ml	1.6
Walnut oil	1 tbsp.	20 ml	1.4
Soybean oil	1 tbsp.	20 ml	1.0
Tofu, firm	½ c.	120 ml	0.7
Soy milk	1 c.	240 ml	0.4
Sardines	2 oz.	60 g	0.3
Oat germ	2 tbsp.	40 ml	0.2
Spinach, cooked	1 c.	240 ml	0.2
Kale, cooked	1 c.	240 ml	0.1
Almond butter	2 tbsp.	40 ml	0.1
Legumes	½ c.	120 ml	0.1
Wheat germ	2 tbsp.	40 ml	0.1

FOOD	SERVING SIZE (COOKED) (OZ.)	(G)	EPA ≤ DHA CONTENT (G)
FOODS RICH IN EPA AND DHA OMEGA-3 FATTY ACIDS			
Farmed Atlantic salmon	3 oz.	90 g	1.8
Herring	3 oz.	90 g	1.7
Wild Atlantic salmon	3 oz.	90 g	1.6
Bluefin tuna	3 oz.	90 g	1.3
Sockeye salmon, canned	3 oz.	90 g	1.3
Atlantic mackerel	3 oz.	90 g	1.0
Farmed rainbow trout	3 oz.	90 g	1.0
Wild rainbow trout	3 oz.	90 g	0.8
Sardines, canned	3 oz.	90 g	0.8
Swordfish	3 oz.	90 g	0.7
Mussels	3 oz.	90 g	0.7
Sole	3 oz.	90 g	0.4
Tuna, white meat, canned	3 oz.	90 g	0.2
Wild catfish	3 oz.	90 g	0.2
Farmed catfish	3 oz.	90 g	0.1
Atlantic cod	3 oz.	90 g	0.1

FOOD	SERVING SIZE (OZ./C./TBSP.)	(G/ML)	LINOLEIC ACID CONTENT (G)
FOODS RICH IN LINOLEIC AND OMEGA-6 FATTY ACIDS			
Walnuts	1 oz.	30 g	11.0
Safflower oil	1 tbsp.	20 ml	10.1
Sunflower oil	1 tbsp.	20 ml	9.2
Soy nuts, roasted	½ c.	120 ml	9.0

Continues >

TABLE 2.6 FOOD SOURCES OF ESSENTIAL FATTY ACIDS *continued*

FOOD	SERVING SIZE (OZ./C./TBSP.)	(G/ML)	LINOLEIC ACID CONTENT (G)
FOODS RICH IN LINOLEIC AND OMEGA-6 FATTY ACIDS, *CONTINUED*			
Corn oil	1 tbsp.	20 ml	7.8
Brazil nuts	1 oz.	30 g	7.0
Soybean oil	1 tbsp.	20 ml	6.9
Pecans	1 oz.	30 g	6.0
Tofu, firm	4 oz.	120 g	5.4
Peanuts	1 oz.	30 g	4.5
Peanut butter	2 tbsp.	40 ml	4.4
Almond butter	2 tbsp.	40 ml	3.8
Almonds	1 oz.	30 g	3.0
Wheat germ	2 tbsp.	40 ml	0.8
Flaxseed, ground	1 tbsp.	20 ml	0.5

SOURCE: USDA NATIONAL DATABASE FOR STANDARD REFERENCE WWW.NAL.USDA.GOV/FNIC/FOODCOMP/SEARCH/.

DIETARY CHOLESTEROL

Dietary cholesterol is found only in animal foods. While excess cholesterol formed in the body is not healthy, we do need some to form hormones such as estrogen, testosterone, and progesterone, as well as other hormones. Cholesterol is in all the membranes of the cells in our bodies, and much of it can actually be made in our bodies. Excess dietary cholesterol can increase levels of blood cholesterol in our bodies, though it does not have as great an effect as saturated fat and trans fat.

To emphasize the best fat choices, you can balance your intake in the following ways:

- Consume fish such as salmon, light tuna, sole, and tilapia twice or more weekly.
- Emphasize soy and canola oils and related products, and use olive oil as well.
- Include green leafy vegetables, walnuts, and ground flaxseed in your diet.
- Choose the leanest cuts of red meat possible and choose grass-fed animals.
- Limit fatty cheeses; choose low-fat or fat-free versions.
- Emphasize poultry, beans, lentils, and soy protein in your diet.
- Control margarine intake and choose products with liquid oil as the first ingredient.
- Avoid processed foods that contain partially hydrogenated oils and trans fats.

CONSUMING FISH OILS SAFELY

Fish is a great source of omega-3 fatty acids, which can reduce disease risk and enhance health by decreasing inflammation in the body. But when you consume fish, take into consideration choices that will minimize your mercury intake. Mercury is present in our air and water and when converted to methyl-mercury can accumulate in fish and humans. Methyl-mercury is a known toxin to developing fetuses, infants, and children and is now considered a potential threat to adults as well. Mercury can damage the brain and nervous system and cause symptoms such as fatigue and hair loss.

The health benefits of eating fish do outweigh these risks, if you make good choices regarding the type and amount of fish consumed. Currently the American Heart Association recommends eating fish twice weekly. Generally you can keep your total fish portions to about 12 ounces weekly, though mercury's effects are somewhat dose-related based on body weight.

Choose types of fish that tend to be low in mercury. Those highest in mercury are shark, swordfish, king mackerel, and tilefish. Other high-mercury fish are fresh tuna, red snapper, orange roughy, and marlin. Some types of fish and shellfish that tend to be lower in mercury are shrimp, salmon, pollock, catfish, tilapia, sardines, and sole. Canned white albacore tuna contains more mercury than canned light tuna and should be limited. Other fish fairly low in mercury are haddock, herring, and whitefish.

Many salmon lovers are also concerned about the cancer-causing polychlorinated biphenyls (PCBs) in fish. Testing indicates that both farmed and wild salmon are contaminated with PCBs, with the farmed varieties containing much higher amounts. Farmed varieties from both the United States and Canada contain lower amounts of PCBs than those from European countries, but the levels present in all farmed salmon are much higher than in wild varieties. When it is in season, choose wild Alaska salmon, which is lowest in PCBs. Canned salmon, which comes almost exclusively from the wild Alaskan variety, is also a good choice. Since 2004, all seafood has been labeled as farmed or wild. The country of origin is also now marked. This labeling requirement should be a great help to consumers who wish to include fish in their diet on a regular basis without ingesting harmful toxins.

Fish oil supplements are another option for obtaining DHA and EPA omega-3 fatty acids in your diet. In fact, it may be safer to take fish oil supplements than to eat the amount of fish needed to obtain the same level of these beneficial substances. Lab analysis has

continues

CONSUMING FISH OILS SAFELY *continued*

shown supplements to be free of mercury, PCBs, and dioxins. Mercury accumulates in the muscle tissue of fish, not the fat tissue that is the source of most fish oil. One exception is cod liver oil, which comes from fish liver, where toxins do accumulate. Fish oils are also processed to remove any toxins. Look for brands that have been "distilled" or "deodorized."

Consider discussing fish oil supplements with your physician. Some individuals with heart disease may be placed on therapeutic doses ranging from 1 to 3 grams daily, but the higher doses require medical monitoring. Large doses can sometimes cause nausea or burping. People who take blood-thinning medications, who have a history of a bleeding stroke, or who are scheduled for surgery should not take EPA and DHA supplements. If you take a fish oil supplement, choose a brand that contains both DHA and EPA at the highest level that you can tolerate in one pill. Supplements are better absorbed when taken with meals.

ATHLETE PROFILE

Improving Diet Quality: **Gary**

Gary is a triathlete who was always eating on the run. He usually ate packaged convenience foods from the grocery store or purchased meals at local fast-food restaurants. Gary knew he was consuming enough energy, carbohydrates, proteins, and fat because of his frequent meal and snack intake; however, he felt that the quality of his diet was lacking. He wanted to prepare some simple yet nutritious meals that could fit into his busy work and training schedule.

Gary often trains twice daily, particularly in the build phase of a training cycle, leading to an important race. Rather than waking early for breakfast, he consumed sports nutrition supplements before early workouts to provide quick and easily digested fuel and utilized sports nutrition products appropriately before, during, and after training.

Gary's main goals were to improve his overall nutritional intake and the quality of his diet, so the focus of his nutrition sessions was on meal planning strategies and specific food choices. He was given breakfast suggestions that provide optimal recovery nutrients from carbohydrates, proteins, and fluids in the form of whole-grain cereal, skim milk, fruit, and fruit juice, as well as high-quality protein sources to start the recovery process after early-morning training sessions. Lunch choices could be consumed at his health club or at home. Healthy lunch choices that could be purchased at or near work were also outlined, as well as ideas for a packed lunch when time and logistics allowed. He was provided with sandwich ideas that include lean proteins along with another whole-grain serving, such as a pasta salad or bean soup, to round out his carbohydrate intake, as well as vegetables and fruits for their high nutrient contents.

Gary also learned to pack nutritious snacks that can be stored in his workout bag and to keep fresh items for the week at work in the communal refrigerator. Most important, he learned to precook simple dinner meals, using lean proteins, whole grains, and vegetables. Planning meals ahead for the week and purchasing groceries weekly on the weekend or for home delivery have been essential to improving diet quality and healthy eating during each training week.

VITAMINS, MINERALS, AND ELECTROLYTES

The Nuts, Bolts, and Spark Plugs of Your Diet

As an endurance athlete, you no doubt have more than a passing interest in getting the vitamins and minerals you need in your diet. These nutrients are important for everyone, but for an endurance athlete they are crucial. Because of your training and the stress it imposes on your body, you may need higher amounts of vitamins and minerals than your sedentary counterparts. And, as an athlete, you have a highly vested interest in keeping your immune system healthy so that illness does not put a halt to training, especially during the peak of race season. Athletes have long been advised by sports dietitians to consume high-quality foods for an optimal nutrient intake, but many advertisers touting their products suggest that athletes require megadoses of specific nutrients. Some endurance athletes rely on high-dose supplementation, and vitamins and minerals are now added to many sports nutrition products such as energy bars and recovery drinks. Are the advertising claims correct? Vitamins and minerals are indeed essential to good health and maximum performance, but how much of these essential ingredients do you need?

Of course, choosing foods that provide you with adequate amounts of vitamins and minerals is necessary for optimal perfor-

Optimize vitamin and mineral intake for good health and performance.

Higher doses of some nutrients may be needed depending on training, metabolism, and health concerns.

Some vitamins and minerals may be toxic in high doses.

Inappropriate supplementation can lead to nutritional imbalances or deficiencies.

Food sources of antioxidants and phytonutrients should be emphasized.

mance. Vitamins and minerals are essential for metabolizing energy, building body tissue, maintaining fluid balance, and carrying oxygen in the body. Vitamins and minerals also play a role in reducing the oxidative stress that is brought on by endurance training. Correcting dietary inadequacies could improve your performance. Depending on your health status, typical dietary intake, and specific nutrient needs, you may need to supplement your diet in an educated fashion. However, research has not conclusively proven that taking "extra" amounts of vitamins and minerals when no deficiency is present will enable an athlete to train harder or longer. In fact, in some cases taking too many supplements can be harmful—large doses of the fat-soluble vitamins A, D, E, and K, for example, can be toxic, and megadoses of even some of the water-soluble vitamins can cause problems.

Although vitamins and minerals—in the correct amounts—are important components of anyone's diet, endurance athletes should be aware of the nutrients that are especially suitable for meeting their unique health and training needs. A well-balanced diet that includes a wide variety of nutritious foods can provide ample amounts of vitamins, minerals, and phytochemicals. And as an endurance athlete, you have higher energy needs than the average sedentary person because of the time you spend training, which means that you can eat more of the nutrient-rich foods your body requires. You should also keep in mind that nutrients exist together in foods in the proper balance, which is not the case with capsules, pills, and specially formulated powders or drinks. This chapter discusses your vitamin and mineral requirements for exercise, the functions of these nutrients in your body, optimal food sources of these nutrients, and appropriate reasons and guidelines for supplementation.

VITAMINS

Vitamins, any of thirteen organic compounds found in small amounts in foods, play important roles in many physiological processes. During prolonged or vigorous exercise, extra demands are placed on your body that intensify these processes—in other words, your body has to work extra hard to train, to perform in competition, and to heal during the recovery phase, and this work draws upon your body's vitamin and mineral reserves. To ensure that these body processes function optimally, you should try to maintain high levels of these nutrient reserves. Although inadequate intake of vitamins is known to result in deficiencies, whether it will adversely impact your performance depends on the extent of the deficiency. Many dietary inadequacies can be corrected by making the proper food choices or supplementing appropriately if indicated.

Athletes most likely to have problems with an inadequate vitamin intake are those following a restricted-calorie diet for weight loss, those who have adopted an extreme or fad diet, and sometimes those on a restrictive vegetarian diet. Overall, however, athletes training and competing in endurance sports can greatly minimize their risk of vitamin deficiency by consuming a wide variety of nutrient-dense foods and adequate calories to match their training needs.

Vitamins play a major role in catalyzing energy-production reactions from body fuel stores. For instance, a number of B vitamins are essential to converting carbohydrates into energy for muscular contraction. Vitamins themselves do not directly provide energy, which must be obtained from consuming carbohydrates, protein, and fat. The vitamins B12, B6, and folic acid play an important role in the development of red blood cells, which deliver oxygen to your exercising muscles. Vitamins are also involved in tissue repair and protein synthesis. Several vitamins, such as E and C, are antioxidants that protect cells from potentially toxic free radicals. Free radicals are unstable molecules produced by oxygen-related reactions in the body and have been implicated in contributing to a number of diseases. Each vitamin is unique in the functions it performs in the body and in how it interacts with other dietary nutrients.

Vitamins are separated into two classifications: fat-soluble and water-soluble. Water-soluble vitamins require only water to be absorbed, and excess can be excreted in the urine, though large doses aren't necessarily harmless. Fat-soluble vitamins require dietary fat to be absorbed and can be stored in body fat; some can build up to toxic levels if taken in excess. Fat-soluble vitamins are not excreted as easily as water-soluble vitamins.

Fat-soluble vitamins include vitamins A, D, E, and K. For the most part, we can store adequate amounts of fat-soluble vitamins if our daily intake is adequate. One exception is vitamin D. Deficiencies or insufficiencies of this nutrient may affect over two-thirds of the U.S. population due to limited food sources and protection from sun exposure—our main source of vitamin D production.

The water-soluble variety—which consists of vitamin C and the eight B vitamins, thiamin (B1), riboflavin (B2), pyridoxine (B6), niacin (B3), cobalamins (B12), folacin (B9), biotin (B7), and pantothenic acid (B5)—are not stored in your body in significant amounts. Harmful effects of excessive intakes of these water-soluble vitamins are not as likely, though there are exceptions. Appendix B provides a list of vitamins, their functions, Dietary Reference Intakes (DRIs), and food sources.

OPTIMAL HEALTH AND DIETARY REFERENCE INTAKES

The Dietary Reference Intake (DRI) system, developed by the Food and Nutrition Board of the National Academy of Sciences in the 1990s, is designed to reflect the health goals of the twenty-first century. It is hoped that rather than merely preventing nutrient deficiencies, these latest guidelines for nutrient intakes will optimize health by reducing the risk of chronic diseases such as heart disease, cancer, and osteoporosis.

The DRI system includes four classifications:

Recommended Daily Allowance (RDA): The RDA is the amount of a nutrient that should decrease the risk of chronic disease for most healthy individuals in a specified age group and gender. It is based on estimating the average requirement plus an increase to account for individual variation. You may also see the term "% Daily Value" or "%DV" on food labels. The Daily Value is a reference number based on the RDA and developed to help consumers determine whether a food contains a little or a lot of a specific nutrient. On the Nutrition Facts label, %DVs are based on a 2,000-calorie diet. If a food contains over 20 percent of the Daily Value in one serving, it is considered to be a good source of that nutrient. The RDA is a good starting point for athletes who wish to determine the nutritional adequacy of their diet. However, athletes of all ages are likely to have energy requirements higher than the average person, and some vitamins and minerals are required to process this energy. Endurance athletes may also have a higher nutrient intake than the average person, however, simply because of their high energy needs and quality food choices.

Adequate Intake (AI): The AI is used when there is not enough scientific evidence to set an RDA. It is a recommended daily intake based on observed or experimentally determined approximations of nutrient intake by a group of healthy people. The AI can be used as a goal for individual intake when an RDA does not exist.

Estimated Average Requirement (EAR): The EAR represents the average nutrient intake required to maintain a specific body function. For example, the EAR for vitamin C is set at a level that prevents scurvy, a deficiency disease. The EAR is used to develop the RDA, assess adequacy of intakes, and plan diets for population groups.

Tolerable Upper Intake Level (UL): The UL is the highest daily intake level of a nutrient, from both food and supplement sources, thought to be within safe limits. This is not a recommended amount, but rather an upper limit. This number can provide guidance to athletes who consume numerous fortified foods, take various vitamin and mineral supplements, and frequently use sports nutrition products that are supplemented with nutrients.

B VITAMINS

Many B vitamins are easily obtained from a variety of carbohydrate-rich foods, such as breads, cereals, brown rice, wheat germ, and vegetables, and certain B vitamins are also found in protein-rich foods that are often staples in the high-energy athlete's diet, such as dairy milk and yogurt, pork, fish, and poultry. Often the intake of the B vitamins easily exceeds the RDAs when an endurance athlete consumes the calories required for training and competing from a healthy diet.

Thiamin and Riboflavin

Thiamin, or vitamin B1, is present in a wide variety of food sources besides whole grains, including nuts, dried peas and beans, and pork. It plays an important role in deriving energy from carbohydrates. A thiamin deficiency is unlikely to occur in athletes. Many athletes with high energy needs likely consume thiamin well above the current RDA of 1.2 milligrams daily.

Riboflavin, or vitamin B2, is also involved in energy production from carbohydrates, proteins, and fats. Vegetarians should pay attention to their riboflavin intake, as milk, meat, and eggs are good sources. Some plant sources are brewer's yeast, wheat germ, soybeans, avocados, green leafy vegetables, and enriched bread and cereals. Training for your sport may slightly increase your riboflavin requirements, but the higher amounts are easily met in a well-balanced diet.

Pyridoxine and Niacin

Pyridoxine, or vitamin B6, is closely linked to protein metabolism, the manufacture of muscle and hemoglobin, and the breakdown of muscle glycogen. It is found mainly in whole-grain cereals, brown rice, wheat germ, bananas, legumes, fish, and poultry. Athletes who consume adequate calories should get plenty of vitamin B6 in their diets. Though most water-soluble vitamins are easily excreted, excess supplementation of B6 can present a problem. Doses of more than 1 gram daily over several months may cause numbness and even paralysis. Symptoms have also been experienced with chronic doses as low as 200 milligrams daily.

Niacin, or vitamin B3, is involved not only in carbohydrate, protein, and fat metabolism but also in glycogen synthesis and cellular metabolism. Good food sources of niacin are meat, whole or enriched grains, nuts, seeds, and dried beans. Because niacin occurs in such a wide variety of foods, it is relatively easy to obtain enough of it in your diet. In fact, excess niacin from oversupplementation can block the release of free fatty acids, resulting in greater use of muscle glycogen and thereby depleting a limited energy source for exercise. Large doses may actually reduce performance.

Vitamin B12

Vitamin B12 (less known by the name cobalamins) plays a major role in red blood cell development, folic acid metabolism, and DNA development, among other important functions. Your vitamin B12 needs are easily met by consuming animal foods, but vegetarian athletes, especially strict vegans, should pay close attention to their B12 intake. If you consume eggs and dairy foods, your intake levels should be fine. The only plant foods that can be counted on for their B12 content are those that have been fortified with this vitamin, such as soy milk, soy burgers, and some breakfast cereals. Plant proteins such as tempeh and miso may not contain the active form of vitamin B12, however. The human intestinal tract does make some vitamin B12, but this form is generally not well absorbed.

Although the Recommended Daily Allowance (RDA) for this vitamin is relatively low, a deficiency can have serious implications and even lead to irreversible nerve damage. Vegans who do not regularly consume fortified foods should take a vitamin B12 supplement providing 100 percent of the Daily Value (DV), and consume foods fortified with B12.

Megadoses of vitamin B12 are not needed or recommended. However, endurance athletes have routinely taken high doses of this vitamin for years, often injecting the nutrient during periods of heavy training. There is no evidence to suggest that this improves performance.

Folacin

Folacin, or vitamin B9, has deservedly received much increased attention from health professionals over the past several years. Folacin is the collective term for folate, folic acid, and other forms of the vitamin. Folate is the form found naturally in foods, and folic acid is the form of the vitamin found most often in your body and added to foods and supplements. Folic acid is actually absorbed twice as well as the folate that occurs naturally in foods.

Since 1998, manufacturers in the United States have been required to add folic acid to all enriched products, including flour, bread, rolls, grits, cornmeal, rice, pasta, and noodles. There is good reason for this fortification. Obtaining enough folic acid in the early weeks of pregnancy can significantly reduce the risk of neural tube defects such as spina bifida in newborns. Initially it was believed that this fortification may not only benefit pregnant women and newborns but could also reduce the risk of heart disease, stroke, and certain cancers. However, a recent analysis of eight clinical trials did not find a reduced risk of cardiovascular disease and cancer.

Many researchers suggest that individuals over the age of fifty take a supplement providing the RDA of folic acid, B12, and B6 (high doses are not advised). Older individuals are also more likely to take medications that interfere with folic acid absorption.

Every athlete should increase the intake of folate-rich foods because of folate's relationship to maintaining red blood cells. Folate deficiencies can lead to alterations in protein synthesis and a type of anemia called megaloblastic anemia. Try to obtain folate from fresh foods, since it is easily destroyed by long storage times and common cooking techniques. Romaine lettuce is a great source; for other examples of folate-rich foods, see Table 3.1.

Biotin and Pantothenic Acid

Biotin (B7) plays a role in glucose production, in carbohydrate metabolism, and in the synthesis of glycogen and proteins. It is found in egg yolks, peanuts, walnuts, pecans, and yeast. Because biotin can be synthesized by bacteria in the intestines, a biotin deficiency

TABLE 3.1 FOLATE-RICH FOODS

FOOD	SERVING SIZE (OZ./C./TBSP.)	(G/ML)	FOLATE CONTENT (MCG)
Lentils, cooked	1 c.	240 ml	358
Yeast, brewer's	1 tbsp.	20 ml	312
Liver, beef	3 oz.	90 g	285
Garbanzo beans, cooked	1 c.	240 ml	282
Kidney beans, cooked	1 c.	240 ml	229
Turnip greens, cooked	1 c.	240 ml	171
Asparagus, boiled	6 spears		131
Beans, white, baked	1 c.	240 ml	122
Orange juice	1 c.	240 ml	110
Spinach, raw, chopped	1 c.	240 ml	108
Mustard greens, cooked	1 c.	240 ml	103
Broccoli, cooked	1 c.	240 ml	78
Romaine lettuce	1 c.	240 ml	76
Endive	1 c.	240 ml	72
Wheat germ, raw	¼ c.	60 ml	70

SOURCE: USDA NATIONAL NUTRIENT DATABASE FOR STANDARD REFERENCE, WWW.NAL.USDA.GOV/FNIC/FOODCOMP/SEARCH/.

is rare. Pantothenic acid (B5) is part of a compound, coenzyme A, that plays an important role in carbohydrate, protein, and fat metabolism. Pantothenic acid is found in a wide variety of foods, with meat, whole grains, beans, and peas being the best sources.

VITAMIN C

Several important functions of vitamin C impact athletes. The vitamin is necessary for the formation of connective tissue, cartilage, bone, skin, and tendons and is involved in the healing of wounds, fractures, and bruises. It also plays a role in the production of certain hormones and neurotransmitters that are secreted during exercise, in iron absorption, and in the formation of red blood cells. Vitamin C is also strongly promoted because of its role as a powerful antioxidant. Symptoms of vitamin C deficiency could impair athletic performance.

Although vitamin C is a water-soluble vitamin that is easily excreted, the human body actually has a pool of vitamin C stores ranging from 1.5 to 3 grams. Serious vitamin

TABLE 3.2 FOOD SOURCES OF VITAMINS C AND E

FOOD	SERVING SIZE (OZ./C./TBSP.)	(G/ML)	VITAMIN C (MG)
Pepper, green	1 large		130
Orange juice	1 c.	240 ml	124
Cranberry juice	1 c.	240 ml	108
Grapefruit juice	1 c.	240 ml	94
Broccoli, cooked	½ c.	200 ml	90
Brussels sprouts, cooked	7		85
Strawberries	1 c.	240 ml	85
Orange, navel	1		80
Kiwifruit	1 medium		75
Cantaloupe pieces	1 c.	240 ml	70
Cauliflower, cooked	1 c.	240 ml	65

FOOD	SERVING SIZE (OZ./C./TBSP.)	(G/ML)	VITAMIN E (IU)
Wheat germ oil	1 tbsp.	20 ml	25
Sunflower seeds	1 oz.	30 g	21
Almonds	1 oz.	30 g	11
Sunflower oil	1 tbsp.	20 ml	10
Wheat germ	1 oz.	30 g	5
Margarine, soft	1 tbsp.	20 ml	3
Mayonnaise	1 tbsp.	20 ml	3
Brown rice, cooked	1 c.	240 ml	3
Mango	1 medium		3
Asparagus	4 spears		2

C deficiencies are rare because fresh or frozen fruits and vegetables are so abundant in our modern food supply. Though vitamin C is readily available from food, athletes often consume vitamin C supplements. Correcting a deficiency clearly improves performance, but research does not demonstrate that vitamin C supplements enhance performance when a vitamin C deficiency is not present.

Nevertheless, because exercise places stress on the body, moderate amounts of vitamin C above the RDA of 75 to 90 milligrams may be appropriate for athletes. Some scientists have recommended 200 to 300 milligrams daily, which can be obtained from a diet abundant in fruits and vegetables. Research indicates that 200 milligrams daily of vitamin C leads to full saturation of this nutrient in the plasma and white blood cells, which supports optimal immune function. Vitamin C supplements may reduce the symptoms and duration of upper respiratory tract infections, which may be more likely to occur following strenuous physical efforts. Vitamin C also plays an important part in the healing process when there is injury or muscle soreness. However, contrary to popular belief, most studies have not found that vitamin C supplementation helps to prevent the common cold.

A diet rich in fruits and vegetables provides ample amounts of vitamin C as well as other healthful substances found in those foods (see Tables 3.2 and 3.3). Avoid excessive intake of vitamin C supplements reaching 1,000 to 3,000 milligrams daily, which can cause side effects such as diarrhea and kidney stones. The safe upper limit is 2,000 milligrams daily.

VITAMIN E

Vitamin E receives much attention from athletes because of its role as a potent antioxidant. It prevents the oxidation of unsaturated fatty acids in cell membranes and protects cells from damage. Vitamin E is widely distributed in foods and stored in the body, so vitamin E deficiencies are rare. Polyunsaturated oils such as soybean, corn, and safflower are the most common sources of vitamin E. Other good sources are fortified grain products and wheat germ (see Table 3.2).

Experiments on vitamin E supplementation at altitude have produced some interesting results, but more research is required to determine whether any real performance benefits are possible. Because of its antioxidant effects, vitamin E may also be beneficial to athletes training in high-pollution areas. Endurance athletes should supplement with vitamin E carefully, however. One study assessed oxidative function in triathletes who supplemented with 800 IU of vitamin E in the weeks leading up to an Ironman triathlon. This level of vitamin E supplementation was actually found to increase oxidation rather than decrease it.

Vitamin E supplements may be recommended for possible prevention of chronic diseases, especially heart disease. Some researchers currently feel that a daily supplement dose of 100 to 200 IU is safe and appropriate, though more research on the highest safety dose is required. Individuals with a bleeding disorder or who are taking an anticoagulant medication or statin medication (designed to lower elevated blood lipids) should be cautious and first check with their physician before taking vitamin E. If you do take a vitamin E supplement, choose one that provides the natural source of the vitamin.

CAROTENOIDS AND VITAMIN A

Beta-carotene is one of 600 carotenoid pigments that give fruits and vegetables their yellow, orange, and red colors. Carotenoids are also abundant in green vegetables. While carotenoids are not vitamins, many act as antioxidants and also protect cells from free radicals.

The carotenoids most commonly found in blood and tissues are alpha-carotene, beta-carotene, lycopene, beta-cryptoxanthin, lutein, and zeaxanthin. Only alpha-carotene, beta-carotene, and beta-cryptoxanthin can be converted to vitamin A in the body. Research is just beginning to determine how specific carotenoids can boost immunity and protect the heart and eyes from chronic disease.

To obtain a variety of carotenoids in your diet, aim for at least five servings combined of fruits and vegetables daily, focusing mainly on yellow-orange, red, and dark green choices. You can easily obtain ample amounts in your diet.

Taking a supplement with carotenoids requires some caution, particularly in the case of beta-carotene supplements, which were

TABLE 3.3 SUPER SOURCES OF CAROTENOIDS*		
	SERVING SIZE	
FOOD	(C.)	(ML)
Apricot, dried	6 halves/pieces	
Broccoli, cooked	½ c.	120 ml
Cantaloupe pieces	1 c.	240 ml
Carrot, raw	1 medium	
Collard greens, cooked	½ c.	120 ml
Grapefruit	½ medium	
Kale, cooked	½ c.	120 ml
Mango	1 medium	
Mustard greens, cooked	½ c.	120 ml
Orange	1 medium	
Papaya	½ medium	
Pepper, red, raw	½ medium	
Pumpkin, cooked or canned	½ c.	120 ml
Spinach, raw	½ c.	120 ml
Sweet potato, mashed	½ c.	120 ml
Tangerine	1 medium	
Tomato sauce	½ c.	120 ml

*Includes alpha-carotene, beta-carotene, beta-cryptoxanthin, lutein/zeaxanthin, and lycopene.

found to increase cancer in smokers. If you do supplement, stay under 3 milligrams daily. Also keep in mind that carotenoids interact with one another. Supplementing with one carotenoid may impair the absorption of others. Carotenoids are converted to vitamin A as the body requires. But vitamin A supplements can be highly toxic at greater than the daily RDA of 5,000 IU. Besides, foods high in carotenoids may provide health-promoting substances not found in supplements. It's quite possible that these protective nutrients work best when they are packaged together. Table 3.3 lists some of the best sources of carotenoids.

VITAMINS D AND K

Because of vitamin D's important role in bone building, it is covered below in the section on calcium, although it also plays other important roles in maintaining good health and possibly athletic performance.

Vitamin K is also essential to bone health and is needed for the formation of pro-thrombin, which is required for blood to clot properly. Good food sources include leafy green vegetables, spinach, broccoli, Brussels sprouts, and cabbage. Vitamin K is also made by bacteria in the gut.

MINERALS

Like vitamins, minerals are involved in energy metabolism and also play important roles in building body tissue; in maintaining and strengthening the skeleton; in enabling the muscles to contract properly; in transporting oxygen as needed throughout the body via the red blood cells; in maintaining the acid-base, or pH, balance of the blood; and in regulating normal heart rhythm—all important for top athletic performance. Weak bones can contribute to the development of stress fractures, and an acid-base imbalance can affect endurance and energy metabolism so that fuel is not utilized as efficiently as possible during training. Minerals are involved in the metabolism of carbohydrates, proteins, and fats and in obtaining energy from an important fuel source, phosphocreatine.

There are two classes of minerals, both important for optimal body functioning. The *macrominerals* are present in relatively large amounts in the body and include calcium, phosphorus, and magnesium. Trace or *microminerals* include iron, zinc, chromium, copper, and selenium. Several minerals also function as electrolytes and play important roles in fluid balance. Sodium, chloride, and potassium are of special interest to the endurance athlete because they are three of the electrolytes lost in sweat. Magnesium and calcium also function as electrolytes and are lost in sweat in smaller amounts. Many of the recommendations for sodium that are made to the general public may not apply adequately to endurance athletes, who lose large amounts of sweat on a daily basis.

Altogether there are twenty-five essential minerals, each with its own unique functions. Minerals are obtained in our diet from the water we drink and from both plant and animal foods. Training-induced mineral losses can occur not only through sweat but through urine and gastrointestinal losses as well.

Three minerals very important to the athlete are calcium, because of its essential role in maintaining healthy bone structure; iron, which plays a crucial role in oxygen transport; and sodium, because of the potential sweat losses of this mineral and the negative performance effects that can result from excess loss.

CALCIUM

Calcium is the most abundant mineral in the body. Ninety-eight percent of calcium is found in bone, a dynamic tissue that is constantly being broken down and rebuilt. The remaining 2 percent of calcium is circulating in your bloodstream and contained in your teeth.

Calcium circulating in your blood has a significant effect on metabolism and physiological functions. It is involved in all types of muscle contraction, including contractions of the heart muscle, skeletal muscle, and smooth muscle found in blood vessels. Calcium also plays a role in both the synthesis and breakdown of muscle and liver glycogen. It is involved in nerve impulse transmission, blood clotting, and secretion of hormones. These physiological functions of calcium take precedence over formation of bone tissue. If a person's diet is low in calcium, it can be pulled from the bone to meet these more urgent needs.

Building and Maintaining Bone Mass
Calcium deficiency can develop from increased calcium excretion or inadequate intake. Strenuous exercise increases sweat loss of calcium. A major health concern associated with inadequate intake of calcium is osteoporosis, a disorder in which bone mass decreases and susceptibility to fracture increases. Optimal bone building takes

place until age twenty-five, but you can continue to build some bone until age thirty-five. After this age, efforts often focus on maintaining your current level of bone mass, but certain food, supplement, and medication strategies can support increased bone mass at any age.

Hormonal status, more specifically estrogen loss, also contributes significantly to the development of osteoporosis, making women more susceptible to this disease after menopause occurs, though men can also develop osteoporosis. Hormonal status in younger female athletes plays an important role in bone health. Extra calcium is recommended for female athletes with absent or irregular menstruation and for postmenopausal athletes. Weight-bearing exercise such as running and weight training enhances calcium skeletal absorption, increases bone mass, and can help prevent bone loss at any age. Calcium recommendations for various ages are provided in Table 3.4.

What Is the Best Way to Get Calcium in Your Diet?

Dairy products are very concentrated sources of calcium and for most individuals provide about three-fourths of their total calcium intake. Vegan athletes and athletes who do not have a high intake of dairy products need to focus on alternative plant sources of calcium and increase their intake of calcium-fortified foods. Choose low-fat options as much as possible. Some good plant sources of calcium are dark leafy greens, broccoli, bok choy, dried beans, and dried figs. Food sources of calcium are listed in Table 3.5. Some good fortified sources are soy and rice milk, orange juice, cereals, tofu processed with calcium sulfate, and some types of energy bars. Look for products marked as "high" or "rich" in calcium or as an "excellent source" of calcium, as they contain more than 200 milligrams per serving.

TABLE *3.4* DAILY CALCIUM AND VITAMIN D REQUIREMENTS		
AGE	CALCIUM (MG)	UPPER LEVEL (MG)
CALCIUM		
19–50 years	1,000 (men and women)	2,500
51–70 years	1,000 men 1,200 women	2,000
71 years and older	1,200 (men and women)	2,000
AGE	VITAMIN D (IU)	UPPER LEVEL (IU)
VITAMIN D		
9–70 years	600	4,000
71 years and older	800	4,000
SOURCE: NATIONAL INSTITUTES OF HEALTH.		

TABLE 3.5 FOOD SOURCES OF CALCIUM

GREAT SOURCES (300 MG PER PORTION)	SERVING SIZE (OZ./C./TBSP.)	(G/ML)
1% milk	8 oz.	240 ml
Skim milk	8 oz.	240 ml
Orange juice, calcium-fortified	8 oz.	240 ml
Collard greens, cooked	1 c.	240 ml
Rhubarb, cooked	1 c.	240 ml
Yogurt	6–8 oz.	200–240 ml
Mackerel, canned	3 oz.	90 g
Sardines, canned, w/bones	3 oz.	90 g
Salmon, canned, w/bones	3 oz.	90 g
Swiss cheese	1 oz.	30 g
Blackstrap molasses	2 tbsp.	40 ml

GOOD SOURCES (200 MG PER PORTION)	SERVING SIZE (OZ./C./TBSP.)	(G/ML)
Bok choy, fresh	1 c.	240 ml
Broccoli, cooked	1 c.	240 ml
Kale, cooked	1 c.	240 ml
Mustard greens, cooked	1 c.	240 ml
Soybeans, cooked	1 c.	240 ml
Turnip greens, cooked	1 c.	240 ml
Soy milk or rice milk, fortified	1 c.	240 ml
Soy yogurt	6 oz.	180 g
Tempeh	1 c.	160 g
Brick cheese	1 oz.	30 g
Cheddar cheese	1 oz.	30 g
Colby cheese	1 oz.	30 g
Edam cheese	1 oz.	30 g
Mozzarella cheese	1 oz.	30 g
Sesame seeds	2 tbsp.	30 g
Instant breakfast drink	1 packet	

FAIR SOURCES (100 MG PER PORTION)	SERVING SIZE (OZ./C./TBSP.)	(G/ML)
Cottage cheese, 1%	1 c.	240 ml
Navy beans, cooked	1 c.	240 ml
Pinto beans, cooked	1 c.	240 ml
Swiss chard, cooked	1 c.	240 ml
Shrimp, cooked	6 oz.	200 g
Lobster, cooked	6 oz.	200 g
Frozen yogurt	½ c.	120 ml
Pudding	½ c.	120 ml
Tofu	½ c.	120 ml
Parmesan, grated	1½ tbsp.	30 ml
Skim milk, powdered	1 tbsp.	20 ml
Figs, dried or fresh	5 medium	
Orange	1 large	

Individuals who are lactose-intolerant can buy specially formulated lactose-free milk or take lactase supplement enzymes before consuming milk products. Yogurt and cheese have lower lactose levels than milk and may be well tolerated. You may also be able to tolerate small amounts of lactose-containing foods.

A well-balanced training diet should provide many of the essential nutrients needed to build and maintain healthy bones; however, a calcium supplement may be indicated if your food intake is not adequate. If you do take a calcium supplement, find one that provides no more than 500 milligrams per pill, and take one pill at a time. Amounts greater than 500 to 600 milligrams will not be fully absorbed. Calcium carbonate should be taken with meals to increase absorption, while the calcium citrate form can be taken at any time. Avoid calcium made from oyster shells, bonemeal, or dolomite as these sources may contain lead.

Vitamin D and Bone Health

Vitamin D recommendations are also provided in Table 3.4 because this vitamin is essential for adequate calcium absorption, which is crucial to bone health. Without adequate vitamin D, we absorb only 10 to 15 percent of the calcium that we consume, compared with the typical 30 percent. Vitamin D may also have an effect on athletic performance because of its role in muscle function and strength, in controlling inflammation, and in the immune system.

Good food sources of vitamin D are limited. They include fatty fish, such as cod, mackerel, salmon, and sardines, and egg yolks. Fortified food sources of vitamin D include milk, soy milk, butter, margarine, and many cereals. If you spend a considerable amount of time in direct sunlight when participating in your endurance training, you could make adequate vitamin D from sunlight. Sunscreen blocks vitamin D production, however, and safe sun exposure without sunscreen is estimated to be only ten minutes in lighter-skinned persons; even twice to three times as much sun exposure is needed in darker-skinned persons. Moreover, sun exposure of any length may not be adequate from October to April in the northern part of the United States and Canada. Not surprisingly, it is estimated that at least two-thirds of the population is likely to have vitamin D insufficiency or deficiency—the figure may even be higher among some ethnic groups. If you tan when outdoors, you should be making sufficient amounts of vitamin D in your skin. But because our ability to make vitamin D from sunlight also decreases as we age, older athletes and individuals with limited sun exposure living in northern climates, as well as vegetarians, may want to consider taking a vitamin D supplement. Vitamin D is often conveniently combined with calcium in supplement form and can also be obtained from a multivitamin.

Other nutrients besides vitamin D and calcium that are an important part of building healthy bones are:

Vitamin C: Helps produce collagen, which holds bone together. A diet with plenty of fresh fruits and vegetables provides ample amounts.

Vitamin K: Activates osteocalcin, which is needed for optimal bone strength. Good sources are dark green leafy vegetables.

Magnesium: Key to bone formation. Good sources are almonds, bananas, avocados, dried beans, lentils, nuts, tofu, wheat germ, and whole grains.

In contrast, some dietary factors are actually harmful to calcium absorption. Excess sodium, protein, and caffeine, for example, increase calcium excretion. Alcohol can also be damaging to bone cells. Try not to consume excessive sources of caffeine. Intakes of phosphorus—namely, from carbonated beverages—should also be limited, because too much of this mineral can upset the calcium balance in the body. Keep your protein intake at an appropriate level for training, but do not consume excessive and unneeded amounts from supplements.

Obtaining adequate calcium in your diet takes planning. Here are some tips for maximizing your calcium intake:

- Have a breakfast every day that includes high-calcium milk, yogurt, or a calcium-fortified soy product.
- Include a high-calcium food with three meals or snacks daily.
- Choose low-fat milk or soy milk smoothies whenever possible.
- Make stir-fried vegetables for dinner that include: bok choy, kale, broccoli, leafy greens.
- Add reduced-fat cheeses to sandwiches.
- Drink a glass of calcium-fortified orange juice on a regular basis.
- Buy tofu, which is high in calcium, for stir-fries and other recipes.

IRON

Iron's role in exercise metabolism is key. Hemoglobin transports oxygen in the blood, and myoglobin transports oxygen in the muscle. Both of these oxygen-carrying molecules require iron for optimal formation. Many muscle enzymes involved in metabolism require iron. Other iron compounds facilitate oxygen use at the cellular level. Poor iron status can impair these functions as well as exercise performance.

The body storage form of iron, ferritin, is used as an indicator of iron stores, as are transferrin and hemoglobin. About 70 percent of the iron in your body is involved in oxygen transport, while the other 30 percent is stored in the body. Iron deficiency that is not corrected can progress to anemia, and anemia causes fatigue and intolerance to exercise.

Iron Deficiency

Iron deficiency is the most common nutrient deficiency in the United States. It is estimated that 22 to 25 percent of female athletes are iron-deficient, with 6 percent having full-blown anemia. When iron stores are low, total hemoglobin drops and the muscles do not receive as much oxygen. Blood work can be interpreted to determine whether you have early iron deficiency or full iron-deficiency anemia. However, remember that endurance training can affect your blood measurements of iron. Training produces an increased blood volume, which dilutes hemoglobin, making it appear low in some athletes when iron stores are adequate. This increased blood volume often occurs at the start of a training program and has no harmful effect on performance. In fact, this increased blood volume means that your heart can pump more blood to your working muscles, enhancing oxygen delivery.

True iron-deficiency anemia *will* impair exercise performance. Although we have less information regarding the performance effects of a low ferritin level, athletes may experience symptoms of fatigue and poor recovery with this condition. It makes sense to treat low ferritin levels so that full-blown iron-deficiency anemia does not develop. Your

---

WHY WOULD ATHLETES HAVE INADEQUATE IRON INTAKE AND IRON STORES?

- Inadequate dietary intake of iron is the most common cause of iron deficiency and anemia.
- Women with heavy menstrual blood loss may experience iron deficiency.
- Strenuous exercise can increase iron sweat loss, precipitate gastrointestinal bleeding, and decrease iron absorption.
- Heavy training may accelerate red blood cell destruction from mechanical trauma such as runners experience when pounding their heels on pavement.
- Training at altitude can place an athlete at risk of developing iron deficiency.
- Iron deficiency is associated with low-calorie diets, vegetarian diets, very high-carbohydrate diets containing only small amounts of animal protein, and various fad and unbalanced diets.

TABLE 3.6 IRON CONTENT OF SELECTED FOODS

SOURCES OF HEME IRON	SERVING SIZE (OZ.)	(G)	IRON (MG)
Liver, beef, cooked	3 oz.	90 g	6.0
Beef, cooked	3 oz.	90 g	3.5
Pork, cooked	3 oz.	90 g	3.4
Shrimp, cooked	3 oz.	90 g	2.6
Turkey, dark, cooked	3 oz.	90 g	2.0
Chicken, breast, cooked	3 oz.	90 g	1.0
Tuna, light	3 oz.	90 g	1.0
Flounder, sole, salmon	3 oz.	90 g	1.0

SOURCES OF PLANT IRON	SERVING SIZE (OZ./C.)	(G/ML)	IRON (MG)
Cereal, iron-fortified	1 oz.	30 g	2–18
Cream of wheat	¾ c.	200 ml	9.0
Soybeans, cooked	1 c.	170 g	8.8
Lentils	1 c.	240 ml	6.0
Instant breakfast drink	1 packet		4.5
Tempeh	1 c.	160 g	4.5
Kidney beans, canned	1 c.	240 ml	3.2
Baked potato, with skin	1 medium		3.0
Prune juice	8 oz.	240 ml	3.0
Spinach, cooked	1 c.	240 ml	2.9
Wheat germ	¼ c.	60 ml	2.6
Raisins	½ c.	72 g	2.0
Apricots, dried	10 halves		1.7
Spaghetti, enriched, cooked	½ c.	120 ml	1.4
Brussels sprouts	1 c.	240 ml	1.1
Bread, enriched	1 slice		1.0

SOURCE: USDA NATIONAL NUTRIENT DATABASE FOR STANDARD REFERENCE, WWW.NAL.USDA.GOV/FNIC/FOODCOMP/SEARCH/.

blood should be monitored by a physician, and any required treatment should be carried out under a physician's supervision.

Obtaining Enough Iron

Iron is obtained from food in two forms. Heme iron is found in animal foods—good sources are lean meat and dark poultry (see Table 3.6). Nonheme iron is found in plant foods—dried peas and beans, whole-grain products, apricots, and raisins are good sources. Nonheme iron absorption is compromised by the phytates, phosphorus-containing compounds, found in many vegetables and whole grains. Consuming meats and plant iron sources together can enhance iron absorption from plant foods. For example, small amounts of red meat in bean chili, spinach with chicken, and turkey with lentil soup combine heme and

BOOSTING YOUR IRON INTAKE

- Incorporate lean meat regularly into your diet. Eat small amounts several times weekly.
- Add small amounts of red meats to your favorite recipes, such as stir-fries, soups, pasta sauces, and casseroles.
- Mix heme-iron foods with nonheme choices, such as bean chili with dark turkey meat.
- Incorporate iron-fortified cereals into your diet. Avoid cereals with a high bran content, as they contain phytic acid, which binds with iron and decreases absorption.
- Increase fish and shellfish in your diet for their iron content.
- Increase your intake of plant iron such as whole-grain cereals, legumes, and green leafy vegetables. Have them with a vitamin C–containing food to improve iron absorption.
- Blanch green leafy vegetables for 5 to 10 seconds to remove the oxalate they contain, which decreases calcium absorption.
- Athletes training at altitude, female athletes, and vegetarians may want to consider a supplement that provides 100 percent of the Daily Values for iron and other trace minerals, such as zinc and copper, to ensure that they obtain adequate amounts of these nutrients. Many multivitamins contain this amount of iron, so check labels.

nonheme iron. Vitamin C–containing foods also enhance plant iron absorption. Try having orange juice or strawberries with fortified cereal, for example.

Checking Iron Stores

As an endurance athlete, you should have your hemoglobin, hematocrit, and ferritin stores monitored regularly. Do not self-diagnose or attempt to treat your own low iron stores; rather, have your blood work evaluated by a physician and follow his or her advice. Sometimes supplementation is advised; however, taking iron supplements carries some risk, especially if you take a supplement containing greater than 100 percent of the RDA for iron. Higher doses of iron—even a daily dose of 25 milligrams—can inhibit absorption of zinc and copper. Excess iron supplementation may also adversely affect individuals who have a genetic predisposition to iron overload, a condition that can result in excess iron deposits in the heart, liver, joints, and various body tissues, with the potential for damaging

WHY SUPPLEMENT?

Athletes training in endurance sports have the advantage of being able to eat more than their sedentary counterparts. With a focus on quality food choices, this generally means a diet filled with variety and nutrients. While a multivitamin and mineral supplement does guarantee that you will obtain all the Daily Values for vitamins and minerals, it is not the same as eating food. Nutrients from foods tend to be optimally absorbed and will provide you with all the phytochemicals, undiscovered or otherwise, that are not in your supplement.

A supplement containing reasonable amounts of a broad range of vitamins and minerals may provide the extra insurance that endurance athletes seek. Athletes who consume fewer than 1,500 calories daily, or who have food allergies that restrict a significant number of choices from one food group, might want to seriously consider taking a vitamin and mineral supplement. Other athletes may have a unique situation that makes it difficult for them to obtain all the nutrients they need from the foods they eat: they may travel frequently, for example, or have disordered eating or erratic diets. These athletes should consider supplementation. Vegans and other vegetarians may need additional vitamin D, zinc, iron, B12, and riboflavin. Each athlete should make this decision based on his or her own situation and medical history.

these tissues. In addition, high levels of iron supplements can lead to gastrointestinal intolerance and constipation.

ZINC

Zinc is an important mineral for athletes who train hard. An adequate amount keeps your immune system strong and promotes healing of wounds and injuries. Zinc is also a component of several enzymes involved in energy metabolism and is involved in protein synthesis. Like iron, though, excess zinc can be too much of a good thing: over-supplementing with zinc can interfere with absorption of other minerals.

Good sources of zinc include red meat, turkey, milk, yogurt, and seafood—especially oysters. The zinc from animal foods is better absorbed than that found in plant foods. Plant sources of zinc include garbanzo beans, lentils, lima beans, brown rice, and wheat germ.

ELECTROLYTES

Several minerals exist as electrolytes, or small particles that carry electrical charges. Major electrolytes in the body include sodium, potassium, chloride, magnesium, and calcium. Electrolytes function in a number of ways to control metabolic activities in the cells. Because electrolytes are lost in sweat, they are of particular interest to endurance athletes. When you lose large

CHOOSING A MULTIVITAMIN MINERAL SUPPLEMENT

- Consider a broad-range, balanced supplement of vitamins and minerals that provides 100 percent of the DV. These doses are known to be safe.
- Avoid supplements that contain an excess of minerals or any one mineral, as these nutrients compete with one another for absorption.
- Choose a supplement with the United States Pharmacopeia (USP) stamp of approval on the label to guarantee that it dissolves properly in your body.
- Choose a supplement in which the majority of vitamin A is beta-carotene, the precursor to vitamin A. Actual vitamin A, or retinol, should not exceed 3,000 IU daily.
- A blend of natural and synthetic supplements is fine. Look for a mix of vitamin E from tocopherols and tocotrienols. Don't pay more for "time-release" or "chelated" products.
- Calcium and magnesium may need to be purchased separately as they are too bulky to be provided in high amounts in a regular multivitamin pill.
- If you take antioxidant supplements, keep doses to 100 to 200 IU vitamin E and 250 milligrams vitamin C.
- Choose a multiple in which the vitamin D source is D3, or cholecalciferol, the type that is best absorbed.
- Take your multivitamin with a meal or snack and plenty of water.
- Don't double up on the daily dose of vitamins. You may get too much of certain nutrients.
- Avoid megadoses, and be sure to account for any vitamins and minerals you may be taking from sports nutrition supplements.
- Individuals over age fifty can opt for iron-free formulas and should look for B6 and B12 content in the higher range.

It is important to keep the use of antioxidant supplements in perspective, as they are strongly marketed to athletes. Diets abundant in foods that contain antioxidant nutrients have been shown to prevent cancer and other diseases, so don't discount the importance of increasing food sources of these nutrients. If you are concerned about the negative effects of free radicals, don't assume that supplementation is the key to solving the problem: the jury is still out on this issue. It is impossible to directly measure free radical production in humans. Although free radical by-products do increase with exercise, trained athletes may dispose of them more effectively as they make advances in their training—that is, their bodies may learn to cope with the negative by-products over time.

continues

CHOOSING A MULTIVITAMIN MINERAL SUPPLEMENT *continued*

Moderate doses of vitamin C, beta-carotene, and other carotenoids are easily obtained with educated food choices. However, one nutrient that may be difficult to obtain at antioxidant levels on a diet that limits fat intake to the recommended 30 percent level is vitamin E. Good sources of this vitamin are high in fat, and one would have to consume large amounts of them to reach even the low antioxidant dose of 100 IU. Researchers still need to determine the optimal doses of antioxidant supplements required for preventing heart disease and cancer.

If you do supplement, do so wisely. A multivitamin and mineral supplement providing 100 percent of the DV should be safe and does not have to be expensive. But keep in mind that the hazards of vitamin and mineral overdosing are real and can be subtle. If you take a supplement, understand the reasons for taking it and consume appropriate doses.

amounts of sweat during periods of heavy training, you can also lose large amounts of electrolytes. Sodium plays key roles in fluid balance, nerve function, muscle contraction, and acid-base balance.

SODIUM

Daily sodium needs vary widely among endurance athletes. The typical American diet contains up to 4,000 milligrams or more of sodium per day, particularly if you consume processed food and eat out frequently. The 2004 DRI recommendations are for North Americans to restrict their sodium intake to 1,500 milligrams daily, with the Tolerable Upper Intake Level (UL) at 2,300 milligrams of sodium per day.

However, endurance athletes lose considerably more salt from sweating than the average American. Sodium concentration in sweat varies widely among athletes, and some athletes are more prone to large sodium sweat losses than others. Heat-related problems during training and competition, such as hyponatremia (low blood sodium levels) and muscle cramping, have been linked to sodium losses in sweat as well as other factors. Most endurance athletes should be encouraged to salt their food, and they should consume sodium-containing foods during periods of heavy training in warm weather conditions. For example, even an acclimatized female endurance athlete with a relatively low sweat rate can lose more than 2,000 milligrams of sodium through sweat loss during a 2-hour training session; sodium losses during long weekend training sessions would be even higher. In contrast, a fitness enthusiast exercising for an hour may lose less than 1,000 milligrams of sodium during a typical exercise session; at this level, there is no risk of sodium depletion even if the individual has a low-sodium diet. The sodium needs of endurance athletes can drop off when sweat losses decrease during the shorter and less intense workouts in a recovery training cycle.

One way endurance athletes can replace lost sodium during a training session is by having sports drinks. But be careful not to overdo it. Individual athletes should discuss the risks of excess sodium intake with their physician, since a family history of heart disease and other factors in each athlete's medical history should be taken into account.

Chloride is also a mineral and an electrolyte, and intake of chloride is often paired with sodium, as table salt is sodium chloride. Chloride losses can also occur during heavy sweating, but a diet with adequate amounts of sodium should also be adequate in chloride.

POTASSIUM, MAGNESIUM, AND CALCIUM

Potassium, magnesium, and calcium are also contained in sweat, though lost in smaller amounts. Some sports drinks contain small amounts of these electrolytes to assist in replacing sweat losses during exercise.

Obtaining plenty of these three minerals in your daily diet is important. Information on calcium in relation to bone health is provided earlier in this chapter, and food sources are listed in Table 3.5. Women and other individuals at risk of osteoporosis should take extra care with their calcium intake in view of possible sweat losses.

Magnesium plays important roles in muscle contraction and glucose metabolism. Some endurance athletes training in hot and humid conditions for extended periods of time could lose fairly high amounts of magnesium in sweat. Consuming ample amounts of magnesium from good food sources such as milk products, nuts, whole grains, and green leafy vegetables is advised to ensure the recommended intakes.

Ample amounts of potassium can be obtained by consuming plenty of fresh fruits and vegetables, low-fat dairy foods, and animal proteins. High intakes of potassium may also help in preventing the development of high blood pressure. A balanced diet can easily provide several thousand milligrams of potassium daily, and the DRI is 4,700 milligrams. Your body stores of potassium are quite large, and while being an athlete increases your daily requirement, your sweat losses are only a small percentage of your total body stores. More information on replacing electrolyte losses is provided in Chapter 5.

PHYTONUTRIENTS

Unlike vitamins and minerals, phytochemicals or phytonutrients are not nutrients but rather plant chemicals that have health benefits. They are found in carbohydrate-containing foods such as fruits, vegetables, and grains. Important functions of phytonutrients include:

- Act as antioxidants or support the work of antioxidants
- Enhance immune function
- Protect against cancer
- Alter estrogen metabolism
- Reduce LDL cholesterol
- Control inflammation
- Reduce blood clotting

Phytonutrients you may have heard about are the allylic sulfides found in garlic, the flavonoids found in citrus fruits, the genistein found in soybeans, the indoles in broccoli and cauliflower, and the phytoestrogens in soy products, to name a few. To take advantage of these phytonutrients, eat plenty of fruits and vegetables, dried peas and beans, and soy products. Brightly colored fruits and vegetables produce anti-inflammatory and antioxidant pigments, and the deeper the color, the more phytonutrients a given food contains. Some of the best choices are green leafy vegetables, cruciferous vegetables such as broccoli and Brussels sprouts, citrus fruits, and deep red and orange fruits. Whole grains, though not colorful foods, are also high in phytonutrients. In the future, probably even more phytonutrients will be discovered.

Allicin: onions, leaks, garlic, and chives
Anthocyanins: blueberries, blackberries, eggplant, red cabbage

Capsaicin: hot peppers, chili

Carotenoids: mangoes, sweet potatoes, winter squash

Catechins: green tea and black tea

Curcumin: mustard, turmeric

Ellagic acid: raspberries, strawberries, red grapes

Flavonols: quercetin, tea, onions, berries, grapes, apples

Indoles and isothiocyanates: cruciferous vegetables, cabbage, broccoli, cauliflower, Brussels sprouts

Isoflavones: genistein, soybeans and soy products

Lignins: flaxseed, pumpkin seeds, whole grains, asparagus, broccoli

Limonoids: citrus peels

Resveratrol: grapes, wine, peanuts

Marty is a marathon runner who hadn't felt good in training for the past month after stepping up his program. He felt tired despite getting enough sleep and increasing his intake of carbohydrates and protein to match the increased training. Thinking that his diet may need tuning, Marty went to see a sports dietitian.

A diet recall and review of his regular eating habits indicated that Marty limited red meat and eggs, as high cholesterol ran in his family. His intake of dried beans was also limited, as were other foods high in iron. Overall, most of Marty's iron intake came from plant iron rather than heme or animal sources, which are better absorbed.

Clearly his diet was barely adequate in iron, yet Marty's iron requirements were likely higher than the average male's. His high training mileage on hard surfaces likely caused damage to red blood cells, and he likely had higher iron losses through sweating. The cause of his fatigue was thus probably inadequate iron rather than inadequate fuel. The sports dietitian referred Marty to his physician to have his iron stores checked.

Testing indicated that Marty's hemoglobin was below normal and that his ferritin concentration was very low, at under 15 nanograms per milliliter. His physician felt that Marty likely was in the early stages of iron deficiency. He began 12 weeks of iron therapy with an over-the-counter iron supplement to boost his iron stores while he improved his diet to better meet his iron needs.

The sports dietitian provided Marty with a list of high-iron foods and reviewed meal-planning strategies for increasing iron intake. Among the foods added to his diet were lean red meat, iron-fortified cereals, dried beans, several eggs weekly, and higher-iron fruits and vegetables combined with vitamin C sources. He has welcomed the increased variety.

At the end of 12 weeks, Marty's ferritin levels had increased to over 50 nanograms per milliliter, so he stopped taking the supplement and continued to consume iron-rich foods, as well as a multivitamin that provided a low dose of iron. He plans to have his iron stores checked again later in the season.

PART II

YOUR TRAINING DIET

Fine-Tuning Your Diet for Top Performance

An endurance athlete's diet begins with essential nutrition practices, as outlined in Part I. But how can a basic well-balanced diet be transformed into a scientifically sound, cutting-edge sports nutrition plan designed to support your endurance training program? Part II looks at the details of sports nutrition with an endurance athlete's specific needs in mind.

Chapter 4 describes the fundamentals of an endurance athlete's daily training diet. To assist you in understanding the nutritional demands of your diet, it reviews the fuel demands of the body's energy systems. The chapter will enable you to understand the role that your current training cycle plays in determining your daily training diet and to see how your nutritional requirements shift as your training program builds in preparation for an event or competition. Tables outlining your nutritional needs, food lists, and estimation of nutritional requirements are provided.

Because the timing of specific food and fluid portions is an essential component of a high-performance diet, Chapter 5 provides specific guidelines for pre-exercise and immediate post-exercise nutrient intake. Guidelines for fuel, fluid, and electrolyte intake during training are reviewed, as are pre-competition meals and nutritional strategies for an event or race training taper.

Chapters 4 and 5 explain sound methods of:

- Consuming sufficient energy, or balance of calories, for recovery from training, for tissue building in masters athletes, and for growth in younger athletes
- Consuming enough grams of carbohydrates to match that day's training and to be adequately fueled for the next training session
- Timing your intake of carbohydrates to expedite muscle glycogen resynthesis

- Consuming optimal amounts of protein for recovery, muscle tissue repair, and the maintenance of a strong immune system
- Consuming healthy fats and good sources of essential fatty acids to balance out the diet and replenish muscle fat levels
- Consuming adequate amounts of fluid and electrolytes, particularly sodium, after training to rehydrate and replenish body fluid levels
- Timing your post-exercise meals and snacks to maximize recovery until the next training session, with special consideration of immediate post-exercise nutrition recovery guidelines
- Practicing recovery nutrition at regular intervals to replenish fuel, fluid, and electrolyte stores

Body composition is also an important consideration for endurance athletes, and Chapter 6 outlines healthy nutritional strategies essential to muscle building and healthy and appropriate weight loss. Because nutritional supplements surrounded by claims of performance improvements are so heavily marketed to athletes, Chapter 7 is devoted to a review of the science, effectiveness, and safety surrounding these "ergogenic aids."

YOUR DAILY TRAINING DIET

Eating for Optimal Recovery

As an endurance athlete you must consume the right amount of energy, or calories, to meet the nutritional demands of your training program. During periods of moderate to heavy training, endurance work can be tough and tiring, and eating enough food is essential to completing longer exercise bouts at the intensities outlined in your program. The intensity and duration of your training also dictate the types of fuel your body demands and the types it will best utilize for energy on a daily basis. Because of their integral role in fueling endurance exercise and the limitations of your body's fuel stores, carbohydrates are the stars of your training diet, with protein and fat playing important supporting roles. Nutritional recovery is simply the process of eating properly, which provides you with the fuel to go from one training session to the next with the energy required. This recovery process may need to take place in 24 hours, or perhaps 12, 8, or 4 hours, depending on your training schedule. Begin by choosing quality foods for your sports diet as covered in Part I. A review of the body's energy systems, also called its power systems, will help you to appreciate the integral role of proper fueling.

Targeted nutritional strategies enhance your body's energy systems.

Starting exercise with low muscle glycogen can lead to early fatigue.

Match carb intake to training for muscle glycogen replenishment.

Use a food journal to identify areas of the diet that need improvement.

Daily energy needs vary depending on training intensity.

A variety of foods provides the proper breakdown of carbs, proteins, and fats for training and recovery.

THE POWER SYSTEMS

Each endurance sport training plan has its own unique mix of body fuel requirements. That is, during the various components of an exercise program, such as focused training cycles and events and competition, the body uses energy in different ways. Appreciating how your body uses fuel for exercise, how your specific training sessions affect energy use and fuel depletion, and how you can best refuel your body to replenish these energy stores is essential to your full nutritional recovery from one training session to the next. Because the way your body uses energy during training directly impacts the nutritional requirements of your sport, runners, cyclists, swimmers, and triathletes can benefit from a basic review and understanding of energy production and the fuel demands placed on the muscles. Specific nutritional strategies can enhance your body's energy systems and muscle-building efforts and thus affect your athletic performance.

Each energy system uses different metabolic pathways to produce energy. How significantly each system will contribute to the energy required for exercise depends on:

- The type of activity, which is determined by your sport and training program
- The intensity or speed at which you train
- The duration for which you train
- Your fitness level (your muscles' ability to use fat improves as a result of training)

Obviously, your training sessions can vary in intensity and makeup depending on whether you are building your aerobic system, endurance, or speed and whether you are swimming, running, or riding. Some training sessions require quick bursts of activity, some require steady activity with periods of faster movement or specific interval training, and others require that your muscles work slowly and continuously.

Each of these types of training uses a different type of energy system. The energy to power intense activity is referred to as *anaerobic*, whereas the energy that powers moderate and steady activity and the recovery process is mainly *aerobic*. Anaerobic energy systems are not dependent on the availability of oxygen to produce energy, while the aerobic system requires the availability of oxygen to produce energy during exercise. In addition to a mix of aerobic and anaerobic training sessions, many endurance sport athletes use weight training or resistance training (a form of anaerobic exercise) to build muscle and strength specific to optimal performance in their sport, and need to follow specific nutritional guidelines for muscle building. While there are some very important and essential nutritional principles related to training, performance, and recovery for all endurance sport athletes covered in this part of the book, there are also nutritional strategies specific to each endurance sport in Part III.

THE THREE ENERGY SYSTEMS

Because the anaerobic system has two major subcategories, your muscles actually have three energy systems from which to obtain energy or fuel:

- The creatine-phosphate (phosphagen) system
- The anaerobic glycolysis (lactic acid) system
- The aerobic system

A high-speed activity such as sprinting demands the all-out effort of the anaerobic *creatine-phosphate system*, which may provide energy for up to 10 seconds. This fuel is quickly depleted. Muscles can also use stored carbohydrates—primarily glycogen—for fuel through the *anaerobic glycolysis system*. This system is called upon when working at high intensities for longer than 10 seconds but also utilizes fuel supplied by the creatine-phosphate system. There are still limits to this fuel supply, which lasts about 90 seconds or slightly longer, and your muscles will still tap into the aerobic system for energy. If your workout increases respiration for longer than a few minutes, the *aerobic system* comes into play, for example, when you bike for several hours or go for a long run during marathon training. Long workouts rely on the aerobic system for fuel because this system burns oxygen to provide energy for much longer periods of time than can be supplied by the anaerobic system.

AEROBIC VS. ANAEROBIC AND EXERCISE INTENSITY

The aerobic system only predominates as a fuel source, however, when you are working at low to moderate intensities. Once the pace picks up and your muscles start working harder, oxygen cannot be supplied quickly enough, and it is back to predominantly the anaerobic system. Eventually the anaerobic system runs low on fuel and you become fatigued. Fuel can also become depleted from the use of the lower-intensity aerobic system, but a well-fed athlete should be able to train at low to moderate levels for several hours.

Well-trained athletes are able to provide plenty of oxygen to their muscles when needed and limit their reliance on the anaerobic system, delaying fatigue. Whether aerobic or anaerobic, these systems work best when they have the right fuels available. Some of these fuels are easier to supply than others. Body fat stores are in abundant supply even in the leanest endurance athletes. Carbohydrates are in much more limited supply and are needed not only as a direct fuel source but also because they allow fat to be burned effectively.

THE ONE POWER SOURCE: ATP

Although three different power systems supply your body with energy for training, ultimately only one source of fuel can be used for muscle contraction: adenosine triphosphate (ATP). You are constantly using ATP for both daily living and training, whether to simply breathe, go to school or work, or train in your sport. ATP is a high-energy chemical compound found in all muscle cells. When it is broken down, the energy released is used for muscle contraction. Because your muscles contain only a small amount of ATP, it must be steadily recharged for training to continue. The rate at which ATP is recharged in your body must meet the demands of the exercise you are performing. Low-intensity exercise requires a slow, steady supply of ATP, whereas high-intensity exercise requires a more rapid supply.

RECHARGING ATP

Because your body stores ATP in only small amounts, you need plenty of stored energy to recharge ATP and keep energy flowing while you train. Body stores of carbohydrates, protein, and fat release varying amounts of ATP at varying rates when they are burned for fuel. Carbohydrates are stored in limited amounts in your blood as glucose and in your muscles and liver as glycogen. Blood glucose is your brain's sole source of energy at rest and during exercise. A steady supply of it keeps you focused while you perfect your swim stroke in the pool or negotiate a tricky turn on your bike.

Liver Glycogen
Blood glucose levels can quickly run low and become unable to meet the energy demands of training. When this occurs, the liver breaks down its supply of glycogen into glucose and releases it directly into the bloodstream to maintain your blood glucose levels. The liver of a well-fed individual can store up to 400 calories' worth of glycogen. But liver glycogen is a relatively short-lived fuel supply that fills up and empties depending on the timing and composition of your last meal. Depending on what you ate and how

much you ate, liver glycogen stores generally last from 3 to 5 hours. You have likely experienced hunger and some of the symptoms that come with low blood glucose levels when you have not eaten for several hours, such as light-headedness, dizziness, and decreased mental focus. These symptoms, which signal the need for fuel, can occur 3 hours after breakfast, in the late afternoon, or anytime that your liver stores run low.

Muscle Glycogen

Both liver glycogen and blood glucose provide a limited supply of fuel. In fact, they can become depleted fairly quickly during certain types of training sessions and during competition. In contrast to your liver glycogen stores, your muscle glycogen is a larger storage supply of energy, providing anywhere from 1,400 to 1,800 calories, depending on your body weight and the makeup of your diet. When you train at any intensity, from easy to hard and from steady to stop-and-go, this glycogen is converted to glucose and used by the muscle fibers for energy. When your muscle glycogen stores run low, as can occur during long training days and during hard high-intensity and interval training sessions, your muscles can also utilize the glucose in your bloodstream for fuel. You are constantly using your glycogen stores when training at most intensity levels, but how much carbohydrate you actually need, and the rate at which you burn carbohydrates (quickly, moderately, or slowly), depend on how hard and how long you train that day.

Endurance athletes benefit greatly from ensuring that their muscle glycogen stores are refueled after training sessions that significantly deplete these stores. Even if your training session does not fully deplete muscle glycogen stores, constant partial replacement of stores can drain your performance efforts. Several days of successive training without adequate glycogen replacement could ultimately result in poor energy levels and poor training.

Table 4.1 demonstrates that your body's supply of carbohydrates is relatively limited. These carbohydrate stores are easily depleted during very high-intensity exercise and long training sessions. You have probably experienced the symptoms of low body carbohydrate stores during a training session. When your blood glucose levels hit bottom during aerobic training, you may feel dizzy and be unable to focus. You may

TABLE 4.1 CALORIES PROVIDED BY BODY FUEL STORES

BODY FUEL STORE	GRAMS	CALORIES
CARBOHYDRATES		
Blood glucose	20	80
Liver glycogen	75–100	300–400
Muscle glycogen	300–450	1,200–1,800
FAT		
Blood fatty acids	<1	7
Serum triglycerides	8	75
Muscle triglycerides	300	2,700
Adipose tissue triglycerides	9,000	80,000
PROTEIN		
Muscle protein	7,500	30,000

Note: These values can vary depending on the size of the individual and his or her body composition, level of fitness, and diet.

have had to stop exercising altogether or slow down considerably in order to consume carbohydrates and get your blood glucose levels back up. Your legs may have felt heavy and sluggish, and normal training may have seemed harder than usual. You can avoid these energy-draining training experiences by starting your exercise session properly fueled and by consuming enough carbohydrates during the session to offset body fuel losses.

Body Fat Stores

Table 4.1 also shows that fat is the body's greatest source of energy even in the leanest athletes, providing more than 50,000 stored calories (though the exact amount depends on individual body composition). During exercise when your muscles require fat for fuel, the fat stored within your muscle cells, known as intramuscular triglycerides, is used for energy. Just like muscle glycogen stores, intramuscular triglycerides must be replenished after training, though this fuel is not as easily depleted as muscle glycogen. Depending on the intensity and duration of the training session, you will also tap into the fat stored in adipose tissue and convert it to fatty acids that can be transported to your muscles. It is these more visible body fat stores that provide a relatively unlimited supply of fat for fuel. These same stores often become the focus of weight-management efforts among both endurance athletes and members of the general public who exercise for their health. Some endurance athletes include specific training sessions in their program aimed at decreasing body fat levels.

Protein Stores

Muscle protein stores can potentially supply several thousand calories' worth of energy. However, breaking down your muscle protein for fuel is not ideal either for recovery or for health, and this process could be detrimental to your performance. Muscle tissue maintains your strength, and constant excess breakdown of this tissue places undue stress on your body and your immune system. Muscle tissue breakdown can best be avoided by maintaining optimal carbohydrate and calorie consumption.

USING BODY FUELS

Fat and glycogen are the main fuels that your body uses for energy during training. Exercise intensity, which can be measured in terms of VO_2max (see the sidebar "Heart Rate and Fuels for Training"), is particularly important in determining which of these two fuels your body favors. Generally, the harder you train, the more carbohydrates you burn. Interval training or intermittent high-intensity training, in which you take your heart rate to higher intensities repeatedly, burns a significant amount of carbohydrates. Training itself activates the energy system that can best meet the fuel demands of the training session. It is your job to ensure that this energy system is well supplied.

Each of the three energy systems supplies the best type and amount of fuel to meet the energy demands of the training session that activates it. In other words, if your body needs carbohydrates quickly, then the glycolysis (lactic acid) system is activated. If your body requires a steady supply of fat, the aerobic system is activated. The creatine phosphate (phosphagen) system can be activated for an all-out sprint effort. Table 4.2 summarizes the characteristics of these energy systems. Besides showing the differences between the two anaerobic energy systems, the table subdivides the aerobic system into two types to distinguish the glycolytic process from the glycolytic/lipolytic process. In reality, there is no strict division between the two types of aerobic processes; rather, they occur along a continuum as low- to moderate-intensity

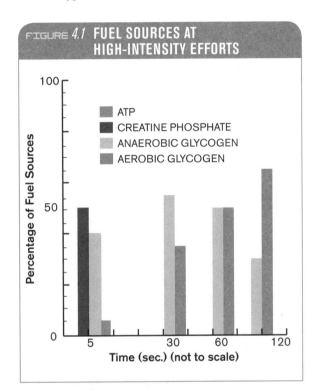

FIGURE 4.1 FUEL SOURCES AT HIGH-INTENSITY EFFORTS

TABLE 4.2 THE BODY'S ENERGY SYSTEMS	
ATP-CP SYSTEM	**ANAEROBIC GLYCOLYSIS (LACTIC ACID SYSTEM)**
ANAEROBIC SYSTEMS	
• Highest rate of ATP production	• High rate of ATP production
• Very limited supply of ATP lasting 6–8 seconds	• Limited supply of ATP lasting 2 minutes
• Highest power output and intensity level	• High power output and intensity level
• Develops explosive power	• Develops lactate tolerance
• Uses ATP and creatine phosphate stored in body	• Uses ATP, creatine phosphate, and muscle glycogen for fuel
GLYCOLYTIC (AEROBIC GLYCOLYSIS) SYSTEM	**GLYCOLYTIC AND LIPOLYTIC SYSTEM**
AEROBIC SYSTEMS	
• 15–90 minutes of exercise	• Greater than 90 minutes of exercise
• Low rate of ATP production	• Lowest rate of ATP production
• High supply of ATP	• High supply of ATP
• Low power production and low intensity	• Lowest power output and intensity level
• 15–30 minutes of exercise: uses muscle glycogen and blood glucose for energy	• Longer than 90 minutes of exercise: uses muscle glycogen, blood glucose, intramuscular fat, and adipose tissue fat for energy
• 60–90 minutes of exercise: uses muscle glycogen, blood glucose, and intramuscular fat for energy	

exercise proceeds. It's also important to realize that although you may specifically train a selected energy system, most training sessions involve both aerobic and anaerobic metabolism. The energy systems do not work in an exclusive fashion, though one may predominate during a particular training session. These two metabolic pathways can work together and complement one another to meet the body's energy demands. Figure 4.1 illustrates the duration of exercise that is possible when maximizing the use of one energy system.

MUSCLE FIBERS AND ENERGY PRODUCTION

Exercise intensity and duration determine not only the predominant fuel system that your body will use to do the work but also the type of muscle fibers it will use to do the work. The three major fiber types, Type I, IIa, and IIb, all have specific training properties. Type I fibers are slow-twitch fibers that predominate in endurance activities. These fibers have a high capacity to produce aerobic energy and store fat for fuel. Type IIa and IIb fibers are fast-twitch fibers that can produce anaerobic energy but differ in some of their characteristics. Type IIa fibers are more of an intermediate fast-twitch fiber and also have the ability to produce energy aerobically. The type of training that you perform affects the aerobic capacity of this fiber, which can behave more like an endurance fiber with aerobic training. The Type IIb muscle fiber is purely fast-twitch and anaerobic and has a high capacity to produce power and store and burn muscle glycogen. The fat-burning, slow-twitch Type I fibers are larger and predominate in top endurance athletes. Type IIa and IIb fibers are narrow and create speed.

HOW ENERGY IS PRODUCED

THE ATP-CP SYSTEM

As its name indicates, the ATP-CP system consists of both ATP and another high-energy compound called creatine phosphate (CP). Because ATP is in such short supply, it must be continuously and rapidly resynthesized to provide energy. Like ATP, CP is an energy-rich compound. When it is broken down, it, too, supplies energy. However, CP's released energy does not directly fuel muscle contraction. Rather, the energy released by CP resynthesizes ATP. Like ATP and the energy released from it, CP is in short supply. Energy from the ATP-CP system can fuel high-intensity efforts for only 10 seconds. Even at 10 seconds' duration, only half of your energy needs come from ATP-CP. Fast-twitch muscle fibers use the ATP-CP system rapidly. This system fuels the initial seconds of sprint events and other events where maximal force is required. It is an important fuel source where single bursts of sustained high-intensity activity are completed. For endurance athletes, any type of workout that involves successive bursts of high-intensity activity intermingled with lower-intensity activity will rely on the ATP-PC system for fuel.

The endurance athlete who has the ability to store more creatine has an advantage during this type of training. Enhanced storage of this important fuel allows you to maintain a higher power output during successive bouts of very high-intensity activity. To improve storage of creatine in your muscle, you must perform activities that focus on this energy system by performing high-intensity movements that are repeated multiple times during an exercise session. Consuming enough calories, carbohydrates, and protein for recovery also improves short-duration, high-intensity performance.

ANAEROBIC GLYCOLYSIS (LACTIC ACID SYSTEM)

Glycolysis is the second metabolic pathway within your muscle cells that is capable of rapidly producing ATP. As its name indicates, this production occurs through the breakdown of glycogen without the presence of oxygen. In glycolysis, a single glucose molecule is broken down from muscle glycogen to produce ATP. Anaerobic glycolysis provides energy for short-duration, high-intensity exercise lasting 10 seconds to several minutes. As exercise continues beyond 1 to 2 minutes, this system will taper off to provide less than half of your energy needs. Anaerobic glycolysis fuels activities such as high-intensity interval training sessions. At the onset of intense exercise, when oxygen cannot be delivered to your muscles quickly enough, this energy system is rapidly ignited to supply ATP.

The predominant source of energy during this type of activity is stored muscle glycogen. When this fuel runs out, your muscles cannot continue to perform at the same intensity and you become fatigued. This anaerobic energy source runs out quickly (after about 90 seconds) and must be followed by a period of rest of about 3 to 5 minutes for your muscles to become replenished with energy. This rest and recovery time is just as important as the high-intensity training time. If you need to run, swim, or cycle at full effort during training or competition, this anaerobic pathway is crucial.

AEROBIC METABOLISM

The aerobic pathway is the primary energy source for lower-intensity, prolonged exercise. This system is glycolytic and lipolytic, as it derives energy from both carbohydrates and fat. This pathway provides half of the energy for exercise lasting longer than 1 minute and the majority of the energy for exercise lasting longer than 2 minutes. When you begin an exercise session, you initially use the anaerobic pathways for energy but then switch to a predominantly aerobic pathway. An adequate supply of oxygen must be delivered to the muscles in order for the oxygen system to release the energy stored in carbohydrates and fats. Protein is not normally used for energy production, but under certain conditions it may become a significant source of energy.

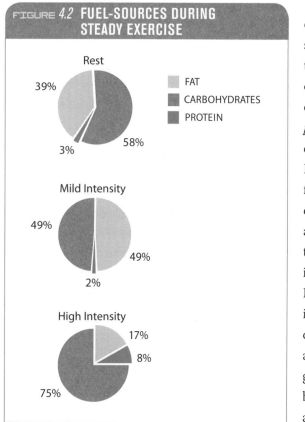

FIGURE 4.2 FUEL-SOURCES DURING STEADY EXERCISE

Rest
39%
3%
58%

FAT
CARBOHYDRATES
PROTEIN

Mild Intensity
49%
2%
49%

High Intensity
17%
8%
75%

Although the aerobic system cannot produce ATP as rapidly as the two anaerobic systems, it can produce much greater quantities at a slower rate. The rate at which the oxygen system produces ATP also depends on whether *aerobic glycolysis* or *aerobic lipolysis* is taking place—that is, whether carbohydrate or fat is being burned for fuel. Figure 4.2 illustrates how carbohydrates, fat, and protein contribute at varying levels of steady-state exercise. Carbohydrates are a more efficient fuel than fat and constitute the predominant fuel for steady exercise lasting more than 2 minutes and up to 3 hours. But one's storage capacity for carbohydrates in the muscles and liver is inadequate for certain endurance events, whereas fat stores are extensive. For the endurance athlete, glycogen depletion can occur during aerobic training as well as during sessions when aerobic training and anaerobic training are combined. For ultraendurance events lasting 4 to 6 hours and for long, low-intensity events, fat becomes the primary fuel source. This aspect of fuel burning applies to many endurance sport athletes during specific phases of their training, such as in long, low-intensity base training sessions or when preparing

HEART RATE AND FUELS FOR TRAINING

What Is VO₂max?

Without oxygen, training is not possible. The harder you exercise, the more oxygen your body requires to function. Eventually you will reach a level beyond which you cannot increase your oxygen use. This point where your oxygen consumption plateaus is called *maximal oxygen consumption*, or VO_2max. An athlete with a high VO_2max is considered to have a greater endurance capacity than an athlete with a lower VO_2max.

VO_2max is actually a measurement of your aerobic capacity, or the amount of oxygen your muscles can extract from the bloodstream. There are different ways of expressing VO_2max. It can be expressed in liters of oxygen used per minute (3.5 L/min.), or it can be expressed relative to body mass as ml/kg/min. (50 ml/kg/min.). Unfortunately, your ultimate aerobic capacity is determined largely by genetics. But you can follow a training program that will enable you to reach your full oxygen capacity potential and subsequently perform at your best. Highly trained athletes can maintain maximal aerobic capacity for only several minutes. Most of the time, you are exercising at a percentage of your maximal aerobic capacity, often called "percentage of VO_2max." Because many athletes have not undergone the scientific testing available to determine VO_2max, exercise intensity is often expressed as a percentage of maximal heart rate. Many athletes are familiar with their maximal heart rate as they train with a heart rate monitor.

What Is Lactate Threshold?

Lactate threshold is a related term. This measurement is usually expressed as a percentage of VO_2max but can also be expressed as a percentage of maximal heart rate. Like VO_2max, the level at which lactate threshold occurs varies among athletes. During exercise of increasing intensity, a by-product called lactic acid is produced. The point at which excess lactic acid begins to accumulate in your bloodstream is referred to as the lactate threshold. Every athlete has his or her own lactate threshold, and it is an important indicator of athletic performance. Basically, it measures an athlete's ability to sustain a high rate of energy expenditure without being limited by fatigue. An athlete with a lactate threshold at 75 percent of VO_2max should have better endurance potential than an athlete with the same VO_2max and a lactate threshold at 70 percent. This is because the higher lactate threshold allows the athlete to work closer to his or her aerobic capacity. In fact, lactate threshold is often a better predictor of endurance performance ability than VO_2max.

continues

HEART RATE AND FUELS FOR TRAINING *continued*

Genetics influences your lactate threshold, but so does training. Good training programs are designed to increase your lactate tolerance and threshold. Both your VO_2max and your lactate threshold can be measured from a graded exercise test on a bicycle or treadmill. Follow-up testing can determine how these performance measurements have responded to your current training program.

Training with a Heart Rate Monitor

When you train with a heart rate monitor, it provides the feedback you need to perform the appropriate training session for that day while staying within a specific heart rate zone. A heart rate monitor can also provide you with feedback on the mix of fuels you burn during exercise.

What fuel do I burn when training under 60 percent of my maximum heart rate?

When you exercise at under 60 percent of your maximum heart rate, training is fueled mainly by your fat stores. As you become more highly trained, adaptations to training allow your fat tissue to release fatty acids into the bloodstream. These fatty acids and the fat stored in your muscle are seemingly in endless supply as they fuel your low-intensity efforts. However, muscle glycogen still provides some of the fuel supply during these low-intensity efforts, and eventually carbohydrate stores will run too low for training to continue.

What fuel do I burn when training at 60 percent of my maximum heart rate?

At about 60 to 80 percent of your maximum heart rate, muscle glycogen and blood glucose stores supply approximately half of your energy needs. The other half of your energy needs comes from fat, with a small amount coming from protein. Your carbohydrate stores also limit exercise maintained at this level. Even at the lower end of moderate-intensity exercise, you eventually run low on glycogen. Depletion may not occur quickly, but it will happen.

What fuel do I burn when training above 80 percent of my maximum heart rate?

As intensity increases, eventually your aerobic system cannot fully meet the demands of your training session. When you train at above 80 percent of your maximum heart rate, fat cannot be utilized as a fuel as effectively and provides less than 25 percent of your energy needs. This is because fat cannot be broken down quickly enough to fuel training. As would be expected, your production of lactic acid increases at this higher intensity. When you exercise at 90 to 95 percent of your maximum heart rate, your body essentially relies on glucose for energy.

How Training Changes the Fuels You Burn

The type of fuel you burn is also determined by your fitness level, and training has many benefits in terms of fuel usage. When you are fit, your body becomes more efficient at producing energy aerobically at a given intensity. Consequently, you burn more fat and less glycogen, sparing your much more limited glycogen stores for a while. This adaptation partly explains how elite athletes can tolerate intense exercise levels without "hitting the wall."

Adaptations in training can also occur with changes in lactic acid accumulation. For example, untrained individuals could begin to accumulate lactic acid at 50 to 60 percent of their maximal aerobic capacity. Training can increase this lactate threshold to up to 70 to 75 percent, or even higher in elite athletes, allowing the well-trained athlete to use more fat and less glycogen at the same exercise intensity. Training programs are designed to increase your lactic acid tolerance in order to help you achieve your competition goals.

Endurance training has one other benefit. It increases your muscle storage capacity of glycogen. Your muscle glycogen is used at a slower rate when you are trained, and if you eat properly, you can begin exercise with higher glycogen stores. All these adaptations result in more stored fuel, more efficient use of fuel, and a higher fatigue threshold.

Regardless of the phase of training and type of training, for endurance athletes, having adequate fuel stores is crucial, and running low on fuel leads to fatigue and poor-quality training sessions. During any type of training session you benefit not only from the right nutrient mix in the daily diet but also from proper nutrient intake immediately before, during, and after training.

for specific events such as an Ironman triathlon, open-water long-distance swimming, or a bicycle road race.

NUTRIENTS FOR ENDURANCE TRAINING

Chapter 2 outlines the health benefits of choosing high-quality, nutrient-rich food sources of carbohydrates, proteins, and fats. But how you time and portion these nutrients specific to your training schedule, for each training session, and within the context of your current training cycle clearly distinguishes your diet as an endurance athlete. Because nutrient timing and portioning are so essential to optimizing the energy available for training and your daily recovery, your nutritional program should be carefully planned each day. Though your nutrient requirements and food strategies can change throughout the season, and even from week to week, there are some essential fundamentals to the role that carbohydrates, proteins, and fats play in your training diet.

ENERGY

As an endurance athlete it is important to appreciate just how much your daily training program affects your energy requirements. On very heavy training days, the number of calories you burn during exercise can easily exceed the number of calories your body requires for basic daily activity, more than doubling your energy needs. To excel at your sport—and to enjoy your training time—you must consume the calories your body needs for both everyday life and training. In short, eating enough food is essential to completing demanding training programs that test your endurance, power, and skill.

HOW MANY CALORIES DO YOU NEED?

In some ways, we can only speculate about the answer to this question. Estimating energy needs is not a precise science, and although many formulas work fairly well, every athlete has a unique energy system with its own tally of energy use throughout the day. In addition, your ideal calorie intake depends on your training and body-composition goals.

Your daily energy requirements are made up of the following components:

Resting metabolic rate (RMR): The amount of energy required to keep your body functioning while at rest. This energy keeps your brain functioning, maintains breathing, and keeps your heart beating. For many North Americans, the RMR accounts for 60 to 75 percent of total energy expenditure for the day. However, this percentage can be far lower for serious athletes who burn a significant number of calories when training. RMR can be estimated using a number of validated formulas, which are used by health professionals such as sports dietitians when estimating your energy requirements. RMR calculators available online also use a standard formula of some sort to estimate this number. But metabolic rate can now be measured outside of strict laboratory conditions with a fair degree of accuracy, allowing athletes and others to more accurately predict their daily energy needs—in other words, all the calories you burn in daily life other than training. Many professional trainers and health-care specialists now provide the testing required to estimate RMR using new portable versions of the RMR testing equipment. RMR can actually vary greatly from athlete to athlete, so this option of direct measurement can be very useful for some individuals, such as an endurance athlete struggling with weight-loss or weight-gain issues. RMR decreases with age, is greater in individuals with greater body mass, increases with greater muscle mass, and decreases with greater body fat stores. Following are some of the factors that affect an individual's RMR.

Growth: The energy needed for physical growth among athletes who are still children or teenagers. This is a major factor for the high-school cross-country runner or swimmer.

Daily physical activity: The energy you burn to carry out everyday activities—for example, the activity required of you at work or school. The number of calories needed for daily activity is generally small unless you have a physically demanding job that requires you to do a lot of walking or lifting, for example. For many individuals, this activity may constitute only about 15 percent of their energy requirements; others may have a higher daily energy expenditure.

Training expenditure: The calories you burn with exercise. This can be a large or small variable for the endurance athlete depending on that day's training intensity and duration. For example, you may have a light 4-mile run early in the week and a long 18-mile run on the weekend when you are preparing for a marathon. Triathletes and cyclists can burn thousands of calories on a long bike ride, whereas a 60-minute gym workout in the evening after a long workday burns significantly fewer calories. Table 4.3 outlines the calories burned during various types of workouts.

TABLE 4.3° CALORIE EXPENDITURE PER MINUTE OF ACTIVITY OF ENDURANCE SPORTS AND TRAINING ACTIVITIES

	WEIGHT OF ATHLETE										
LBS. KG	100 (45)	110 (50)	120 (55)	130 (59)	140 (64)	150 (68)	160 (73)	170 (77)	180 (82)	190 (86)	200 (91)
SWIMMING											
25 yards/min. (23 m/min.)	4.0	4.4	4.8	5.2	5.6	6.0	6.4	6.8	7.2	7.6	8.0
35 yards/min. (32 m/min.)	4.8	5.4	5.9	6.4	6.8	7.3	7.8	8.3	8.8	9.2	9.7
50 yards/min. (46 m/min.)	7.0	7.7	8.5	9.2	9.9	10.6	11.3	12.0	12.8	13.5	14.2
RUNNING											
5 mph (8.5 km/hr.)	6.0	6.6	7.3	7.9	8.5	9.1	9.7	10.3	10.9	11.6	12.2
7 mph (11.6 km/hr.)	8.5	9.3	10.2	11.0	11.9	12.8	13.6	14.5	15.4	16.2	17.1
9 mph (15 km/hr.)	10.8	11.9	12.9	14.0	15.1	16.2	17.3	18.4	19.5	20.6	21.7
CYCLING											
15 mph (25 km/hr.)	7.3	8.0	8.7	9.5	10.0	10.9	11.6	12.4	13.1	13.8	14.5
20 mph (32 km/hr.)	10.7	11.7	12.8	13.9	14.9	16.0	17.1	18.1	19.2	20.3	21.3
25 mph (40 km/hr.)	13.5	15.0	16.3	17.7	19.0	20.5	21.8	23.0	24.5	25.9	27.2
WEIGHT TRAINING											
	5.2	5.7	6.2	6.8	7.3	7.8	8.3	8.9	9.4	9.9	10.5
AEROBIC CONDITIONING											
	4.7	5.2	5.7	6.1	6.5	7.0	7.5	7.9	8.3	8.9	9.4

Thermic effect of food: The calories required just to digest and absorb the food you consume. This number is always quite small but can vary with the type of meal or snack that you consume.

STRATEGIES FOR ESTIMATING ENERGY NEEDS

Although determining energy needs is not a precise science, some general indicators can help you to appreciate just how low, moderate, or high your calorie needs may be for daily recovery from one training session to the next. Of course, many athletes want to consider the proper calorie adjustments to be made for their body-composition goals, whether for muscle building, fat loss, or both. More specific nutritional information on changing body composition is provided in Chapter 6.

Calories per Pound (or Kilogram) Based on Activity Level

One method of estimating daily calorie needs is based on the amount of calories you require per pound of body weight as directly related to the amount of training you complete that day. These calculations take resting metabolic rate, daily energy needs, and energy for training into account. When in serious training mode and preparing for an important day of running, cycling, or swimming, it is best not to fall short on calorie requirements. Several days in a row of not recharging your batteries fully may result in some unplanned rest days, days off, or poor-quality training sessions, all of which can hamper your competition goals.

The calorie descriptions listed here show how your activity can affect your total calorie needs for the day. Energy needs are not consistent every day. A 160-pound (73 kg) adult who trains for 90 minutes one day would require 18 to 24 calories per pound (40–53 kilocalories per kilogram [kcal/kg]) of body weight, or 2,880 to 3,840 calories, to meet his or her total energy needs, while that same adult completing 3 hours of training would require 24 to 29 calories per pound (52–63 kcal/kg) of body weight, or up to 4,640 calories for the day.

Calories per Pound (Kilogram) Weight Based on Training Level

To estimate his or her caloric needs more specifically, an athlete could categorize the training sessions by intensity.

- Mild activity, with no purposeful exercise or training, or even on a rest day from training, you need only 12 to 14 calories per pound (26–31 kcal/kg) of body weight.
- Up to 1 hour of moderate exercise, you need 15 to 17 calories per pound (33–37 kcal/kg) of body weight for the day.
- High-activity day, with 1 to 2 hours of moderate-intensity exercise, you need 18 to 24 calories per pound (40–53 kcal/kg) of body weight.
- Very high level of activity, with several hours of training, you need 24 to 29 calories per pound (53–63 kcal/kg) of body weight.

Calories = RMR + Daily Activity + Training Requirements

You can also estimate the number of calories you need for a particular day by adding together the amount needed for your estimated or measured RMR, the amount needed for your daily activity outside of training, and the amount needed for your particular sport for the amount of time that you train that day. Teenagers and pregnant women would also need to factor in the amount needed to meet their special requirements.

- RMR is generally estimated at 11 to 12 calories per pound (24–26 kcal/kg) of body weight, but it can be lower or higher in some individuals. Fine-tune this number by having your RMR tested by a professional.

- Daily calorie expenditures outside of training may add another few hundred calories.
- The amount of calories you burn can add up with heavy training, as indicated in Table 4.3.

The calorie expenditures supplied in Table 4.3 are listed per minute of activity for the endurance sports reviewed in this book. These figures represent averages, however. Seasoned athletes can become much more efficient in their sport—that is, they can move and use their muscles more efficiently than less experienced athletes, which results in conserving energy. They therefore burn fewer calories when training. Conversely, athletes who are new to an endurance sport are not as efficient in their movements and can burn more calories when training.

Endurance athletes often train with a heart rate monitor to track the number of calories they are burning. When a heart rate monitor is used to measure energy expenditure, it is based on an average linear relationship between heart rate and oxygen consumption. However, particular heart rate levels may not correspond to the same levels of oxygen consumption in every individual. Because of this individual variability, the monitor can provide only an estimation of calories burned. Even when you key your weight into the heart rate monitor and estimate your heart rate, you will receive only an estimate of the calories burned based on a one-size-fits-all equation.

Using a Formula Appropriate for Athletes

First, determine your resting metabolic rate (RMR). There are three ways that you can do this. The Mifflin–St. Jeor equation is the most accurate for the general population. The Cunningham equation, which uses lean body mass and requires that you have your body composition tested, works best for athletes. Alternatively, you can have your RMR measured with portable equipment such as that made by New Leaf.

Estimate your energy requirements using the following as a guide:

1. **Resting Metabolic Rate**

   To use the equations, you will need to convert your weight from pounds to kilograms, by dividing your weight by 2.2. Example: 160 lb. = 73 kg. You will need to convert your height in inches to centimeters by multiplying by 2.54. Example: 68 inches = 173 cm.

   a. The Mifflin–St. Jeor equation:

$$Men: RMR = (9.99 \times wt \, [kg]) + (6.25 \times ht \, [cm]) - (4.92 \times age) + 5$$
$$Women: RMR = (9.99 \times wt \, [kg]) + (6.25 \times ht \, [cm]) - (4.92 \times age) - 161$$

   b. The Cunningham equation:

$$RMR = 370 + (21.6 \times lean \, body \, mass \, [kg])$$

2. **Daily Activity**

   If you have a desk job or sedentary job, this will not significantly impact your calorie intake—it will likely constitute no more than 10 percent of your total calorie intake. Every mile you walk in your daily life throughout a workday burns about 100 calories. You can also multiply your RMR by 1.2 to 1.3 for a sedentary job. Another option is to wear a pedometer.

3. **Training Requirements**

   Training requirements usually represent the largest calorie factor for endurance athletes, and on high-volume training days can even exceed their RMR. Refer to Table 4.3 for the caloric expenditure of various types of endurance exercise.

4. **Carbohydrate/Protein/Fat Requirements**

   Table 4.4 on page 96 outlines daily carbohydrate, protein, and fat requirements.

5. **Example**

   Estimate RMR:

   Triathlete Jack weighs 165 lb. and has 8 percent body fat.

$$Fat \, pounds \, are \, 165 \times .08 = 13.2$$
$$Lean \, mass \, or \, fat \, free \, mass \, is \, 165 - 13.2 = 151.8 \, lb.$$
$$151.8 \, lb. \, lean \, mass = 69 \, kg$$

$$RMR = 370 + (21.6 \times 69) = 1,860 \, calories$$

   Add in daily activity:

   Jack has a desk job so he multiplies his RMR by 1.2.

$$1,860 \times 1.2 = 2,232 \, calories$$

   Training for that day is a 60-minute high-intensity swim in the morning and a 90-minute moderate-intensity run in the evening.

TABLE 4.4 DAILY NUTRIENT REQUIREMENTS FOR TRAINING		NUTRIENT REQUIREMENTS	
NUTRIENT	TRAINING	GRAMS PER LB.	GRAMS PER KG
Carbohydrates	Moderate training (under 1 hr. at moderate intensity or several hrs. at low intensity)	2.3–3.0	5.0–7.0
	Heavy training (1–3 hrs. at moderate/high intensity)	2.7–4.5	6.0–10.0
	Very heavy training (3–4 hrs. at moderate/high intensity)	3.6–5.5	8.0–12.0
Protein	Moderate training	0.5	1.0
	Heavy training	0.5–0.8	1.1–1.6
	Very heavy training	0.8–0.9	1.8–2.0
	SPECIAL CONSIDERATIONS:		
	Strength training phase of training, experienced	0.5–0.7	1.0–1.5
	Strength training phase of training, novice	0.8	1.8
	Growing teenage athlete	0.8–0.9	1.8–2.0
	Athlete restricting calories	0.8–0.9	1.8–2.0
	Maximum recommended for extreme exercise loads	1.0	2.2
Fat	Moderate training	<0.5	1.0
	Heavy training (over 4 hrs.)	0.5–0.6	1–1.2
	Very heavy training (over 6 hrs.)	0.5–0.8	1–1.6

According to Table 4.3,

Swim: 700 calories

Run: 1,200 calories

Calculate total energy requirements:

2,232 + 700 + 1,200 = 4,132 calories

CARBOHYDRATES: THE RECOVERY FUEL

You may or may not have experienced the symptoms of glycogen depletion during a single training session. It is possible, however, that you experienced it over a longer period without realizing it. The symptoms of gradual glycogen depletion can occur over successive days of training and can be much more subtle than simply "hitting the wall." Symptoms of glycogen depletion can creep up over a week's time or longer, producing feelings of sluggishness and heaviness. Besides experiencing general lethargy, you may not be able to put out an increased or even normal effort during training, or you may find it difficult to maintain your usual intensity and duration of training. The more muscle

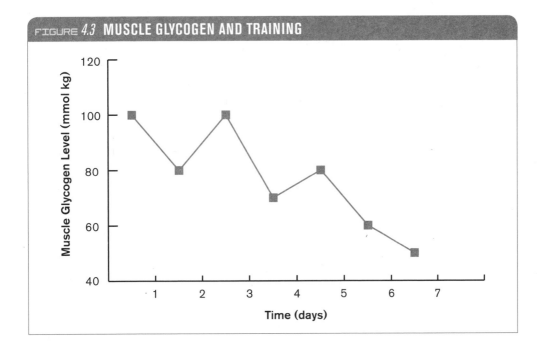

FIGURE *4.3* MUSCLE GLYCOGEN AND TRAINING

glycogen stored in your body, the better the quality of your interval training sessions and the better your energy levels during a long run or bike. Figure 4.3 illustrates how gradual glycogen depletion due to the combination of daily training and inadequate daily carbohydrate intake can occur slowly over a period of several days.

Numerous scientific studies have shown that a diet adequate in carbohydrates is superior for building, maintaining, and replenishing muscle glycogen stores. The amount of carbohydrate you consume in your diet directly affects the amount of glycogen you store in your muscles and liver. Inadequate intake of carbohydrates leads to partial replenishment of muscle glycogen stores. If this incomplete replenishment occurs from one day to the next, your glycogen stores gradually become depleted over a period of a week or more, and your training will suffer. Adequate recovery allows you to start the next training session, whether it is 4, 8, 12, or 24 hours away, with optimal fuel to complete the exercise at the desired duration and intensity spelled out in your training program.

DAILY CARBOHYDRATE REQUIREMENTS: MATCHING INTAKE TO TRAINING

Carbohydrate recommendations are often expressed as a percentage of total calories. This is appropriate for general recommendations for nonathletes, when the goal is usually to decrease unwanted fat intake and increase wholesome carbohydrates from whole grains and fruits and vegetables. However, for endurance sport athletes, it is more appropriate to express carbohydrate targets as grams per pound (or kg) of weight based on the intensity and duration of the training session or sessions for that day. Regardless of the type of training session, your muscles require an absolute amount of carbohydrate to recover sufficiently, particularly after intense exercise sessions that are endurance-based or that include plenty of high-intensity efforts, which can quickly deplete carbohydrate stores.

The ceiling for daily carbohydrate consumption—that is, the point at which your muscle storage capacity has been reached—is 4.5 to 5.5 grams of carbohydrates per pound (10–12 g/kg) of weight. Depending on the size of the athlete, this translates to anywhere from 500 to 700 grams of carbohydrates daily. Higher levels may not resynthesize muscle glycogen stores any faster, however. Most endurance athletes who meet both their energy and carbohydrate needs can average about 50 to 65 percent carbohydrate calories in their training diet. But depending on whether you are restricting calories for weight management or have very high energy needs, the percentage of carbohydrates consumed may vary. Typically, as an athlete you will have to consume greater quantities of carbohydrates than most people, including athletes participating in sports that do not have as high a fuel demand as endurance sports and individuals exercising for general fitness. Table 4.4 outlines your carbohydrate targets based on training time and intensity.

PHASES OF GLYCOGEN REPLENISHMENT

Because any cycle of your training program and every type of workout uses some amount of the more limited fuel supply of muscle glycogen, carbohydrate foods are the foods to focus on for recovery nutrition. There are several phases of glycogen replenishment. If you train only every 24 hours, you simply need to consume the proper amount of carbohydrate between training sessions. However, many endurance athletes train again in 12, 8, or even 4 hours. If training sessions are scheduled in these time frames, and if you have multiple workouts outlined in your training schedule, it is important that you take advantage of the early phases of muscle glycogen recovery. Initially there is a very rapid phase of recovery that lasts for the 30 to 60 minutes after exercise when muscle glycogen stores are very low. The rate of muscle glycogen resynthesis then remains somewhat elevated for the first 6 hours after training, after which it slows down. Nutritional strategies regarding food and fluid choices, portions, and timing presented in Chapter 5 are designed to maximize muscle glycogen resynthesis after training.

PROTEIN AND DAILY RECOVERY REQUIREMENTS

Although carbohydrate intake should receive the most emphasis in your endurance training diet, the demands of endurance training and training for power and strength also increase your need for protein. Protein needs are highest in endurance athletes who follow very intense training programs and who incorporate resistance training into their program. Intense training can also entail significant wear and tear on the muscles and ligaments, requiring protein for repair. Endurance sport athletes who engage in strength training can rely on glycogen for fuel during this mode of exercise and, most importantly, should consume enough carbohydrates so that protein is not utilized for fuel during training.

Elevated protein requirements are easily met by a well-planned sports diet. What distinguishes a sports diet is how you time protein intake, particularly around resistance training (see Chapter 5). Most North Americans consume a diet that easily meets the protein needs of an athlete participating in a demanding training program. Inadequate protein intake may be a concern only for athletes who follow a poorly planned vegetarian diet, who restrict their calories, or who have very specific food dislikes. Consider how simple it is to meet your daily protein requirements. Having some peanut butter and cereal with milk for breakfast, a turkey sandwich for lunch, and a stir-fry of lean red meat and rice for dinner supplies about 90 grams of protein. You can obtain additional protein from between-meal snacks. Foods such as whole grains and vegetables, which are not as concentrated in protein, still contribute to total protein intake and can provide moderate amounts over the course of a day, supplementing your intake of more concentrated protein foods.

FAT REQUIREMENTS

Endurance athletes should consume approximately 0.5 gram of fat per pound (1 g/kg) of body weight to obtain adequate amounts of essential fatty acids. Fat can provide 15 to 30 percent of the day's calories depending on the carbohydrate, protein, and especially energy needs for that day's training. Once carbohydrate and protein requirements are met for your training program and recovery, fat can make up the remainder of the calories appropriate for your weight and body-composition goals.

The most important strategy regarding fat intake is to consume enough healthy fats high in essential fatty acids, as outlined in Chapter 2. For athletes who need to monitor their weight closely to prevent unwanted weight gain, especially during specific training cycles when endurance athletes have lower energy needs, too much fat in the diet may present a problem. This is more likely to happen with athletes who frequently eat out or travel. Some athletes may be accustomed to eating out and frequenting fast-food establishments. A high-fat diet is often very calorie-dense and leaves less room for quality carbohydrates. Weight-conscious athletes should keep fat calories at 20 to 25 percent of total intake. (For more on body-composition strategies, see Chapter 6.)

Recent research regarding fat requirements for athletes in ultraendurance training has shown that athletes who complete training sessions of more than 4 hours when preparing for an Ironman, ultrarunners, ultraswimmers, and ultracyclists can actually deplete their muscle stores of fat, or muscle triglycerides. While more research regarding the fat requirements of ultraendurance athletes is needed, it is speculated that a diet too low in fat could lead to inadequate replenishment of these intramuscular triglycerides. Just how much fat is needed for these long training sessions has not been definitely determined. But a diet with less than 20 percent of total calories from fat, or less than 0.5 gram of fat per pound (1 g/kg) of body weight, could be inadequate for replenishment purposes following these types of training sessions. Fat replenishment is especially important when endurance athletes train for long sessions on consecutive days. Table 4.4 provides a summary of an endurance athlete's carbohydrate, protein, and fat requirements.

FLUID REQUIREMENTS

As explained in Chapter 1, water and fluid are essential components of your daily training diet. Thirst is not a good indicator of when you need to drink; it only signals that body fluid levels are already low. Significant weight fluctuations on the scale could signal inadequate daily hydration and poor rehydration efforts when not training. The color of your urine can also indicate the success of your daily hydration efforts: pale or lemonade-colored urine indicates adequate hydration; darker urine indicates that you need to increase your fluid intake. Specific guidelines for hydrating during exercise and immediately post-exercise are reviewed further in Chapter 5.

PERIODIZING YOUR TRAINING DIET

Because training cycles vary in specificity, volume, and intensity, general nutritional requirements for each training cycle also vary. Each individual athlete has unique nutritional needs throughout the season. Your nutritional requirements vary with your training program, body-composition goals, and level of aerobic and anaerobic training as you fine-tune the program that best fits your sport and your goals for the season. There are some specific nutritional considerations for each training cycle, however, that are helpful for many endurance athletes (see the sidebar "Training Periodization" and Table 4.5).

TABLE 4.5 NUTRITIONAL PERIODIZATION

TRAINING CYCLE	NUTRITIONAL REQUIREMENTS	MALE, 160 LBS. (72 KG)	FEMALE, 140 LBS. (64 KG)
Preparation	3.0 g/lb. (6.5 g/kg) carbohydrates	480 g carbohydrates	420 g carbohydrates
	0.5 g/lb. (1.1 g/kg) protein	80 g protein	70 g protein
	0.5 g/lb. (1.0 g/kg) fat	80 g fat	70 g fat
		2,960 calories	2,590 calories
Build	4.5 g/lb. (10.0 g/kg) carbohydrates	720 g carbohydrates	630 g carbohydrates
	0.8 g/lb. (1.8 g/kg) protein	128 g protein	112 g protein
	0.6 g/lb. (1.3 g/kg) fat	96 g fat	84 g fat
		4,260 calories	3,720 calories
Transition	2.5 g/lb. (5.5 g/kg) carbohydrates	400 g carbohydrates	350 g carbohydrates
	0.6 g/lb. (1.3 g/kg) protein	96 g protein	84 g protein
	<0.5 g/lb. (<1.0 g/kg) fat	80 g fat	70 g fat
		2,700 calories	2,370 calories

Let's take a look at Jack again. We estimated his energy needs using a formula for athletes, along with his daily activity and training energy requirements. But it is also important to calculate Jack's daily nutritional prescription for carbohydrates, proteins, and fats.

Calculate carbohydrate requirements (2.5 hours of total training):

165 lb. × 4.5 g/lb. = 740 g

740 g × 4 cal/g = 2,960 calories from carbohydrate, or 71 percent total calories

Calculate protein requirements (heavy training day):

165 lb. × 0.8 g/lb. = 132 g

132 g × 4 cal/g = 528 calories, or 13 percent total calories

Calculate fat requirements:

0.45 g/lb. = 74 g

74 g × 9 cal/g = 666 calories, or 16 percent total calories

How Jack distributes his carbohydrates, proteins, and fats for the day is a function of that day's training schedule. There are specific timing and portioning strategies to follow before, during, and after training that can optimize fuel for training and recovery between training sessions. Read more about these strategies in Chapter 5.

FUELING FOR THE PREPARATION CYCLE

Because the preparation cycle is low to moderate in intensity and higher in volume as you build your training foundation, your body relies on a fairly even mix of carbohydrates and fat for fuel during training. During this training cycle, longer workouts tend to be lowest in intensity and consequently burn a greater percentage of fat. Strength training workouts in this phase of training also deplete muscle glycogen stores for fuel. Your protein requirements are only slightly higher than normal at this point, though the timing of your protein intake around weight training sessions is very important (for more information on nutrition for weight training, see Chapter 6). Your energy needs are based on the volume of training, and fat can round out your caloric intake after you have consumed adequate carbohydrates and protein. The following list summarizes carbohydrate, protein, and fat needs for training:

CARBOHYDRATES   2.5–3 g/lb. (5.5–6.5 g/kg)   1–2 hours, low intensity
3–4.5 g/lb. (6.5–10 g/kg)   3–4 hours
Requirements can increase even more for the ultraendurance athlete.

PROTEIN   0.5–0.6 g/lb. (1.1–1.3 g/kg)
Ultraendurance athletes can increase protein intake to 0.8 g/lb. (1.8 g/kg).
Proper timing of protein intake around weight training is very beneficial.

FAT   0.4–0.5 g/lb. (0.9–1.0 g/kg)
Round out energy needs with healthy fats. Ultraendurance

athletes require a minimum of 0.5 g/lb. (more than 1 g/kg) to replace muscle fat.

Calories can be adjusted down for weight loss or increased for a focus on muscle building. This is the best time in the training cycle to decrease weight and body fat without a significant compromise in recovery. Here are examples of estimations of the energy needs of some endurance athletes:

MALE TRIATHLETE, 170 LBS. (77 KG)

Training session: Cycling, 90 minutes, low intensity

Carbohydrate requirements	510 g (3 g/lb.) × 4 kcal/g	=	2,040 calories
Protein requirements	102 g (0.6 g/lb.) × 4 kcal/g	=	408 calories
Fat requirements	85 g (0.5 g/lb.) × 9 kcal/g	=	765 calories
Total caloric intake			3,213 (19 kcal/lb.)

FEMALE RUNNER, 140 LBS. (64 KG)

Training session: Running, 75 minutes, 8.5 miles

Carbohydrate requirements	350 g (2.5 g/lb.) × 4 kcal/g	=	1,400 calories
Protein requirements	63 g (0.45 g/lb.) × 4 kcal/g	=	252 calories
Fat requirements	70 g (0.5 g/lb.) × 9 kcal/g	=	630 calories
Total caloric intake			2,282 (16 kcal/lb.)

MALE SWIMMER, 130 LBS. (59 KG)

Training session: Endurance workout, 85 minutes

20 minutes, warm-up

30–45 minutes, base/endurance pace

10 minutes, quick speed

10 minutes, cooldown

Carbohydrate requirements	358 g (2.75 g/lb.) × 4 kcal/g	=	1,432 calories
Protein requirements	78 g (0.6 g/lb.) × 4 kcal/g	=	312 calories
Fat requirements	52 g (0.4 g/lb.) × 9 kcal/g	=	468 calories
Total caloric intake			2,212 (17 kcal/lb.)

TRAINING PERIODIZATION

Every endurance athlete, whether preparing for a marathon, looking ahead to a summer of bike racing, or building to a late-season half- or full Ironman race, separates training into different phases, or cycles, each of which has a specific set of goals. This concept of progressive training cycles building to an important competition or event is referred to as *periodization*. Periodization is a training strategy designed to improve athletic performance by varying your training specificity, volume, and intensity, with rest and recovery incorporated at specific times during your training year to prepare you to do your best at an event or competition.

A *macrocycle* is the largest training cycle and typically lasts one full year. Looking at the macrocycle, an endurance athlete plots out his or her competition and events for the year. At the next level, the training program is broken up into four **mesocycles**, which can last several weeks or months depending on the athlete's goals, his or her strengths and weaknesses, and the number of events on the calendar. Each mesocycle, in turn, is broken down into smaller training cycles, or **microcycles**. These microcycles typically last 1 week but could last up to 4 weeks. They require the athlete to complete a specific daily training schedule. Though the terminology describing these cycles can vary somewhat, the mesocycles are commonly referred to as follows:

The Preparation Cycle (also called a base cycle or foundation cycle): This training mesocycle, which generally begins a macrocycle, is designed to develop aerobic endurance, muscular strength, and flexibility. An athlete in this phase attempts to overload the aerobic system in order to improve aerobic capacity and power. Endurance workouts are relatively long and of low to moderate intensity. This period generally lasts from 16 to 20 weeks and may consist of four or five 4-week training blocks. For athletes preparing for summer racing and events in the Northern Hemisphere, this training cycle typically begins in the late fall or early winter. However, it would take place earlier in the year for athletes living in a temperate climate who are preparing for an early-season race. As this training cycle nears completion, training intensity can increase, but the focus remains on the aerobic system.

If training is decreased to 1 hour on specific days, then the athlete's carbohydrate and protein intake can be shaved down slightly. A longer weekend training session of 2 hours would require a slightly higher carbohydrate intake.

The Build Cycle (also called an intensity cycle): In this cycle, intensity is increasing and volume is decreasing as an athlete builds power very specific to his or her sport, whether it is an individual sport like swimming, running, or cycling or involves a multisport focus, as in triathlons and adventure racing. This pre-race cycle typically lasts 8 to 12 weeks and focuses on improving VO_2max and lactate threshold. Training includes lactate threshold– and VO_2max–specific intervals, such as hill repeats for cycling and running, as well as strength training with heavier weights and fewer repetitions to emphasize explosive power. There is also an emphasis on sport-specific speed and technique. Your training volume can still remain fairly high. For summer racing, this period can take place during late winter and early spring. As your race or event day approaches, training intensity increases, workouts are shorter, and overall training volume decreases. Both high-intensity training and adequate recovery from these workouts are essential. This training cycle also includes a decrease in training, or a "taper," before races and events that are of lesser importance to your season goals and simply a part of your training program.

The Race Cycle: This cycle includes a race taper, or specific decrease in training volume and intensity before a race, and the race itself. This cycle can be short, moderate in length, or long. For example, a taper for a sprint-distance triathlon would be short, whereas a taper for a marathon would be moderate and a taper in preparation for an Ironman triathlon might last several weeks. This race cycle focuses on the most important events or races of your season and demands very specific nutritional guidelines.

The Transition Cycle (also called an off-season cycle): The transition cycle is designed to provide 4 to 8 weeks of active recovery. Initially this period may require some real rest and recovery, which may last for 2 to 4 weeks after the last important race or event of the season. This mesocycle can then last 4 to 12 more weeks before another preparation cycle begins. The purpose of this training cycle is to maintain aerobic conditioning and to improve on your weaknesses and technique. The volume and intensity of exercise are lower in this cycle than in any other training cycle. This is a good time of year to work on your swim stroke or pedaling skills.

FUELING FOR THE BUILD CYCLE

During this training cycle you will build intensity, while overall volume will slightly decrease. Your calorie requirements will increase so that you can recover from the higher level of training, and strong attempts to decrease weight could result in insufficient recovery from training due to inadequate glycogen repletion, compromised lean body mass, and decreased energy. It is also important to take in adequate nutrition for recovery so that your body can meet the demands of the increased training and you can develop your ability to handle lactic acid. Speed sessions that take place at high intensity deplete muscle glycogen stores during training much faster than slow, steady training sessions. Your protein needs will also increase because of the stress placed on your muscles during higher-intensity training and the increased weights used during resistance training sessions.

CARBOHYDRATES	3–4.5 g/lb. (6.5–10 g/kg)	90 minutes–2 hours, moderate to high intensity
	2.5–3 g/lb. (5.5–6.5 g/kg)	60–90 minutes, low to moderate intensity
	3–3.5 g/lb. (6.5–8 g/kg)	45–75 minutes, moderate to high intensity
	On specific training days, ultraendurance athletes such as Ironman triathletes may need to increase their carbohydrate intake to 5–5.5 g/lb. (11–12 g/kg).	
PROTEIN	0.6–0.8 g/lb. (1.3–1.8 g/kg)	
	Increased protein requirements are easily met with a balanced diet. Protein should be timed properly before and after intense weight training sessions. Very heavy training microcycles may require 0.9 g/lb. (2 g/kg) of protein.	
FAT	0.4–1 g/lb. (1–2 g/kg)	
	Higher fat intakes are related to increased energy requirements and are especially appropriate for ultraendurance athletes who are still experiencing fairly high training volumes.	

Caloric intake should be adequate to sustain energy levels for training. Even easy training sessions designed for recovery should be adequately replenished. Your body fat may decrease with training during this cycle, but you should not actively try to lose weight quickly. Even with your increased energy requirements you should focus on healthy food choices and keep treats to moderate levels. Here are two examples:

FEMALE CYCLIST, 150 LBS. (68 KG)

Training session: Interval session, 90 minutes

10–15 minutes, warm-up

5 minutes, short accelerations (20–30 seconds)

Intervals: 2 × 20 minutes tempo, with 5–10 minutes easy recovery

10–15 minutes, easy cooldown

Carbohydrate requirements	450 g (3 g/lb.) × 4 kcal/g	=	1,800 calories
Protein requirements	105 g (0.7 g/lb.) × 4 kcal/g	=	420 calories
Fat requirements	90 g (0.6 g/lb.) × 9 kcal/g	=	810 calories
Total caloric intake			3,030 (20 kcal/lb.)

MALE RUNNER, 180 LBS. (82 KG)

Training session: Track workout, 60 minutes

10–15 minutes, warm-up

5–10 minutes, drills and short builds

Main set: 10–20 × 30 seconds to 2–5 × 4 minutes at high intensity

10–15 minutes, cooldown

Carbohydrate requirements	540 g (3 g/lb.) × 4 kcal/g	=	2,160 calories
Protein requirements	126 g (0.7 g/lb.) × 4 kcal/g	=	504 calories
Fat requirements	72 g (0.4 g/lb.) × 9 kcal/g	=	648 calories
Total caloric intake			3,312 (18 kcal/lb.)

FUELING FOR THE RACE CYCLE

When you are preparing for a race or event that is the highlight of your season, there are specific nutritional strategies that you can follow to make sure you arrive with a full stock of stored muscle fuel for race day. Often referred to as your training taper, this structured decrease in training volume and intensity requires a decrease in energy intake while you consume enough carbohydrates to superload your muscles with glycogen. This training cycle may last several weeks when preceding a very long event such as an Ironman, or it can last just several days for a shorter triathlon. More on this training cycle and the required "carb-loading" is covered in Chapter 5.

FUELING FOR THE TRANSITION CYCLE

Active rest and recovery are important parts of preparing for your next athletic goal. During this annual period of rest, you train to maintain your aerobic conditioning. The level of training might be just one-quarter of what you did during the preparation cycle. This is also a good time of year to try new activities and sports for fun and variety.

CARBOHYDRATES   2–2.5 g/lb. (4.5–5.5 g/kg)   Light to moderate intensity
If you are going easy but still enjoy some volume, aim for
3 g/lb. (6.5 g/kg). Choose high-quality carbohydrates,
as portions are lower.

PROTEIN   0.5–0.6 g/lb. (1.1–1.3 g/kg)
These protein requirements are easily met on a
well-balanced diet.

FAT   Less than 0.5 g/lb. (1 g/kg)

A decrease in calories is the biggest adjustment of this training cycle. Because you are used to eating ample calories during the periods of more structured training, it is easy to gain weight during this training cycle. Here are two examples of the lower calorie requirements that an endurance athlete would encounter in the transition cycle:

MALE SWIMMER, 160 LBS. (73 KG)

Training session: Aerobic "dry-land" training in gym, 60 minutes

Carbohydrate requirements	400 g (2.5 g/lb.) × 4 kcal/g	=	1,600 calories
Protein requirements	96 g (0.6 g/lb.) × 4 kcal/g	=	384 calories
Fat requirements	70 g (0.44 g/lb.) × 9 kcal/g	=	630 calories
Total caloric intake			2,614 (16 kcal/kg)

FEMALE TRIATHLETE, 125 LBS. (57 KG)

Training session: Run, steady, 60 minutes

Carbohydrate requirements	250 g (2 g/lb.) × 4 kcal/g	=	1,000 calories
Protein requirements	63 g (0.5 g/lb.) × 4 kcal/g	=	252 calories
Fat requirements	63 g (0.5 g/lb.) × 9 kcal/g	=	567 calories
Total caloric intake			1,819 (14.5 kcal/lb.)

CREATING THE OPTIMAL TRAINING DIET: YOUR DAILY MEAL PLAN

As an endurance athlete who strives for optimal training and recovery, it is essential for you to translate sound scientific recommendations into everyday food choices that replenish your body's fuel stores and leave you feeling satisfied with your diet. Much of the success of your daily eating plan hinges on consuming adequate calories and carbohydrates that match your training program for that day (and the next day) and rounding out your meals and snacks with the correct balance of healthy proteins and fats.

Meal planning can seem complicated at first, but there are several strategies that can simplify this process. In fact, you will be amazed at how quickly you can adopt some new food strategies and incorporate them into your daily life of training and eating once you have a program and some structure in place. You will find that planning and organization make this part of your training program easier and more effective. Just as you plan ahead to ensure that all the necessary equipment and clothing are available for your workouts, you must also plan to ensure that the optimal foods and required sports nutrition supplements are available to support your training.

Table 4.5 lists the nutritional requirements of two athletes during different phases of their training—a 160-pound (72 kg) male and a 140-pound (64 kg) female. These two examples demonstrate how nutritional requirements can vary from training cycle to cycle, and within a training cycle, as the types of workouts, the duration of the workouts, and the intensity of the workouts vary.

PRACTICAL CARBOHYDRATE ISSUES

Eating adequate amounts of carbohydrate at specific times in portions that allow you to prepare for training, recover from training, and arrive in good shape for competition can be a challenge. Obtaining wholesome carbohydrates conveniently is difficult enough in our society, but consuming them in the proper amounts at the right times takes a concerted effort. Some endurance athletes can easily meet their carbohydrate requirements on specific training days with plenty of well-chosen, wholesome carbohydrates. But on some training days the amounts required for fuel may exceed appetite. At these times, it is important to focus on carbohydrate-rich foods that are appealing, convenient, and easy on your stomach and digestive system.

Food tables that list carbohydrate portions for 30-gram servings are provided to give you a framework for meal planning (see Table 4.6 and Appendix A). You can use such

TABLE 4.6 CARBOHYDRATE CONTENT OF FOODS

FOOD		SERVING SIZE (OZ./C./TBSP.)	(ML)
30 GRAMS CARBOHYDRATE SERVINGS			
Breads	Bagel	½ large, or 2 oz.	60 g
	Bread	2 slices, or 2 oz.	60 g
	Bread crumbs	½ c.	120 ml
	Breadstick	2 oz.	60 g
	Cornbread	1 square, or 2 oz.	60 g
	Dinner roll	2 oz.	60 g
	English muffin	1 whole, or 2 oz.	60 g
	Hamburger bun	1 whole, or 2 oz.	60 g
	Pita pocket	1 round, or 2 oz.	60 g
Cereals	Bran cereal	⅔ c.	160 ml
	Cereal, cold, unsweetened	1½ oz.	45 g
	Cream of Wheat, cooked	1 c.	240 ml
	Granola, low-fat	½ c.	120 ml
	Grape-Nuts™ cereal	⅓ c., or 5 tbsp.	100 ml
	Grits, cooked	1 c.	240 ml
	Oatmeal, cooked	1 c.	240 ml
	Puffed cereal	3 c.	720 ml
	Shredded Wheat	¼ c., or 1½ oz.	45 g
Grains	Amaranth, cooked	⅔ c.	160 ml
	Barley, cooked	⅔ c.	160 ml
	Buckwheat, cooked	1 c.	240 ml
	Bulgur, cooked	1 c.	240 ml
	Couscous, cooked	⅔ c.	160 ml
	Crackers	1½ oz.	45 g
	Millet, cooked	⅔ c.	160 ml
	Muffin, low-fat	3 oz.	90 g
	Pancake mix, dry	⅓ c.	80 ml
	Pancakes, 4-in. diameter	3 cakes	
	Pasta, cooked	1 c.	240 ml
	Pretzels	1½ oz.	45 g
	Quinoa, cooked	⅔ c.	160 ml
	Rice, white or brown, cooked	⅔ c.	160 ml
	Saltines	8 crackers, or 1½ oz.	45 g
	Tortilla, corn or flour	2 tortillas	
	Waffles, toaster or frozen	2 small waffles	
	Wild rice, cooked	1 c.	240 ml
Starchy Vegetables	Baked beans, cooked	¾ c.	180 ml
	Corn, cooked	¾ c.	180 ml
	Kidney beans, cooked	¾ c.	180 ml
	Peas, cooked	1 c.	240 ml
	Potato, baked	1 medium, or 5 oz.	150 g
	Sweet potato, baked	4 oz.	120 ml

FOOD		SERVING SIZE (OZ./C./TBSP.)	(G/ML)
30 GRAMS CARBOHYDRATE SERVINGS, *CONTINUED*			
Fruit	Apples, dried	7 rings	
	Apples, fresh	2 small	
	Applesauce, sweetened	½ c.	120 ml
	Applesauce, unsweetened	1 c.	240 ml
	Apricots, fresh	8 medium	
	Banana	1 large	
	Blackberries	1½ c.	360 ml
	Blueberries	1½ c.	360 ml
	Cantaloupe, raw pieces	2 c.	480 ml
	Cherries, fresh	12 cherries	
	Dates, dried	1 medium	
	Figs, dried	3 medium	
	Fruit salad	1 c.	240 ml
	Grapefruit	1 large	
	Grapes	30 grapes, or 1 c.	240 ml
	Honeydew melon, cubed	2 c.	480 ml
	Kiwifruit	2 medium	
	Mango	1 medium	
	Nectarines	2 small	
	Oranges	2 medium	
	Papaya	1 medium	
	Peaches	2 medium	
	Pear	1 large	
	Pineapple, fresh, pieces	1½ c.	360 ml
	Plums	3 medium	
	Raisins	⅓ c., or 3 tbsp.	60 ml
	Raspberries	2 c.	480 ml
	Strawberries	2½ c.	600 ml
	Watermelon	3 slices, or 3 c.	720 ml
Fruit and Vegetable Juices	Apple juice	8 oz.	240 ml
	Carrot juice	10 oz.	300 ml
	Cranberry juice cocktail	8 oz.	240 ml
	Grape juice	8 oz.	240 ml
	Grapefruit juice	8 oz.	240 ml
	Orange juice	8 oz.	240 ml
	Pineapple juice	8 oz.	240 ml
	Vegetable juice cocktail	24 oz.	720 ml
Sweets, Baked Goods, and Snack Foods	Angel food cake	1/12 whole	
	Cake, flour type	1/12 whole	
	Chocolate milk	8 oz.	240 ml
	Cookies, fat-free	4 small	
	Fruit spreads, 100% fruit	2 tbsp.	40 ml
	Gingersnaps	6 cookies	

Continues >

TABLE 4.6 **CARBOHYDRATE CONTENT OF FOODS** *continued*

FOOD		SERVING SIZE (OZ./C./TBSP.)	(G/ML/L)
30 GRAMS CARBOHYDRATE SERVINGS, *CONTINUED*			
	Graham crackers	6 squares	
	Granola bar, low-fat	1 medium	
	Honey	2 tbsp.	40 ml
	Hot chocolate	2 packages	
	Ice cream	1 c.	240 ml
	Jam or jelly	2 tbsp.	40 ml
	Muffin, low-fat	4 oz.	120 g
	Pie	⅛ whole	
Sweets, Baked Goods, and Snack Foods, *continued*	Popcorn, no fat added	6 c. popped	1.4 L
	Pretzels	1.5 oz.	45 g
	Pudding, regular	½ c.	120 ml
	Sherbet	½ c.	120 ml
	Sorbet	½ c.	120 ml
	Syrup, regular	2 tbsp.	40 ml
	Trail mix, fruit-based	2 oz.	60 g
	Vanilla wafers	10 cookies	
	Yogurt, frozen, fat-free	1 c.	240 ml
	Yogurt, frozen, low-fat	⅔ c.	160 ml

FOOD		SERVING SIZE (OZ.)	(ML)
10–30 GRAMS CARBOHYDRATE SERVINGS			
	Almond milk	8 oz.	240 ml
	Buttermilk, 1%	8 oz.	240 ml
	Chocolate milk	8 oz.	240 ml
	Milk, 1%	8 oz.	240 ml
	Milk, 2%	8 oz.	240 ml
Dairy Products and Substitutes	Milk, nonfat	8 oz.	240 ml
	Rice milk	8 oz.	240 ml
	Soy milk, original or chocolate	8 oz.	240 ml
	Yogurt, low-fat	8 oz.	240 ml
	Yogurt, nonfat	8 oz.	240 ml
	Yogurt, with fruit	8 oz.	240 ml

FOOD		SERVING SIZE (C.)	(ML)
10 GRAMS CARBOHYDRATE SERVINGS			
	Artichoke	1 medium	
	Asparagus, boiled	1 c.	240 ml
	Beans, green, boiled	1 c.	240 ml
	Beet greens, cooked	1¼ c.	300 ml
Vegetables	Broccoli, boiled	1 c.	240 ml
	Broccoli, raw	2 c.	480 ml
	Brussels sprouts, boiled	¾ c.	180 ml
	Cabbage, cooked	¾ c.	180 ml

Continues >

FOOD		SERVING SIZE	
		(C.)	(ML)
Vegetables, *continued*	Carrots, cooked	⅔ c.	160 ml
	Carrots, raw	2 medium	
	Cauliflower, cooked	¾ c.	180 ml
	Kale, boiled	1¼ c.	300 ml
	Mushrooms, cooked	1 c.	240 ml
	Mustard greens, cooked	1½ c.	360 ml
	Peppers, sweet, raw	2 c.	480 ml
	Spinach, boiled	1½ c.	360 ml
	Summer squash, cooked	1 c.	240 ml
	Tomato, raw	2 medium	

lists to make sure you are getting the correct total grams of carbohydrates required for training on a given day. A 180-pound triathlete training for 3 hours one day may require a full 700 grams of carbohydrates, whereas a runner of the same weight completing a shorter run may require only 400 grams of carbohydrates daily. Consuming 400 grams of carbohydrates in a given training day is much easier than consuming 700 grams—attaining the higher amount requires more structure and planning.

The food system outlined in this chapter provides you with the flexibility to emphasize various carbohydrate sources from one day to the next depending on your food preferences, fuel needs, training schedule, and training cycle. Food lists are a helpful tool as you strive to meet your carbohydrate requirements. They can make one of the most important nutrients in your training diet more accessible and manageable because they spell out precise daily servings and portions. During periods of high training volume and/or intensity, consuming adequate amounts of carbohydrate can be challenging. During lighter training cycles, downsizing your diet to more moderate portions can also be challenging because it requires a shift in meal planning. In practical terms, individualized plans can differ from athlete to athlete depending on medical history, food preferences, schedule, and culinary skills; the charts can help you to individualize the general recommendations to suit your unique needs and situation.

FOOD LISTS FOR PLANNING YOUR TRAINING DIET

Table 4.6 outlines the portion sizes of various foods that supply 30, 10, or 10 to 30 grams of carbohydrates per serving. If you are just learning to keep track of your carbohydrate consumption, using this list on a daily basis can simplify meal planning for your training

PRACTICAL CARBOHYDRATE STRATEGIES FOR HEAVY TRAINING

On training days that demand a very high carbohydrate intake, timing and tolerance issues can complicate your efforts to meet specific nutrition goals. Consuming enough carbohydrates takes planning, as the amounts you require often exceed what is found in an everyday diet. But if you leave your diet to chance, your intake may be inadequate. Fortunately, it becomes easier if you follow some simple practical suggestions.

Use sports bars and energy bars with enthusiastic caution.
- They are a concentrated and convenient source of carbohydrates, supplying up to 50 grams per serving.
- They travel well and can be consumed quickly between training sessions or on the way back to class or work.
- Remember that these bars are often vitamin- and mineral-fortified. Do not consume doses of these nutrients that are too high simply by overconsuming sports bars.
- Energy bars should not replace fruits, vegetables, and whole grains in your diet, but they can supplement a high-energy, high-carbohydrate diet based on fresh foods.
- Get the right amount of fiber.
- Too much fiber can be hard on your digestive system on intense training days. Adding lower-fiber carbohydrate foods to the mix may be more practical when carbohydrates must be consumed in very large amounts.
- Concentrated lower-fiber choices include large bagels, calorically dense cereals, fruit juices, jams, honey, and syrup.

diet and make it more effective. Make sure you choose carbohydrates from several food groups: the bread, cereal, and grain group; the fruit and fruit juice group; the vegetable group; and the milk, yogurt, and soy group. Then, supplement these on high-intake days with miscellaneous carbohydrate foods provided by snack items, desserts, and the like.

CARBOHYDRATES

Grains and Starches

On days when your carbohydrate needs are especially high, grains and starches are likely to make up a good portion of your diet because they are such concentrated food sources,

Try yogurt, shakes, and smoothies.

- A tasty snack of yogurt with fruit, a low-fat milk shake, or a fruit smoothie can up your carbohydrate intake considerably and provide needed fluid.
- High-carbohydrate supplement drinks or meal replacements are also convenient sources of carbohydrates, easy to carry, and quickly consumed.
- Desserts can be part of a nutritious diet in reasonable amounts. Some carbohydrate-dense choices are sherbet, sorbet, and frozen yogurt topped with fruit.

Try snacking and grazing.

- Meeting your daily carbohydrate intake often requires consuming between-meal snacks and "grazing" throughout the day.
- Carbohydrate-rich foods should comprise at least half of your meals and snacks.
- Low-fiber choices may be tolerated better than high-fiber choices when you are eating close to the start of your training session.

Limit hidden fat.

- Try to watch for carbohydrate foods that are also high in fat (often unhealthy fats), such as croissants, creamed or deep-fried vegetables, doughnuts, French toast, fried rice, scones, muffins, pancakes, pastries, potato chips, snack crackers, and popcorn popped with oil.

providing 30 grams of carbohydrates per serving in the portion sizes supplied in the table. As discussed in Chapter 2, try to choose only lightly processed or whole-grain sources as much as possible. Many items from the grain group, such as pretzels and crackers, also make good snack choices.

Fruits and Juices

Fresh fruits, dried fruit, and fruit juices, which also provide 30 grams per serving in the listed amounts, are your next great source of carbohydrates. Because of the abundant nutrients they supply, they are excellent food choices for maintaining good health. Vegetables also provide carbohydrates—though, at about 10 grams per serving, not as much per portion as grains and fruits. However, few foods can match vegetables for their high nutrient content.

Low-Fat Dairy Foods

Dairy milk and yogurt, as well as other milks such as soy milk and rice milk, are also good sources of carbohydrates, ranging from 10 to 30 grams per serving in the amounts listed. Yogurt can be especially high in carbohydrates when mixed with fruit and sugars.

Sweets and Desserts

One last source of concentrated carbohydrates is sweets and desserts, which also supply 30 grams per serving in the portion sizes listed in the table. Sweets should not routinely replace more wholesome carbohydrate choices in your diet, but they are a source of additional carbohydrates. They offer the advantage of being more dense and less filling than some higher-fiber, more wholesome choices, and when your carbohydrate requirements are especially high, exceeding 500 grams daily, they do come in handy. For very heavy training days, you can also consider adding some sports nutrition products high in carbohydrates to your food plan.

PROTEINS

Of course, endurance athletes cannot live—and should not live—on carbohydrates alone. Choosing quality proteins and healthy fats will provide you with essential nutrients and balance out meals and snacks. Proteins and fats also keep you full longer and even out blood glucose levels during the day. The protein foods listed in Table 4.7 are ranked according to their fat content to aid you in ensuring you do not exceed healthy limits of total fat and saturated fat in your diet. Plant proteins and milk and dairy sources should be emphasized for vegetarian athletes.

A well-balanced diet with adequate calories and with up to 15 to 20 percent of those calories from protein provides enough protein for the muscle growth and repair that endurance athletes engaged in hard training need. It also should be enough for those who do strength training. Protein consumed in excess of your requirements is simply stored as fat—though, as explained earlier, it may also be burned for energy. Converting protein to fuel for exercise is inefficient, however, when compared with burning carbohydrates.

Consuming excess protein can result in other negative effects. Protein from both food and supplements increases your need for fluid, as your kidneys require more water to eliminate the end products of protein metabolism. A high protein intake should be accompanied by a high fluid intake. Individuals with liver or kidney problems are also susceptible to the negative effects of excessive dietary protein. Excess dietary protein leads to a short-lived increase in the urinary excretion of calcium, an important mineral for building healthy bone tissue. Thus, high protein intakes should also be accompanied by adequate amounts of calcium. And although food sources of protein are best, they can contribute substantial amounts of fat and cholesterol to the diet. Consuming excess protein can therefore increase your risk of heart disease and other health problems. You should be selective regarding the type of protein foods you eat. There are plenty of low-fat animal protein food sources to choose from and plenty of healthy plant proteins as well. When planning meals, it is important to remember that the grains and vegetables that you consume also contribute to your daily protein intake.

Your protein needs for daily training, muscle repair, and other important protein functions are easily met through a well-planned diet adequate in calories. The key is to obtain adequate amounts of quality lean or low-fat protein sources throughout the day and to consume enough calories so that protein is not burned for energy.

FATS

Table 4.8 outlines sources of fat in 5-gram servings according to the type of fat each food provides. Again, you can use the table as a guide in making your own individual food choices. Emphasize healthy essential fatty acids and foods high in monounsaturated fat. During periods of very high training volume, these healthy fats are a needed source of additional calories and add flavor and variety to your meals.

PERSONALIZING THE FOOD TABLES

As you use these food tables—and the sample menus provided in Appendix E—you will discover how to follow my general guidelines while making adjustments to suit your own health goals and personal tastes. For example, if you do not like dairy products or are lactose-intolerant, you can easily emphasize other choices and keep dairy to a minimum. You could add servings of fruits and juices, or substitute soy milk for cow's milk. Or, on some training days you may wish to have fewer grain servings and increase the number of servings of fruits and fruit juices to match your carbohydrate requirements. On light

TABLE *4.7* FAT CONTENT AND PROTEIN CHOICES

VERY LOW-FAT PROTEINS (‹2 G FAT/OZ., OR 30 G)	LOW-FAT PROTEINS (3–4 G FAT/OZ., OR 30 G)	MEDIUM-FAT PROTEINS (4–5 G FAT/OZ., OR 30 G)	HIGH-FAT PROTEINS (6–8 G FAT/ OZ., OR 30 G)	VERY HIGH-FAT PROTEINS (›8 G FAT/OZ., OR 30 G)
FISH				
Whitefish, such as: Tilapia Halibut Haddock Shellfish, such as: Shrimp	Darkfish, such as: Salmon Mackerel Sardines	Tuna and salmon packed in oil		Any fried fish product
CHEESE				
Fat-free cheeses Cottage cheese, 1% Cottage cheese, 2%	Low-fat cheeses	Feta cheese Mozzarella, part-skim Grated Parmesan	Mozzarella Neufchatel	Regular cheeses, such as: American Cheddar Muenster Swiss
BEEF				
Round, choice, 90% lean	Round, choice, 85% lean Ribeye, choice Flank steak, choice Porterhouse, choice	Round, choice, 73% lean Round, choice, 80% lean	Roast beef Meat loaf	Short ribs Corned beef Prime cuts
PORK				
Ham, lean, 95% fat-free Pork tenderloin Boneless sirloin chop Top loin chop	Sirloin roast Center loin chop Boneless rib roast Center rib chop Blade steak Canadian bacon	Pork butt	Italian sausage	Pâté Pastrami Bacon Pork sausage
LAMB				
Leg, top round Leg, shank, half	Loin chop Loin roast Rib chop	Roast lamb		Ground lamb
LEGUMES (PER C.)				
Black beans Kidney beans Lentils Lima beans Pinto beans	Garbanzo beans	Tofu	Soybeans	
POULTRY				
Turkey breast Chicken, white, no skin Turkey, dark, no skin	Chicken, dark, w/ and w/o skin Turkey, dark, w/skin Duck, roasted, no skin	Ground turkey, mixed meat/skin	Duck, roasted, w/skin	
OTHER				
95% fat-free lunch meat Egg whites Egg substitute	86% fat-free lunch meat Egg substitute	Eggs	Lunch meat Bologna Turkey/chicken Hot dogs Salami	Knockwurst Bratwurst Beef/pork hot dogs Peanut butter

training days, your carbohydrate needs may be lower than on others, and you can adjust your choices accordingly. The point is, these plans can and should be modified to suit your needs. However, regardless of your personalized food plan and preferences, for optimal performance and recovery you need to reach the recommended carbohydrate amounts in total grams. You should also keep in mind that your choices must also supply you with all the nutrients described in Part I.

Let's take a look at how a high-performing triathlete can obtain carbohydrates by consuming foods from the various groups on a heavy training day.

Jack consulted the food tables to determine how many servings of grains and starches, fruits, vegetables, and milk/yogurt servings he would require to obtain his carbohydrate target of 740 grams daily. While some of this carbohydrate intake would be obtained from fueling during training, mainly in the form of a sports drink, Jack aimed for 540 grams of this carbohydrate amount to come from food and fluids consumed before, after, and between the two training sessions.

Based on 540 grams of carbohydrate, Jack decided to aim for:

> 4 fruit servings (120 g carbohydrate)
> 12 grain servings (360 g carbohydrate)
> 1 milk serving (12 g carbohydrate)
> 2 yogurt servings (40 g carbohydrate)
> Total carbohydrate intake from food: 532 g

Leave 188 grams carbohydrate for 2.5 hours of training or 75 grams carbohydrate per hour.

Read more about Jack's specific nutrition strategies in Chapters 5 through 7.

FOOD JOURNALS: TRACKING YOUR INTAKE

Even with the food tables, some athletes find it difficult to keep track of how many calories they have consumed throughout the day. By late afternoon, with all the distractions of everyday life, you may have forgotten how many grams of carbs you have taken in so far or how much protein you ate. Besides, most of your attention is being focused on the training itself. A useful tool for overcoming this problem is a food journal. Keeping a

TABLE 4.8 SOURCES OF FAT

SOURCE		SERVING SIZE (TSP./TBSP.)	(ML)
MONOUNSATURATED FAT (5 GRAMS PER SERVING)			
Almond, cashew, and peanut butter		2 tsp.	12 ml
Avocado, medium		⅛ whole	
Nuts	Almonds	6	
	Brazil nuts	2	
	Cashews	6	
	Hazelnuts	5	
	Macadamias	3	
	Peanuts	10	
	Pecans	4 halves	
	Pistachios	16	
Oil: avocado, canola, hazelnut, olive, peanut		1 tsp.	6 ml
Olives, black		8 large	
POLYUNSATURATED FAT (5 GRAMS PER SERVING)			
Margarine (trans fat free)	Stick, tub, or squeeze	1 tsp.	6 ml
	Reduced-fat	1 tbsp.	20 ml
Mayonnaise	Regular	1 tsp.	6 ml
	Reduced-fat	1 tbsp.	20 ml
Nuts: walnuts, pine nuts		1 tbsp. or 4 halves	20 ml
Oil: corn, grapeseed, cottonseed, safflower, soybean, sunflower, flaxseed, walnut		1 tsp.	6 ml
Salad dressing	Regular	1 tbsp.	20 ml
	Reduced-fat	2 tbsp.	40 ml
Seeds: flaxseed, pumpkin, sesame, sunflower		1 tbsp.	20 ml
Tahini or sesame paste		2 tsp.	12 ml
SATURATED FAT (5 GRAMS PER SERVING)			
Bacon, cooked		1 slice	
Butter	Stick	1 tsp.	6 ml
	Whipped	1 tsp.	6 ml
	Reduced-fat	1 tbsp.	20 ml
Coconut, shredded		2 tbsp.	40 ml
Cream, half-and-half		2 tbsp.	40 ml
Oil: coconut, fractionated poly kernel, palm, palm kernel		1 tsp.	6 ml
Shortening or lard		1 tsp.	6 ml
Sour cream	Regular	2 tbsp.	40 ml
	Reduced-fat	3 tbsp.	60 ml

food journal helps you determine whether you are meeting your energy and nutrient requirements over the course of each day or week. To reap the most benefits, it is best if you write down your food choices and portions while you are still eating or immediately afterward. Don't forget to note snacks, supplements, and fluids consumed. With help from the food lists provided, you can assess a number of items regarding your food intake:

- Add up the number of carbohydrate grams you consumed during the day and determine whether your intake matches your training efforts. Note carbohydrate amounts from food labels, and use the food lists provided to estimate the amount of carbohydrate per serving. You can also tally your total serving intake from the carbohydrate-containing food lists and see how your choices match up with the meal plans provided. You can determine not only whether your daily totals are adequate but also whether the amount of carbohydrate you consumed before and after exercise was appropriate to support your training and recovery efforts.
- Record the amounts of fluids and carbohydrates that you consume before, during, and after your workout. By looking back over your records, you can learn whether you have been meeting the recommended fluid amounts and taking ample opportunity to consume fluids and carbohydrates during breaks in training. Note how your energy levels during training may fluctuate depending on your carbohydrate and fluid intake.
- Look through the day's intake to ensure that you are consuming the right amount of concentrated and high-quality lean protein. If you are vegetarian, check that your plant proteins are amply portioned so that your body receives all the required amino acids (see the sidebar "Protein and the Vegetarian Athlete"). Check that protein is included in your recovery foods and fluids and that you also consume high-quality protein before and after weight training.
- Determine whether the fats you consume are derived from healthy monounsaturated oil, liquid unhydrogenated polyunsaturated oil, and omega-3 fatty-acid food choices. Be sure to include good sources of essential fatty acids in your diet.
- Measure your intake of hydrating fluids for the day, including before and after training. Ensure that you are well hydrated before exercise and that you consume enough fluids to replace sweat losses after exercise.
- Check for hidden fats, such as those found in muffins, pastries, and high-fat crackers. Minimize your intake of these foods whenever possible.

• Pay attention to your eating patterns. Note if you become too hungry at some times during the day, and adjust your mealtimes accordingly. Pay attention to any eating that may occur due to boredom, stress, or other issues not related to hunger.

See Table 4.9 for examples of the number of servings of each food type that can combine to make up a well-balanced sports nutrition diet at different levels of calorie intake. Then, check your food journal to see if any adjustments should be made to improve your overall mix.

LABEL-READING TIPS

Nutritional information on labels can help you determine the nutritional breakdown of foods. First, check the ingredients list. You may want to include more whole-wheat flours and other whole grains in your diet. Ingredients are listed on the labels by weight, from the item weighing the most to the one weighing the least.

Pay attention to the serving size on the label and compare it with the amount that you actually eat. Portions you consume may be double those on the package, and you should adjust the nutrition information accordingly. You can also use the label to evaluate if a food will significantly impact your carbohydrate intake by checking the total grams of carbohydrates listed. You can then determine what portion of that particular food would provide 30 grams or more of carbohydrates to help you meet your training requirements.

Total fat grams, as well as calories from fat, are also listed. To determine the percentage of calories from fat, divide the fat calories per serving by the total calories per serving and

TABLE *4.9* SERVING RECOMMENDATIONS FOR VARIOUS CALORIE LEVELS					
FOOD GROUPS	2,000 CALORIES	2,400 CALORIES	2,900 CALORIES	3,400 CALORIES	4,000 CALORIES
Grains	6	7	8	10	12
Vegetables	2	3	3	3	3
Fruits	3	3	4	5	6
Dairy	2	2	2 (milk) 1 (yogurt)	2 (milk) 1 (yogurt)	3 (milk) 1 (yogurt)
Protein	6	6	6	7	8
Fats	3	4	5	6	8
Nutrient breakdown	315 g carbs. 84 g protein 45 g fat	350 g carbs. 112 g protein 60 g fat	450 g carbs. 114 g protein 70 g fat	550 g carbs. 120 g protein 80 g fat	650 g carbs. 150 g protein 89 g fat

multiply by 100. Keep higher-fat foods in perspective. Your fat intake needs to be considered in the context of an entire day. Your total day's intake should provide 20 to 25 percent fat calories, which allows for some healthy foods that may be a bit higher in fat. Some foods, such as dried pasta, are low in fat, while others, such as margarine, provide a high amount of fat.

The Daily Values (DVs) for various vitamins and minerals provided on the nutrition label are based on a 2,000-calorie intake. The percentage of DV can tell you whether a food is high or low in a nutrient such as calcium, fiber, iron, or vitamin C. A food is considered to be a good source of a nutrient if it provides 20 percent of the DV. Besides increasing your intake of foods high in specific nutrients, you can use the DV to avoid excess fat, saturated fat, and cholesterol.

PROTEIN AND THE VEGETARIAN ATHLETE

Vegetarianism and veganism can certainly provide a basis for a healthy diet, and many athletes are successful in their sport while maintaining a vegetarian diet. However, endurance athletes do have increased protein requirements, and vegetarian athletes should appreciate that a quality plant is not as concentrated a source of protein as an animal protein. It is possible, however, to compensate for the reduced number of protein grams in vegetable sources. The first key for vegetarian endurance athletes is to consume enough carbohydrate calories so that the protein they do consume is not processed for energy. Second, vegetarians should emphasize high-quality and concentrated plant protein sources. Certain grains, dried peas and beans, lentils, nuts, and seeds are some of the best sources. Soy products such as tempeh and tofu are almost equivalent to animal protein in quality.

Although it is not necessary to combine or complement various plant proteins at the same meal (as was once thought), vegetarians should make a concentrated effort to obtain an adequate combination of plant proteins in their diet throughout the day. Your body will make its own complete proteins over the course of the day if you consume enough calories from a variety of sources. If your calorie intake falls short, some of the protein you consume may be processed for energy rather than utilized for important functions that only protein can accomplish.

Protein Tips for Vegetarians

- Include a protein-rich food at all meals and snacks.
- Add milk or a fortified soy milk or yogurt equivalent to every meal and snack.
- Use nut butters, hummus, and low-fat cheeses (soy or regular) for toppings on breads, bagels, and crackers.
- Add nuts and seeds to a fruit-and-yogurt snack.
- Eat tofu and tempeh—both make good elements of a stir-fry.
- Experiment with quick-and-easy bean recipes such as burritos, casseroles, and salads.
- Make thick soups and stews with beans and lentils.
- Experiment with various meat-replacement products on the market, such as tofu dogs and burgers.

Meal-Planning Tips for Vegetarians

- Health food stores provide a wide variety of vegetarian food choices and convenience items; more and more supermarkets are broadening their selection of these items as well, and some have special health food sections. Take the time to browse these markets and discover new products.

- The number of textured vegetable protein products has increased significantly. You can now buy high-protein products that resemble and taste like hot dogs, burgers, and breakfast sausages. These can be used to make quick and easy lunches.

- Tofu can be substituted for chicken in most recipes. Seasoned tofu is available, and you can also season the recipe to spice up tofu's milder taste.

- Substitute vegetable broth when recipes call for beef or chicken stock. Vegetable broth is available in many supermarkets and health food stores.

- Canned lentils, garbanzo beans, and other beans are a quick and nutritious vegetarian option. Many bean and lentil recipes can be batch-cooked and frozen for later use.

- Purchase calcium-fortified soy and rice milks if you drink these products instead of dairy milk.

- Purchase iron-fortified cereals, and consume them with products high in vitamin C such as orange juice.

ATHLETE PROFILE

Undereating: *Nick*

Nick has competed several times in Olympic-distance triathlon and has decided to complete a half-Ironman for the upcoming season. This required him to increase some of his training distances in all three disciplines and his overall weekly training time from 8 hours to over 15 to 20 hours. While completing 12 training sessions a week, Nick felt good early in the training cycle and was enjoying the longer workouts, but he started to struggle 6 weeks into his base training cycle and complained of general fatigue and low energy during the end of long training sessions.

When the sports dietitian looked at Nick's training schedule and food journals, she found that he had not sufficiently increased his energy and macronutrient intake to match his increased training volume. He also needed to take better advantage of opportunities to eat and drink before, during, and after training sessions in order to provide fuel for each session and start the recovery process for the next session, which was often less than 8 hours away.

The sports dietitian started by estimating Nick's energy requirements. At a weight of 165 pounds and working at a desk job, his daily activity needs are about 2,300 calories. During moderate-intensity training Nick typically burns anywhere from 650 calories (60 minutes running) to 850 calories (60 minutes of cycling) per hour. On days when he completes 3 hours of training, his energy needs can reach 4,650 calories.

The sports dietitian provided Nick with a nutrition plan for 4,600 calories and the proper balance of carbohydrate, protein, and fat. She reviewed the 30-gram carbohydrate servings and encouraged Nick to eat two to four carbohydrate servings at meals, and one or two servings at snack times. She also instructed Nick on consuming carbohydrate during training sessions lasting over 75 minutes and showed him how to time and portion his carbohydrate before training based on the timing of the session for optimal fueling. Post-training carbohydrates were also encouraged to take advantage of the early phase of glycogen replacement. Finally, Nick's meals and snacks were rounded out with the proper servings of lean proteins and healthy fats.

FOOD AND FLUID INTAKE FOR TRAINING AND COMPETITION

Timing Is Everything

Competition or endurance events are your big day, reflecting hours of training and dedication. But in order to arrive at a competition or event fully prepared, you must be aware of the physiological issues that can slow you down and develop nutritional strategies for squashing them in their tracks. Your strategies will help you prevent or limit these fatigue factors, increase the quality of your training day to day, and ultimately put you at the starting line feeling fresh and well prepared.

WHAT IS ATHLETE FATIGUE?

For an endurance athlete, fatigue is the inability to sustain speed, endurance, strength and power, skills, and mental focus. Fatigue can be dramatic, such as hitting the wall during a long run, or more subtle, as you find the quality of your workouts slowly diminishing.

From a nutritional perspective, fatigue can be related to a number of factors, including:

- Depleted body fuel stores
- The rate of fluid loss and accumulation of body heat
- Low blood sodium
- Gastrointestinal disturbances

How you prepare for and recover from training (or competition) affects these fatigue factors. Nutritional fatigue can be manifested in several ways, and two common terms to describe it are *hitting the wall* and *bonking*. The wall refers to the feeling of heaviness or deadness in your legs and is likely due to muscle glycogen depletion. Bonking usually refers to low blood glucose levels and produces a central nervous system or brain effect of poor focus, dizziness, and mental fatigue.

PREVENTING NUTRITIONAL FATIGUE WITH FINE-TUNING

Think of your daily training diet as a 24-hour outline of your carbohydrate, protein, and fat requirements. The guidelines described in Chapter 4 help you determine how much and what type of fuel your body needs each day. These amounts and types of fuel will change from day to day depending on your daily training session and your training cycle. You can fine-tune your diet even more, however, through specific timing of your food and fluid intake. Matching your intake patterns to the specific fuel demands of your training schedule optimizes your energy for training, enhances your recovery from training, and helps you to meet your body-composition goals. Timing is especially important for endurance athletes who have a full schedule of training built around work or school. One of the biggest nutritional mistakes an athlete can make is to undermine his or her own performance by not taking in enough of the foods needed to provide fuel for training. Failing to time this fuel intake properly is another big mistake. The wrong timing can have a detrimental effect on your performance. This conclusion is backed up by plenty of solid research that has paved the way for specific nutritional strategies that endurance athletes can practice in the hours before, during, and after training.

TIMING FOOD AND FLUID INTAKE AROUND TRAINING

Ideally, your training and recovery diet will take you in top nutritional form from one training session to the next. However, real life can sometimes (or perhaps often) get in the way of recharging your fuel stores to the optimal levels required for quality training. A hectic training schedule, especially when combined with work or school, often leaves limited time for meals and snacks, let alone meal preparation. Daily training sessions and other life commitments can easily get in the way, leaving only brief windows of time for meal preparation and eating the recommended amounts of fuel. Nevertheless, it is safe to say that all athletes can benefit from careful timing. Even an athlete with an ideal daily training diet can obtain a clear performance boost by paying attention to the foods and fluids he or she consumes during the 4-hour period before training and the 4-hour period after training.

Our bodies run well on a steady supply of fuel throughout the day. Each time you consume a meal or snack, you add some carbohydrate stores to your liver and ensure optimal blood glucose levels for the next several hours. When you overconsume fuel at any given meal or snack, the excess—whether from carbs, protein, or fat—is simply sent to your fat stores (though carbs and proteins must be converted to fat first, of course). For this reason, eating several times daily seems to work well not only from a weight-management perspective but also from a fueling perspective. As you consume foods and fluids throughout the day, you allow your body to both prepare for and recover from training, often more than once daily.

MATCHING INTAKE TO OUTPUT

What you consume in the hours before, during, and after training should match up with the fuel depletion that occurs during the training session. When training for your endurance sport, the longer and harder your training session, the greater the risk of developing glycogen depletion and dehydration. Remember that a full supply of glycogen provides anywhere from 1,400 to 1,800 calories' worth of fuel. During steady exercise at a moderate to high intensity, you burn through this fuel in less than 90 minutes. During high-intensity training, such as when completing a session focusing on speed work and interval training, you can burn through fuel quickly and experience significant glycogen depletion in less than an hour. Once you experience muscle glycogen depletion, fatigue sets in and you cannot respond to the demands of training. Even with plenty of fat stores remaining, you may need to decrease your exercise intensity. In fact, you may not even be able to complete the training session. Your fat stores cannot supply fuel quickly enough to sustain the high intensities in some types of workouts, and consequently your muscle fibers don't receive the fuel they need to contract during exercise.

How quickly you deplete your body fuel stores depends on the nature of your training. When you bike at a steady, moderate rate, you steadily burn both fat and carbohydrates. Speed workouts at the track can deplete your carbohydrate stores in under an hour. Indoor gym workouts that incorporate cardiovascular work and resistance training are also glycogen depleting. Glycogen depletion from just one training session can be significant. But glycogen depletion can also occur gradually over several days' time or even over one or several weeks' time.

Blood glucose provides a very limited amount of fuel during exercise. It is your brain's only fuel source and is supplied and maintained by your liver glycogen stores. When you run low on blood glucose, you cannot focus on the exercise task at hand. You may experience light-headedness, poor concentration, and irritability, and you may not perform the skills for your sport as easily as you know you can. Exercise will seem much harder, and coordination will suffer. Your judgment can also become impaired, and this can affect your technique. You may have to slow down considerably or stop exercising altogether, because the blood glucose supplied by your liver is also an important fuel source for your muscles when they become depleted of glycogen.

Other body nutrient stores can also become depleted. Fluid depletion is an important concern and can impede your training efforts. Dehydration can slow down both moderate- and high-intensity efforts, impair your mental concentration, decrease muscular endurance, and result in overheating, possibly to dangerous levels in hot weather. Excess sodium losses can also adversely affect your performance and increase health risks during exercise.

NUTRITIONAL STRATEGIES BEFORE TRAINING

Endurance athletes who want to complete their training program or compete at their best can benefit from several pre-exercise nutrition strategies designed to minimize the fuel, fluid, and electrolyte depletion that can occur during training. Making the most of specific food and fluid choices before training or competition offers several important performance advantages:

- It allows you to start training or competition with optimal fluid levels, helping to delay or at least minimize dehydration.
- It refills liver glycogen stores and decreases your risk of developing hypoglycemia during exercise.
- It tops off your muscle glycogen stores and delays glycogen depletion while training and competing.
- It provides you with fuel and fluid during the early part of exercise.
- It ensures that your stomach is settled and prevents hunger pains during exercise.
- It provides a psychological edge and certain level of comfort to know you've consumed a well-tested pre-competition meal.

Clearly, stocking your liver and muscle glycogen stores is essential prior to demanding training sessions. The nutritional strategies recommended below are specific about how to time your pre-exercise meals and snacks. The guidelines are flexible enough, however, to allow some variations due to schedules dictated by work, school, and practice times. Often an appropriately portioned and timed pre-exercise meal is just what an endurance sport athlete needs to fuel his or her training session, restore fuel depleted from a previous training session, and replenish fuel stores after the overnight fast that takes place during sleep. The recommended portions and suggested foods and fluids to be consumed are directly related to the timing of your pre-exercise meal. Metabolically speaking, there are two distinct time periods for pre-exercise eating: 2 to 4 hours before exercise, and 30 to 60 minutes before exercise. When you eat is often a matter of practicality and scheduling. What you eat is truly a matter of metabolic, gastrointestinal, and personal tolerances.

3 TO 4 HOURS BEFORE EXERCISE

Many seasoned athletes have identified the window of time occurring 3 to 4 hours before training as an optimal period for pre-exercise eating. During this time, you can consume a moderate to large meal and still have plenty of digestion time. The main focus of this pre-exercise meal should be to replenish your liver glycogen stores and even to store fuel in your muscles for later release. With the right timing and portions, eating 3 to 4 hours before exercise provides the following benefits:

- Restores liver glycogen to normal levels. Liver fuel stores are important if you train early in the morning, since they are depleted overnight.
- Enables your body to store carbohydrates in the muscle to be used as needed, if portions are large enough.
- Allows you to store some carbohydrates in the gut for absorption and release during exercise, while maintaining a placid GI system.
- Prevents you from feeling hungry during training.

Metabolically and physically, you can consume a substantial amount of carbohydrate in the 3- to 4-hour period prior to training. Consuming carbohydrates within this time frame does elevate blood insulin levels and favor the use of carbohydrates as a fuel. But because you can consume a good amount of carbohydrate during this time, blood glucose levels remain nice and steady. Research indicates that eating during this period enhances performance. Not eating during this period before training could put a drain on your training sessions.

Pre-exercise eating portions should be appropriate for your tolerances, but try to consume the upper limits for a fuel and performance benefit. For every hour that you allow between the time you eat and the start of your event or race, or your pre-race digestion time, consume just under half a gram of carbohydrates for every pound (approximately 1 g/kg) of body weight. Using this formula:

- 4 hours before exercise, you can safely consume 2 grams of carbohydrates per pound (4 g/kg).
- 3 hours before exercise, you can safely consume 1.5 grams per pound (3 g/kg).

Eating 3–4 Hours Before Exercise: Food Choices

If you decide to eat a large meal or snack 4 hours before a long run or hard training ride, 2 grams of carbohydrates per pound (4 g/kg) for a 160-pound (73 kg) athlete would translate to 320 grams of carbohydrates. It would probably be easiest on your stomach if a portion of this fairly substantial meal consisted of dense, low-fiber foods and even some liquid carbohydrate sources. The more intense the workout, the more carefully you want to pay attention to specific food tolerances and timing.

For easy digestion, you can obtain 300 grams of carbohydrates by consuming one large bagel topped with 2 tablespoons of jam, followed by a fruited yogurt and 32 ounces of a sports drink. With the full 4 hours of digestion time, you may also find that 1 cup of granola, 8 ounces of skim milk, one large banana, and 12 ounces of juice accompanied by two slices of toast and 2 tablespoons of jam, all providing 200 grams of carbohydrates, are also well tolerated. This pre-exercise meal could be topped off with 12 ounces of a high-carbohydrate energy drink to provide a total of close to 300 grams of carbohydrates. Of course, some athletes can only tolerate smaller meals even with 4 hours of digestion time. Every athlete needs to iron out his or her individual tolerances in regard to foods and portions when eating in the 3- to 4-hour period before training.

EATING 2 HOURS BEFORE EXERCISE

Consuming food 3 to 4 hours before training may not always be possible because of scheduling conflicts and very early start times (rising at 5:00 a.m. to eat prior to an 8:00 a.m. workout does not sound very appealing). Thus, eating 2 hours before training may be your preferred choice. One good rule for pre-exercise eating is that the closer to exercise you plan to eat, the smaller the meal you should consume. Keep the following points in mind:

- Limit your intake of carbohydrates to 1 gram per pound (2 g/kg) of body weight in this time interval. For example, a 160-pound (73 kg) athlete could consume up to 160 grams of carbohydrates.
- Liquid carbohydrate choices are attractive because they are more quickly digested. Breakfast shakes, liquid meal replacements, smoothies, and sports supplements often provide more than 50 grams of carbohydrates per serving. A juice smoothie may work well, as do easily digested energy bars.
- Eating 2 hours prior to exercise could be the best timing for an early or mid-morning training start time.
- It can also work well for tricky early-afternoon training times. Following a large breakfast that is well digested, a small to moderate snack 2 hours before training works well for many athletes who plan ahead for afternoon or evening start times.

EATING 1 HOUR BEFORE EXERCISE

A variety of scenarios could create the need for food 30 to 60 minutes prior to exercise. Rising in the extreme early hours of the morning simply to eat food and fuel up for an early training time may not be feasible or desirable. Other scheduling scenarios could mean a large time gap between the last sizable meal and the start of a training session, making hunger and limited fuel during training an issue. Or you may prefer to eat closer to longer training sessions because the added fuel can provide a performance benefit.

Consuming Carbohydrates 1 Hour Before Exercise

Whether to consume carbohydrates 30 to 60 minutes prior to exercise depends on your tolerances and training schedule. You will likely benefit from ingesting fuel 30 to 60 minutes prior to exercise when the carbohydrates you consume replenish compromised fuel stores. Consider consuming carbohydrates within an hour before exercise if you have not eaten for 4 hours or more before training, or prior to early-morning training when liver glycogen is low. Eating an hour before intense training sessions can prevent hunger and provide needed extra calories for athletes who have very high energy requirements.

Consuming carbohydrates in this 30- to 60-minute window prior to exercise will have different metabolic results than consuming them several hours before exercise. When you eat at the later time, there will be marked increases in your blood glucose and blood insulin levels prior to training. A decline in blood glucose during training follows, and your liver decreases the amount of glucose it sends into your bloodstream.

Owing to these metabolic effects, some controversy has surfaced over the years regarding carbohydrate consumption in the hour before exercise. The concern has been that carbohydrate consumption at this time can result in hypoglycemia, or a decrease in blood glucose levels, during exercise, which produces negative symptoms and can have an adverse effect on performance. In fact, however, many studies have confirmed that consuming carbohydrates in the hour before exercise does not impair performance and can actually help performance. These studies used exercise test protocols that mimicked steady-state endurance training, not the high-intensity, moderate-intensity mix that would have better mimicked some of your training sessions. But what was also interesting about these studies was the variation in individual blood glucose responses seen in the test subjects. Results showed that although blood glucose may drop during the early part of training, it quickly corrects itself to normal levels, and the majority of athletes experience no adverse symptoms or performance effects. A small number of subjects, however, did experience some hypoglycemia and a negative effect on performance.

THE CARBOHYDRATE-SENSITIVE ATHLETE

If you are concerned that you may be a carbohydrate-sensitive athlete during the hour prior to training, you may find a few sensible strategies useful. Consuming a high enough number of carbohydrates may simply offset any lowered blood glucose levels and hypoglycemic symptoms. Amounts of 70 grams or more seem to maintain blood glucose levels in individuals susceptible to exercise hypoglycemia. Individuals not susceptible to hypoglycemia can consume only 50 grams of carbohydrates and still obtain a performance benefit, but they may be able to consume more than 70 grams just as well. Athletes can often tolerate up to 100 grams of carbohydrates in the hour prior to training. Choices and amounts are a matter of preference and GI comfort. Practical choices include carbohydrate gels, energy bars, and carbohydrate or sports drinks, which often provide 30 to 50 grams of carbohydrates per serving. Endurance athletes can choose one of the items or any combination of them in portions that are tolerated.

Regardless of your training schedule, a pre-training meal or snack can provide some performance benefit. While the main part of your nutritional intake will be carbohydrates, small amounts of protein, and perhaps fat, may be tolerated if appropriately timed. Determine your optimal pre-exercise meal through experimentation during training. The recommended carbohydrate amounts for various pre-exercise meal times are summarized later in this chapter (see Table 5.5).

THE GLYCEMIC EFFECT

Some endurance athletes may choose to incorporate foods that are low to moderate on the glycemic index into their pre-training meal in order to maintain steady blood glucose levels over the next few hours and through training. In other words, these foods might produce less of a metabolic jostle and soften the degree to which the ingested carbohydrates result in greater use of carbohydrate and less use of fat for fuel.

Although research regarding pre-exercise eating and low-glycemic foods does not fully back this strategy, choosing low-glycemic foods in the several hours before training certainly does not hurt performance. However, many of these studies did not provide carbohydrate during the performance test, which would more closely mimic real-life training conditions. Of course, intake of carbohydrates during training may be more challenging during some workouts than others.

In one study, runners who consumed a low-GI meal 3 hours before exercise were able to run 8 minutes longer than after consuming a high-GI pre-exercise meal. Often the decision to choose these lower-glycemic foods is a matter of personal preference and tolerance; athletes can find what works best for them through experimentation. For this runners study lentils were the pre-exercise meal. Experiment with consuming low- to moderate-glycemic-index foods (see Appendix A) and determine what choices work best for you.

As was discussed in Chapter 2, adding protein and a small amount of fat to a meal can blunt the glycemic effect of the meal. Small amounts of lean protein and easily digested sources of fat can help to maintain steady blood glucose levels and prevent hunger during exercise, and these foods are often well tolerated when consumed 2 to 4 hours prior to training. Many low-glycemic carbohydrate options, such as unprocessed grains and fruits, are also good sources of fiber, and timing can be an important issue with these foods before training. However, in the 30 to 60 minutes prior to training, many well-tolerated options are not likely to be whole, unprocessed foods but rather sports nutrition supplements. Frequently these products have a higher glycemic index than whole foods, though as new products become available this may change.

Athletes should also consider that consuming a carbohydrate source during training (more on that strategy later in this chapter) can offset any drop in blood glucose, making the types of carbohydrates that you consume before exercise less important.

The bottom line is that you should focus on pre-training nutrition strategies that are appropriate for your training times, schedule, and tolerances and that are based on smart experimentation. Table 5.1 offers some pre-exercise meal suggestions in various carbohydrate amounts.

HYDRATION BEFORE TRAINING

Dehydration is one of the most significant performance-related problems that can occur during training (and competition). It can put a halt to your training long before you feel the effects of fuel depletion. Despite your best attempts to keep up with sweat losses during training, it is possible that you are not going to match 100 percent of your fluid losses. Depending on the type of training session, you may have limited opportunity to drink during training.

Just as strategies to maximize muscle and liver glycogen stores offer a performance advantage, so do techniques for maximizing fluid stores before training. Pre-hydrating is not considered to be as effective as drinking during exercise to offset dehydration and its detrimental performance effects. However, if you anticipate that it may be difficult to drink plenty of fluids during training, either because there is no way to carry enough fluids with you or because there will be little opportunity to drink during the training session, pre-hydrating could be a very important and practical strategy. Even when training sessions allow time and opportunities for replenishing fluids and replacing sweat losses, and an athlete is consciously making an effort to hydrate during exercise, only up to 80 percent of sweat losses are usually replaced.

TABLE 5.1 PRE-EXERCISE MEAL SUGGESTIONS

CARB RANGE	SAMPLE MEALS		
100	1 ½ c. concentrated carbohydrate beverage (360 ml) 1 slice of toast **90 g carbohydrates** **380 calories**	1 carbohydrate gel 24 oz. of sports drink (720 ml) **95 g carbohydrates** **380 calories**	2 slices toast or small bagel (60 g) 1 large banana 2 tbsp. jelly (40 ml) 8 oz. juice (240 ml) **120 g carbohydrates** **520 calories**
200	Chicken, 2 oz. (60 g) Bread, 2 slices (60 g) Fruit juice, 16 oz. (480 ml) Pretzels, 2 oz. (60 g) Carbohydrate supplement, 16 oz. (480 ml) **220 g carbohydrates** **1,030 calories**	Fruit smoothie: 8 oz. yogurt (240 ml) 8 oz. milk (240 ml) 8 oz. juice (240 ml) 1 c. fruit Bagel, 1 large (120 g) Jam, 2 tbsp. (40 ml) Energy bar, 1 whole **225 g carbohydrates** **1,185 calories**	Pasta, 2 c. cooked (480 ml) Marinara sauce, 1 c. (240 ml) Bread, 2 slices (60 g) Frozen yogurt, 12 oz. (360 ml) Fruit juice, 8 oz. (240 ml) Margarine, 2 tsp. (24 ml) **235 g carbohydrates** **986 calories**
300	Pancakes, 4 medium Fruit topping, ½ c. (120 ml) Syrup, ½ c. (120 ml) Fruit juice, 8 oz. (240 ml) **270 g carbohydrates** **1,200 calories**	Cooked cereal, 2 c. (480 ml) Instant breakfast drink, 1 serving Banana, 1 large Orange juice, 8 oz. (240 ml) Carbohydrate beverage, 24 oz. (720 ml) **300 g carbohydrates** **1,410 calories**	Rice, 3 c. cooked (720 ml) Cooked vegetables, 1 c. (240 ml) Shrimp, 4 oz. (120 g) Sorbet, 1 c. (240 ml) Soft drink, 12 oz. (360 ml) Oil, 2 tsp. (14 ml) Carbohydrate beverage, 16 oz. (480 ml) **300 g carbohydrates** **1,600 calories**

TIMING			
	3–4 hours before exercise	2 g carbohydrate/lb. (4 g/kg)	
	2 hours before exercise	1 g carbohydrate/lb. (2 g/kg)	
	1 hour before exercise	0.5 g carbohydrate/lb. (1 g/kg)	

At all costs, avoid starting training in a dehydrated state. Your goal during training is to keep up with sweat losses as much as possible, so starting out dehydrated already puts you behind on your fluid-intake efforts. It is important to plan ahead and begin your next training session as well hydrated as possible.

To prepare for the next day's training:

- Consume 16 ounces (480 ml) of fluid before bedtime.
- Your early-morning intake should consist of 16 to 24 ounces (480–720 ml) of fluid.
- Prior to training, try to consume 8 to 10 ounces (240–300 ml) more of fluid every hour during the day.
- About 1 hour before training, consume 16 to 32 ounces (480–960 ml) of fluid. At this time, fluids providing carbohydrates and small amounts of sodium, such as sports drinks, are likely to be the best choice and may have some hydration advantages over water.

- Fill your fluid stores further by drinking 8 to 16 ounces (240–480 ml) more 20 minutes prior to training.

You should be adequately hydrated in preparation for training if you focus on these simple guidelines.

HYDRATION AND FUELING STRATEGIES DURING TRAINING

Even when you start training well fueled, you can significantly drain your fluid stores, carbohydrates, and even electrolytes during moderate- to high-intensity training and during very prolonged training sessions. That's why consuming adequate fluid, carbohydrates, and electrolytes during training and competition is beneficial to your performance. This practice brings you several benefits:

- Delays and minimizes dehydration
- Maintains blood glucose levels
- Offsets muscle and liver glycogen depletion
- Provides fuel for your brain
- Offsets electrolyte losses, particularly sodium

DANGERS OF DEHYDRATION

Dehydration can develop when you train both indoors and outdoors, and it can negatively affect your performance long before fuel depletion begins to drain your efforts. In cold and hot weather, during the peak of the racing season or during the off-season months, it can develop sooner than you might think and can affect you in ways you may not realize.

When you train, heat is a major by-product of your working muscles. As this heat builds up, your body temperature rises. Water then acts as a coolant to keep the body from overheating. During exercise, sweating is the body's primary mechanism for getting rid of excess heat. Sweat losses can easily reach anywhere from 16 to 32 ounces (500–960 ml) and sometimes even 48 ounces (1.5 L) or more per hour, depending on environmental conditions, exercise intensity, and the sweat rate of the individual athlete. Sweat losses can reach 64 ounces (approximately 2 L) or more per hour in some endurance athletes, especially during hot-weather training.

Even losing as little as 2 percent of your body weight through sweating can impair your ability to exercise. When you sweat, your blood volume goes down and stress is placed on your cardiovascular system, which reduces your ability to take in and utilize oxygen. Muscular endurance ability is also impaired with dehydration, and your heart rate may increase at a given level of intensity. When fluid losses through sweat are not replaced, your body temperature rises further and exercise becomes harder. Clearly, not meeting your fluid needs hinders your athletic goals.

SIGNS AND SYMPTOMS OF DEHYDRATION

Unfortunately, thirst is not a good indicator of the amount of fluid that your body requires, either during exercise or at rest. Some early signs and symptoms of dehydration are light-headedness, headache, decreased appetite, dark-colored urine, and fatigue. By the time you are thirsty, you have already lost 1 percent of your body weight through fluid loss. Even fluid losses of 1 to 2 percent of your body weight can adversely affect performance. When fluid losses reach more than 2 to 4 percent of your body weight, increased thirst and symptoms such as irritability and nausea may occur. Dehydration can also result in GI upset.

Consequently, when you make the effort to drink more after you have become dehydrated, your rehydration efforts can result in stomach discomfort. At losses of 5 to 6 percent of body weight, there will be an increase in heart rate and breathing regulation, and body temperature regulation will be significantly impaired. Remember, too, that dehydration can affect your mental concentration and ability to perform the skills required for your sport. Clearly, dehydration does not support your top performance if it affects movement control, decision making, and concentration.

The longer and harder you train, the greater the risk that your sweat losses will impair your performance. Your sweat losses are also affected by your genetic makeup, fitness level, and acclimatization to the temperature in which you are training. Although you will have greater sweat losses in the heat than in cooler weather, your hydration can also be compromised in the cooler weather because you are working so hard. By preventing dehydration, you will likely avoid the following detrimental physiological effects:

- Increased heart rate
- Raised body temperature
- Decreased blood volume
- Decreased cardiac output

- Decreased skin blood flow
- Heightened perception of effort
- Compromised mental concentration
- Compromised fine-motor skills
- Delayed stomach emptying of fluids
- Greater risk of gastrointestinal upset

SERIOUS CONSEQUENCES OF DEHYDRATION

Of course, dehydration can result in serious health risks, including heat exhaustion and heatstroke. Those suffering from heat exhaustion may feel weak, may have cold and clammy skin, may have a weak pulse, and may experience faintness, fatigue, and nausea. When depletion of body fluid is severe, an athlete may even stop sweating; in this case, his or her skin may feel cool and dry. The athlete may be semiconscious and have reduced blood flow to the brain. This condition requires immediate medical attention. Heatstroke is an even more serious condition and is characterized by hot and dry skin and a very high body temperature. Heatstroke is most likely to occur from overexertion in extreme heat accompanied by poor hydration strategies. Previous illness, poor preparation for training in the heat, and even certain medications can increase risk of heat illness.

MINIMIZING DEHYDRATION

It is important to gauge your sweat losses during various types of training sessions in a number of environmental conditions. Athletes cannot train themselves to adapt to or tolerate dehydration. Preventing or minimizing it as much as possible is therefore essential. Just as sweat rates vary greatly among athletes, however, there is also much variability in efforts to replace fluids during exercise. Ideally, endurance athletes should try to match their fluid intake to their fluid losses; most athletes fall short of this goal, however, replacing only 50 to 80 percent of their fluid losses during their training sessions even under the best of conditions. Even if you do make a strong effort to match your fluid losses, your gastrointestinal system can only absorb a certain volume of fluid per hour. Practical considerations, however, may be the main obstacle to adequate fluid replacement during exercise. Consuming the recommended amounts can be challenging because of the logistics of obtaining fluid when training and competing, limited opportunities to drink, taste preferences, and GI tolerances.

When you regularly train in the heat, your body does adapt, or acclimatize. As your conditioning improves, your sweat rate increases and there is greater blood flow to your muscles and skin. Your heart is able to pump more blood, and sweating begins at a lower core body temperature. Your core temperature will not rise as quickly or increase to as high a level when you are in an acclimatized state. Thus, when you are acclimatized you actually sweat more, not less. It is best if your skills at hydrating during exercise keep pace with your adaptation to heat so that you are adept at replacing these increased fluid losses.

At any level of training and in any environmental condition you need to assess drinking opportunities and fluid availability. Training and preparing for your sport in the gym simply require that you bring fluids with you. Matching fluid intake to sweat losses should not be a problem in most indoor training situations. Outdoor workouts may prove more challenging. Clearly, it is much easier to drink fluids when you are on your bike than when you are on a run. During swim practices you can keep a bottle of fluid at the end of your lane, as well as at the track during run speed workouts.

Refer to the sidebar "Estimating Your Sweat Losses" for guidelines on estimating your fluid losses during training and gauging your efforts to rehydrate. Once you have come up with the best fluid strategies for the various types of training sessions that you engage in, it is up to you to make the most of your opportunities to drink during training. Regardless of your fluid-replacement strategies, you are more likely to consume fluids that taste good and are the proper temperature for your training conditions.

Not only do you need to focus on how much fluid to consume, you should also be aware of the most optimal and appropriate fluid choices for training in various environments and conditions. Commercial sports drinks are often used by endurance athletes not only because of their flavor but also because they provide fuel and electrolytes in the form of carbohydrates and sodium chloride.

FUEL REQUIREMENTS DURING EXERCISE

Due to the sheer length of many endurance sport workouts, and the high-intensity, intermittent nature of speed and interval training, fuel replacement can be an important consideration. Carbohydrates consumed during training can maintain blood glucose levels and provide fuel to glycogen-depleted muscles In addition, carbohydrate consumption during interval training may allow your body to store glucose in the muscle fibers during the time those fibers are at rest. For example, as you exercise at low intensity between hard efforts, the muscle fibers that fuel the high-intensity efforts can be replenished.

Your brain can also benefit from carbohydrate intake during long, intense training sessions, as consuming only water can result in lowered blood glucose levels. Because your brain counts on glucose for fuel, lowered blood glucose can have some negative effects on your central nervous system. Having adequate blood glucose to fuel your brain helps you maintain the high level of skill required by your endurance sport. Carbohydrate intake can prevent or reverse symptoms of glucose deprivation such as fatigue, perception of increased effort, and poor coordination. Carbohydrates are thought to prevent the increase in brain serotonin levels that can occur during prolonged exercise. Serotonin produces feelings of drowsiness and fatigue and is helpful at bedtime, but not in the middle of a workout when you want to make the most of the time available to reach your fitness goals.

Much of the research on carbohydrate intake during exercise has centered on steady-state endurance activity. But studies also demonstrate that besides providing performance benefits for exercise lasting 90 minutes or longer, carbohydrates may improve performance during high-intensity exercise lasting about 60 minutes. Several studies over the past decade measured the performance effects of consuming a sports drink during exercise performed at 80 to 90 percent VO_2max and lasting about 1 hour. Results indicated that the sports drink provided a performance benefit.

Several additional studies measured the performance effects of carbohydrates on intermittent, high-intensity exercise lasting about 1 hour. This exercise more closely resembled the type of training conducted in interval or speed workouts. The bottom line was that athletes who consumed a sports drink at rest intervals were able to work out longer than those who consumed a placebo. Researchers speculated that the carbohydrate drinks provided fuel for the fast-twitch muscle fibers, which operate at high intensities, by replenishing them during the rest intervals between high-intensity efforts. The performance benefits may also come from the effect of the carbohydrates on the brain. Although these results are not conclusive, and more research of this type is needed, consider consuming a sports drink during long training sessions, and even during short sessions if they are high in intensity, to both meet the demands of reduced muscle glycogen and boost fluid reserves.

SPORTS DRINKS

Much research has gone into the development of sports drinks in an effort to come up with the ideal fluid for athletes to consume during their workouts. The basic theory—

ESTIMATING YOUR SWEAT LOSSES

This technique for estimating sweat losses is fairly accurate, especially in warm-weather training. Use it to check your sweat losses for various types of training sessions, whether indoors or out, to better estimate fluid needs.

- Check your weight on the scale before and after training. Because you will want to know your actual weight without shoes and clothing, both weigh-ins should be done in the nude, and after training be sure to towel-dry to eliminate most of the sweat on your body. Then, calculate your weight loss from the exercise session by subtracting the post-training weight from the pre-training weight. For example, an athlete who started a 2-hour workout session at 160 pounds and ended it at 158 pounds (going from 73 to 72 kg) has experienced a 2-pound (0.9 kg) loss of water weight during training. This is not the final answer, however, because the athlete may have taken in fluids by drinking during the workout or lost fluids through urination. To account for these factors, follow the next steps.
- Keep track of the amount of fluid that you consumed during a training session. Fifteen ounces of fluid weigh about 1 pound (1,000 ml of fluid equals 1 kg). You can weigh the bottle before and after your training session to determine the actual weight of the fluid you consumed during training. You can use a graduated bottle during these workouts for more precise calculations.
- Let's say the hypothetical athlete mentioned above consumed 60 ounces (1,800 ml) of fluid during a 2-hour training session, and this fluid weighed or was the equivalent of 4 pounds (1.8 kg).
- Add the amount of weight lost to the amount of fluid consumed. For example, the athlete who had a 2-pound weight loss during training and drank 4 pounds of fluid during training would add 2 and 4. Since 2 plus 4 equals 6, this means he lost 6 pounds of fluid (or 0.9 + 1.8 kg = 2.7 kg).
- Record any urine volume that occurred between the weigh-ins and subtract this number (translated into pounds or kilograms) from the result obtained in the previous step.
- Divide the weight of total fluid lost by the exercise time. For example, 6 pounds, or 90 ounces of fluid, divided by 2 hours equals 45 ounces per hour for sweat losses (2.7 kg equals 2,700 ml fluid, divided by 2 hours equals 1,350 ml lost per hour).

continues

This procedure can be translated into a formula:

Sweat rate = (body weight pre-training − body weight post-training +
fluid ingestion − urine volume) ÷ exercise time

Sweat rates in athletes can vary from 24 ounces, or 3 cups (720 ml), of fluid per hour to 80 ounces, or 10 cups (2,400 ml), or more.

You can check your sweat rate for various workouts and throughout the season at different temperatures. A blank "Sweat Loss–Worksheet" is provided in Appendix F.

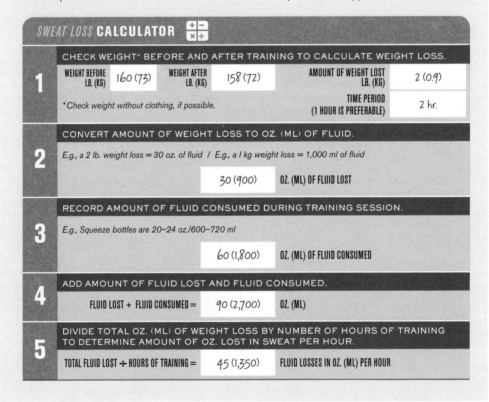

SWEAT LOSS CALCULATOR

1 CHECK WEIGHT* BEFORE AND AFTER TRAINING TO CALCULATE WEIGHT LOSS.

| WEIGHT BEFORE LB. (KG) | 160 (73) | WEIGHT AFTER LB. (KG) | 158 (72) | AMOUNT OF WEIGHT LOST LB. (KG) | 2 (0.9) |

*Check weight without clothing, if possible.

| TIME PERIOD (1 HOUR IS PREFERABLE) | 2 hr. |

2 CONVERT AMOUNT OF WEIGHT LOSS TO OZ. (ML) OF FLUID.

E.g., a 2 lb. weight loss = 30 oz. of fluid / E.g., a 1 kg weight loss = 1,000 ml of fluid

30 (900)   OZ. (ML) OF FLUID LOST

3 RECORD AMOUNT OF FLUID CONSUMED DURING TRAINING SESSION.

E.g., Squeeze bottles are 20–24 oz./600–720 ml

60 (1,800)   OZ. (ML) OF FLUID CONSUMED

4 ADD AMOUNT OF FLUID LOST AND FLUID CONSUMED.

FLUID LOST + FLUID CONSUMED =   90 (2,700)   OZ. (ML)

5 DIVIDE TOTAL OZ. (ML) OF WEIGHT LOSS BY NUMBER OF HOURS OF TRAINING TO DETERMINE AMOUNT OF OZ. LOST IN SWEAT PER HOUR.

TOTAL FLUID LOST ÷ HOURS OF TRAINING =   45 (1,350)   FLUID LOSSES IN OZ. (ML) PER HOUR

that athletes need a convenient way to take in both fluids and carbohydrates in order to maintain hydration and fuel stores during exercise—is sound. Sports drinks can deliver the right ingredients to your body in a timely and well-tolerated manner. A high-quality sports drink passes easily through the digestion and absorption process, emptying from your stomach quickly, entering your small intestine, and then getting absorbed into the bloodstream. The carbohydrates from the drink are then available to maintain blood glucose levels, supply energy to exercising muscles, and replenish muscle fuel stores. The fluid from your sports drink also maintains blood volume and offsets sweat losses.

In an effort to develop scientifically sound formulations, sports drink researchers have looked at each of the steps in digestion and absorption to see where the flow may actually slow down or speed up. If your sports drink gets bogged down in any of these steps, it takes the fluid and carbohydrates that much longer to reach your bloodstream and muscles. Consequently, the sports drink is not as performance-enhancing as it could be. Researchers have concluded that two main factors determine how quickly a drink leaves your stomach: the concentration of carbohydrates in the drink and the volume of fluid in your stomach.

Concentration

Finding the ideal formulation for a sports drink involves striking a delicate balance. Although researchers agree that carbohydrates are essential ingredients, they have had to experiment to determine how many carbohydrates to include in the mix. Research has determined that a concentration of about 6 to 8 percent carbohydrates empties from the stomach very efficiently. Thus, most sports drinks fall into this range. This drink concentration allows fluid to reach your bloodstream pretty much as quickly as water but still deliver performance-boosting carbohydrates. Drinks of this type also seem to be well tolerated by most athletes, and tolerance to these products can improve with practice. In contrast, drinks of 10 to 12 percent carbohydrates, such as soft drinks and fruit juices, empty more slowly from the stomach. Although they do provide carbohydrates and energy, these drinks are not as hydrating as sports drinks and should be diluted if they are consumed during exercise.

Volume

The volume of fluids in your stomach affects the degree of stomach distention and consequently affects gastric emptying. Increased stomach distention will result in liquids emptying from your stomach more quickly, with about 50 percent of stomach contents being emptied every 10 minutes. Too, the more dehydrated an athlete becomes, the slower the rate of gastric emptying. Once an athlete reaches a very slow rate of gastric emptying, attempting to drink more fluid only exacerbates the condition and can even result in nutritional upheaval, such as vomiting, particularly during very demanding races like the Ironman. Of course, mental stress can have a significant impact upon the gastrointestinal system. Being keyed up for an important training session or race can also slow down the rate of gastric emptying.

To maximize emptying, start exercise with a comfortably full stomach and drink at regular intervals of about 10 to 15 minutes, if possible. How much fluid an athlete can empty from his or her stomach is highly variable. However, emptying rates of 24 to 40 ounces, or 3 to 5 cups (720–1,200 ml), per hour are commonly seen. The most important strategy is to consume fluid whenever the opportunity presents itself. Aim to consume at least one 20-ounce (600 ml) squeeze bottle for every hour of a workout. Refill your bottle as needed whenever possible, depending on the duration and nature of the training session, and the sweat rate that you have calculated in various conditions.

Intestinal Absorption: It's All About the Optimal Carbohydrate Mix

Studies measuring intestinal absorption rates have determined that sports drink solutions are as readily absorbed as water. Different forms of carbohydrates are absorbed across the intestinal wall via various transport mechanisms that carry different carbohydrates across the intestine, or allow them to pass through the intestinal wall. Although the majority of early sports drink research has demonstrated that the maximum amount of carbohydrate that an athlete can comfortably absorb is about 1 gram per minute, a decade of newer research has looked at the effect of two or three sources of carbohydrates on intestinal absorption, and there are measureable performance benefits for endurance athletes.

Multiple Carbohydrate Sources

Mixing carbohydrate sources has been measured to allow for faster absorption rates, increased from 1 gram per minute with glucose only to 1.5 grams per minute with a carbohydrate mix of either glucose and fructose or sucrose and fructose. These multiple carbohydrate mixes result in more carbohydrates being available as fuel for training and competition rather than sitting in the gut and causing GI problems. This strategy could be especially important in events that require the athlete to maximize fuel absorption in order to keep up with the fuel burned during competition, such as long-distance triathlons, cycling road races, and ultraendurance runs. This improved absorption has also been shown to translate into improved performance.

Sports drink brands that provide at least two sources of carbohydrates are worth trying. Refer to Appendix C for sports drink brands and their carbohydrate sources. It is also helpful to know that most of these carbohydrate mixes appear to have a moderate to high glycemic index, which gives them the ability to quickly raise blood glucose levels and supply a quick burst of both brainpower and energy. Just as with various food choices, the glycemic index of a sports drink is not necessarily related to whether the drink is a "simple" or "complex" carbohydrate. The number of sports drinks with a lower glycemic index is limited, and the glycemic index of many sports drinks has not been measured.

Refer to the sidebar "Sifting Through the Sugars" for the latest practical application of various carbohydrate sources in sports drinks. Endurance athletes need to experiment with different brands or mixes of brands and flavors to determine which sports drinks and carbohydrate concentrations they tolerate best and like best for different types of training sessions. It is also in athletes' best interests to test out the drink offered on the race course, as they may be limited in how much they can pack and carry for the event.

Temperature

During exercise, cooler fluids empty from your stomach more quickly than warmer fluids. Of course, during training sessions in hotter weather, cooler fluids are more palatable and appealing as well. You are more likely to drink greater volumes of fluid if it is cool. Prepare bottles ahead of time and make sure that you start with a cold drink.

Amount and Timing

General guidelines for the consumption of sports drinks during exercise are the same as the water-intake guidelines described previously, or about 4 to 8 ounces (120–240 ml) every 15 to 20 minutes. Drink at regular intervals during training or whenever there is adequate opportunity to drink. Performance benefits occur when an athlete takes in about 30 grams of carbohydrates per hour. However, 50 to 60 grams may be even better during high-intensity exercise, particularly after some muscle glycogen depletion has already occurred. Every athlete has his or her own personal tolerances and carbohydrate requirements that maintain optimal energy levels during training.

Check the labels and instructions of your sports drinks. Then determine what volume you would need to consume to obtain 30 to 60 grams or more of carbohydrates

SIFTING THROUGH THE SUGARS

Reading labels of sports drinks and making sense of the various carbohydrate sources can be confusing. Following is a list of various carbohydrate sources and combinations provided in many commercial sports drinks:

Glucose: A simple carbohydrate that can be absorbed at the rate of 1 g per minute or 60 g per hour.

Maltodextrin: Often referred to as glucose polymers, which are long chains of glucose molecules. It does not offer any absorption advantages over glucose but often has a milder taste. May be promoted as a "complex carbohydrate," but it is still a manufactured carbohydrate with a high glycemic index.

Fructose: A simple carbohydrate often added as a second carbohydrate source to sports drinks. Usually not used as the sole or main carbohydrate amount in sports drinks. May not be tolerated in large amounts by athletes who have a fructose intolerance.

Glucose-fructose combination: Appears to be the most effectively absorbed carbohydrate mix, as several transport mechanisms can be used simultaneously. Generally drinks provide a 2:1 glucose:fructose ratio. Absorption is at 1.5 g per minute or up to 90 g per hour, an amount that favors fueling for longer events.

Glucose-sucrose combination: Essentially fuels like a glucose-fructose combination, as sucrose is a two-molecule carbohydrate that breaks down into glucose and fructose.

per hour. Experiment to determine what consumption volume best enhances your performance and hydration levels. More sport-specific and training- and race-distance–specific carbohydrate guidelines are provided in Part III.

As far as timing is concerned, large single feedings and smaller regular intakes of a sports drink are both beneficial. Basically, drink whenever possible as the nature of your training session permits. Consuming carbohydrates after depletion has set in can help, but it is more prudent to consume the carbohydrates early on in order to prevent fatigue. Don't wait until the signs and symptoms of a low fuel tank register before consuming your carbohydrate sports drink.

Other Sources of Carbohydrates: Liquid to Solid, and Somewhere in Between

In recent years the sports nutrition industry has developed new options for refueling in the form of bites, wafers, blocks, gels, and energy bars. In addition to sports drinks, which offer carbohydrates in liquid form, these products offer carbohydrates in semiliquid and solid form. These sports supplements may be consumed before, during, and/or after exercise. Tolerances to these products can vary, however, depending on the intensity of exercise and the timing of the carbohydrate supplement. Obviously, carbohydrate drinks offer the advantage of supplying both hydration and fuel, and for this reason they are more practical than the supplements. But many endurance athletes may appreciate the more concentrated carbohydrate gels or similar products, especially in situations where energy needs outweigh the desire for fluid. They are a convenient carbohydrate source. Nevertheless, these products should be consumed with some fluid. More solid items, such as energy bars, may take the edge off hunger during training, though most athletes prefer to avoid solid items during high-intensity training sessions.

Basically, fluid and carbohydrate choices can be somewhat individualized. Keep in mind that your body may need fluids much more than it needs carbohydrate supplementation when training outdoors in hot weather. However, your carbohydrate needs may be a greater priority at the end of an intense workout. At that point, a gel taken with water or a more concentrated sports drink may provide the shot of energy you need to maintain performance.

Protein During Training

Some sports drinks now on the market contain small amounts of protein. Studies attempting to evaluate whether these drinks offer an advantage over traditional sports drinks have had conflicting results due to variations in research design and testing protocols. In the case of endurance exercise, particularly ultraendurance exercise, some

REFUELING DURING EVENTS

Carbohydrate consumed during longer workouts and events can provide an additional fuel source for the brain and muscles. Both running and cycling studies have found that fuel intake during exercise improves endurance (how long you can train before you fatigue) and performance (allowing you to finish a race faster). Below are some guidelines for refueling during specific exercise times:

Under 45 minutes: probably not needed
Can consider carbohydrate replacement if the workout is very high-intensity or there has been limited refueling on a multiple-session training day.

45–75 minutes: up to 30 g carbohydrate per hour
Carbohydrate is most beneficial when consumed during an early-morning workout before breakfast or when the workout begins several hours after the last meal.

1–2.5 hours: 30–60 g carbohydrate per hour
Practice and refine a fueling plan that fits with your hydration requirements and gut tolerances.

Over 2.5 hours: 80–90 g carbohydrate per hour
Products that provide multiple carbohydrates are required to absorb this high rate of carbohydrate. The athlete should experiment with maximum levels of sports drinks that fit his or her sweat losses and add additional products such as gels and blocks as needed.

athletes may add small amounts of protein to their race nutrition plan. It is not recommended, however, that you consistently consume a protein-containing product during training and competition. Rather, focus on products and strategies that replace fluid, carbohydrate fuel, and sodium. Research does indicate that protein stores and muscle are less likely to be utilized as a fuel source if carbohydrate intake is optimal.

The Electrolyte Edge

Though your sweat consists mainly of water, it does contain a number of electrolytes, including sodium, potassium, and calcium.

A quart of sweat (960 ml) can contain the following level of electrolytes:

- 500–1,800 milligrams of sodium
- 700–2,100 milligrams of chloride
- 150–300 milligrams of potassium
- 40 milligrams of calcium

Clearly, the main electrolyte lost in sweat is salt, or sodium chloride, though electrolyte losses in sweat vary widely among individual athletes. Because electrolytes are the major solid component of sweat, much research has focused on the replacement needs of these nutrients during exercise. Sodium and potassium have been the most frequently studied electrolytes, though chloride is also a consideration. Sodium is an important consideration for athletes who train in the heat and humidity. Those who are prone to developing low blood sodium levels, or hyponatremia, and muscle cramping are especially interested in the subject because sodium levels seem to be related to these conditions. Some athletes continue to have high losses of sodium in their sweat even when they are acclimatized to warm weather. This may be due to genetic or other influences.

At the same time, we often hear about the dangers of consuming high levels of sodium. While restricting sodium may be a useful health strategy in sodium-sensitive and

CARBOHYDRATE MOUTH RINSE STUDIES: THE BRAIN CONNECTION

New research indicates that carbohydrate doesn't have to reach our brain to provide a performance effect. To date, seven studies have had subjects rinse a carbohydrate solution in their mouths, rather than swallowing the drink. Five have found a performance benefit, and two have not. While the mechanisms are not perfectly clear, it is believed that this "carbohydrate mouthwash" may activate the reward centers of the brain and stimulate an improvement in performance that is related to the central nervous system, rather than connected to blood glucose levels and fueling for the muscle. In other words, even if the fuel doesn't arrive, the brain acts as if it did. More research is needed.

sedentary individuals and in anyone susceptible to high blood pressure, it may not be the best strategy for the endurance athlete susceptible to muscle cramping or prone to moderate to high sodium losses through sweating.

Several hours of sweating daily during training can add up to significant sodium losses in some athletes, particularly ultraendurance athletes. These sodium losses need to be replaced during training, quite often with a diet adequate in salt. Sports drinks have varying levels of sodium, and athletes prone to high sodium sweat losses and cramping can choose those higher in sodium. Some physiology laboratories can measure sodium losses in individual athletes, but determining whether you have high sodium content in your sweat does not have to be expensive or difficult. Often there are clear markers to indicate high sodium sweat losses, such as salt rings and marks on your skin and workout clothing. Acclimatization to heat should result in a decrease in the salt content of sweat, though as mentioned above, this may not occur as efficiently in some salty sweaters.

Preventing Hyponatremia

Hyponatremia, or an abnormally low blood sodium level, is a condition that can develop during and after long training sessions, and particularly during competition. Many endurance athletes experience mild or moderately lowered blood sodium from time to time. But severe hyponatremia can be dangerous and even fatal. The lower the blood sodium level drops, the more serious and life-threatening the symptoms. Symptoms of hyponatremia include headache, confusion, nausea, cramping, bloated stomach, and swollen extremities. At the very least, this condition can slow down your competitive efforts and is best prevented.

Don't overdrink! There are multiple causes of hyponatremia. The main instigators, however, are excess fluid intake, in which the blood sodium is diluted, and a high rate of sodium loss from sweating. Endurance athletes who naturally have a high concentration of sodium in their sweat, or who simply sweat a lot, are especially susceptible to the condition. But usually when athletes develop hyponatremia during an endurance event, it is because they were drinking too much water. In addition, for reasons that have not been clearly defined, there seems to be a higher incidence of hyponatremia among female athletes. The condition also seems to be particularly common in marathon running. Drinking excessively during a race taper in the two to three days before competition may set the stage for hyponatremia. Drinking in excess of fluid needs during the race can lower blood sodium levels further, and replacing sweat losses with plain water, rather than a sodium-containing sports drink, aggravates the condition even more. Slower finishers are at increased risk of developing hyponatremia because of the relative ease with which they can consume excess fluid, and athletes who are not well prepared for an event and poorly acclimatized are also at increased risk.

Match or Minimize Your Sweat Losses and Consume Sodium During a Race

Although fluid overload often characterizes hyponatremia, restricting water intake is not the answer—athletes competing in ultraendurance events who do this will end up finishing their event both dehydrated and sodium-depleted. Thus, unless it is medically contraindicated, endurance athletes should consume some salt in their diet. Athletes with special health considerations—for example, older athletes who have questions about how salt intake may affect their blood pressure or heart health—should consult with a physician on these matters. In addition, although it is best to maintain good hydration levels prior to competition, athletes should be sure not to overhydrate. During a race taper, sweat losses from training decrease considerably. Drink regularly, and monitor your urine color to assess your hydration status. During a race it is important to match your fluid intake with sweat losses and not overdrink. Athletes who know they are prone to hyponatremia because of their sweat rate or content should always consume sports drinks that contain sodium, and these athletes can reach for sports drinks with higher sodium levels. Endurance athletes with exceptionally high sodium requirements may even take salt or electrolyte tablets during training to offset high sodium sweat losses. These tablets should not be consumed in excess, however, and they should be taken with fluid. High-sodium foods such as pretzels and chicken broth are often offered on ultraendurance race courses such as an Ironman or ultramarathon. Though individual requirements can vary, ultraendurance athletes can aim for about 1,000 milligrams of sodium per hour during training and competition to maintain normal and safe blood sodium levels.

Fluid, Fuel, and Electrolyte Replacement Strategies

Obtaining adequate fuel and fluid during training sessions, and replacing high sodium losses if needed, takes practice, experience, and experimentation. Each athlete should develop an individualized plan for various training sessions and races. Here are some practical tips for making the most of your fuel and fluid intake during exercise:

Have a plan and drink on a schedule. Have a squeeze bottle of fluid ready and available for training so that you can consume fluid during breaks or regular intervals during training. Check your intake every hour to determine whether you are keeping up with the required fluid amounts.

Consume 4 to 8 ounces (120–240 ml) of fluid during every 15 to 20 minutes of exercise. Practice drinking at regular intervals so that you become skilled at consuming enough fluid during training. Take big gulps, as larger volumes empty from your stomach more quickly. For many athletes this fluid intake is a good starting point for minimizing dehydration.

Know your sweat losses by monitoring your weight before and after training. It is not necessary to consume more fluid than your body requires, but do try to consume adequate fluid during practice to minimize sweat losses. If you lose more than 2 pounds (approximately 1 kg) during a workout lasting an hour or more, you need to drink more. Gaining weight during workouts indicates that you are consuming too much fluid relative to your sweat losses.

Start exercise well hydrated. Drink 16 to 20 ounces (480–600 ml) of fluid in the hour before exercise, and start your training with a comfortably full stomach. This will speed up gastric emptying, as will drinking fluid every 15 to 20 minutes. This is especially important if the nature of your training session will not allow for frequent drinking opportunities.

Avoid "catch-up" drinking. Once you are dehydrated, fluids empty from your stomach more slowly. In extreme situations, dehydration may lead to GI upset, including a bloated stomach. Because fluids are emptying slowly, you will feel dehydrated and compensate by attempting to drink more, further aggravating stomach upset.

Start fueling early on during your training session. Greater performance benefits are seen when you use a sports drink from the start.

Develop a taste for various sports drinks. Although you likely have a favorite brand and flavor, practice with products and flavors that will be available on the race course and get used to their taste and feel during training. This allows for greater flexibility and improved drinking on competition day.

Fluids should be accessible. Keeping a squeeze bottle on hand allows you to drink an ample amount of fluid whether you are training indoors or out. Or, if you have a training route or loop, plan where you can purchase or place additional sports drinks.

Use a sports drink during moderate- to high-intensity workout sessions lasting longer than 60 minutes. Research indicates that this combination of fluid and carbohydrates improves performance by replacing sweat losses and providing carbohydrate fuel for your muscles. Even high-intensity workouts lasting just under 60 minutes may benefit from carbohydrate intake due to the effect on the brain.

Consume at least 30 to 60 grams of carbohydrates per hour from a sports drink that has multiple carbohydrate sources during moderate- to high-intensity training. This will ensure that you do not become dehydrated and will also provide fuel as glycogen stores become depleted. Optimally, you can absorb over 0.5 gram of carbohydrates for every pound (1 g/kg) and up to 0.7 gram per pound (1.5 g/kg) of body weight over a 1-hour period of exercise. Most sports drinks provide 14 to 20 grams of carbohydrates per 8-ounce (240 ml) serving. One full 20-ounce (600 ml) squeeze bottle will provide 35 to 50 grams and should be consumed over a 1-hour workout.

Consume 60 to 90 grams of carbohydrate per hour for training sessions lasting over 3 hours. Fueling needs are higher for longer workouts, and a combination of sports drinks and foods may be required.

Experiment carefully with other sources of carbohydrates. During intense training sessions or sessions where carbohydrate requirements outweigh fluid considerations, a more solid form of carbohydrate, such as a gel, may be appealing and provide needed carbohydrate fuel to prevent depletion. Gel servings usually provide up to 25 to 50 grams of carbohydrates per gulp. Just remember to consume gels with 8 to 16 ounces (240 to 480 ml) of water; otherwise they empty from your stomach slowly because they are so concentrated. Research indicates that gels may lead to gastrointestinal problems when consumed during running, though they are often well tolerated on the bike. Gel block and energy bars should also be consumed with plenty of water.

Know your sweat losses in different environmental conditions and at different times during the season. Monitor your weight before and after training in various temperatures and types of training sessions and at different times of the year. Condition yourself to drink the proper volumes to replace sweat losses in various situations. As your conditioning improves, your sweat rate will actually increase. Sweat rates also increase with acclimatization, though the sodium concentration of sweat should decrease. The plan needs to be personalized. A plan that only minimizes sweat losses in the hot summer months could lead to overhydration during cold-weather winter training.

Have a squeeze bottle or back-mounted hydration system at each training session, and consume fluids from it regularly. Have a plan to replenish supplies as needed.

Pay attention to signs of dehydration. Frequent gastrointestinal problems may indicate that you are not drinking enough. Gastric emptying is delayed when you are dehydrated. It may appear that you do not tolerate a particular product, when what is actually occurring is that the product is unable to empty from your stomach, and further drinking causes bloating.

Note the signs and symptoms of hypoglycemia. If you feel dizzy or light-headed or experience an inability to focus, your blood glucose levels are probably running low. Be proactive and increase your intake of carbohydrates with sports drinks or gels.

Refine your drinking technique. Practice drinking in all types of training situations. Know your limits regarding exercise intensity and your ability to tolerate certain volumes of fluid ingestion. Push your limits and maximize your fluid intake to maintain fluid balance.

Increase your sodium intake if you are susceptible to muscle cramping or are a salty sweater. Emphasize salty foods, and salt your foods to taste during periods of heavy training, particularly in hot weather. Choose higher-sodium sports drinks for training and competition. If you plan to use electrolyte replacement tablets or mixes in competition, experiment with them first in training and consume them with plenty of fluid. Salt also makes drinks tastier and encourages drinking.

NUTRITIONAL RECOVERY STRATEGIES AFTER EXERCISE

What you eat and drink from one training session to the next has a significant impact on your nutritional recovery. Consuming the total amounts of carbohydrate, protein, and fat that you require for your 24-hour nutritional recovery is essential. But for up to 4 to 6 hours after moderate to hard training, you can make the most of your nutritional recovery because the rate at which you can replace muscle fuel, specifically muscle glycogen, is accelerated at that time. Making the most of this accelerated recovery window is especially important when you need to train again in less than 24 hours, and especially when you have less than 12 hours of recovery. Paying attention to recovery nutrition in the hours after training can also improve rehydration efforts. Nutritional strategies for recovery are designed to promote:

- Replacement of the fluid and electrolytes lost in sweat
- Replenishment of muscle glycogen stores
- Support of the immune system
- Repair of muscle damage

After you determine what your recovery mix should be, or how much carbohydrate, protein, fluid, and electrolytes, focus on consuming the optimal amount of each nutrient at the right time. Chapter 4 summarizes the amount of daily carbohydrate that should be consumed to replenish muscle fuel stores.

CARBOHYDRATES AND IMMEDIATE RECOVERY

Because of the daily demands placed upon muscle glycogen, carbohydrate intake should be one of your primary nutritional considerations immediately after training. How long and hard you train directly affects how much glycogen was used and how much needs to be replaced before the next workout. The two main considerations for glycogen replacement are how much to consume and when to consume it. Muscle glycogen can be stored at a rate of about 5 percent per hour, so in 24 hours you can fully replenish fully depleted stores.

It is important to take in carbohydrates shortly after hard training. Delaying carbohydrate intake after a tough training session by even 2 hours can slow down the replenishment process. Several scientific studies have concluded that athletes should consume anywhere from 0.5 to 0.7 gram of carbohydrates per pound (1–1.5 g/kg) of body weight within 30 minutes of completing intense exercise to take advantage of this optimal time for muscle glycogen replacement. One study demonstrated that subjects fed carbohydrates a full 2 hours after exercise synthesized the carbohydrates into glycogen 45 percent more slowly than subjects fed carbohydrates immediately after exercise. It appears that muscle glycogen storage is slightly enhanced for up to 2 hours after exercise, during which time the muscle has a greater capacity to take up blood glucose. This strategy is worth taking advantage of when recovery needs are high and refueling time is short.

Studies have also shown that both liquid and solid carbohydrates are adequate in refueling the body after hard exercise. However, emphasizing higher-glycemic carbohydrate foods that elicit a higher insulin response, such as sports nutrition supplements and breads and cereals, may enhance glycogen resynthesis. A list of high-glycemic foods is provided in Appendix A.

If you have less than 8 hours of recovery time and the next workout requires good carbohydrate stores, you should not only consume carbohydrates immediately after hard training but also consume the same recommended carbohydrate amount (following the grams-per-pound formula) again in 2 hours. This allows you to continue to take advantage of the recovery process and stimulate muscle glycogen resynthesis. Glycogen resynthesis does slow down over time, but it is still relatively elevated in the 4 hours after training.

If you have a full 24 hours of recovery time, you can wait a bit longer for the next meal or snack. This may be more convenient and allow you to choose nutrient-dense options rather than what is just quick or convenient.

For the rest of the day, carbohydrates can be consumed as a series of snacks or a few larger meals, depending on your training schedule, food preferences, and total daily carbohydrate requirements. Both eating styles will promote glycogen recovery if the total amount of carbohydrate consumed is adequate. Eating a balanced mix of low-, moderate-, and high-glycemic carbohydrates throughout the day will support the glycogen recovery process. Fructose, which is found mainly in fruit, fruit juices, and some sports drinks, does more to enhance liver glycogen storage than it does muscle glycogen. But consuming an adequate amount of total carbohydrate grams from a variety of foods over the 24-hour period is a very important carbohydrate recovery strategy.

MUSCLE DAMAGE AND REFUELING

Muscle damage mainly from eccentric exercise, which often makes you sore a day later, can lead to a delay in replenishment of muscle glycogen stores. For example, after completing a marathon, runners often have only partial fuel stores in the week following the race. That's because disruption and damage to your muscle fibers can physically interfere with their muscle glycogen storage capacity. This impediment to muscle glycogen replenishment can last 24 to 48 hours after a tough run or race. You may need to up the ante on your carbohydrate intake to make up for the impaired replenishment.

PROTEIN AND IMMEDIATE RECOVERY

Early on, a fair amount of debate focused on the benefits of adding protein to the recovery carbohydrate snack immediately after exercise. In some studies, the results could be invalid because any benefit seemingly derived from the protein may have been due to the fact that the protein simply provided additional calories over the foods given to the carbohydrate-only group. Studies where researchers provided the same amount of calories when comparing a carbohydrate-only dose with a carbohydrate-and-protein combination dose indicate that carbohydrates alone can promote optimal recovery. What is certain is that having protein contribute about one-fourth of your recovery snack will not compromise your muscle glycogen recovery, and it may well contribute to it. Consuming some protein immediately after exercise may also speed up the repair of muscle tissue and provide important nutrients for your immune system. It will also send you on your way to optimizing your protein intake until the next training session, whether that session is the next day or even later the same day. Even if you completed endurance exercise rather than a specific weight training session, protein intake supports the production of muscle cells, hormones, enzymes, and other proteins after exercise.

Whether you consume carbohydrates alone or a carbohydrate-and-protein combination may be a matter of convenience. Packing and transporting high-carbohydrate items may be easier than including items containing protein. But if you do wish to include protein in your post-training snack, keep in mind that recovery protein should be from high-quality sources such as whey, dairy and soy milk, yogurt, and lean meats. A variety of commercial recovery products are also available. Although these are not necessary, they can be very convenient for replenishing your body immediately after training. Experiment with a low-fat shake or smoothie recipes made from cow's milk, yogurt, soy milk, or juice and fresh or frozen fruit for a hydrating carbohydrate-and-protein combination.

Ten to 20 grams of high-quality protein is more than adequate for your immediate protein intake, with the protein response leveling off at 20 to 25 grams. While protein may not need to be part of your immediate recovery snack, it should be part of your next meal and snack and go toward meeting your total protein requirements.

FLUID AND IMMEDIATE RECOVERY

Rehydration is a top priority after moderate to hard training, as athletes typically replace only three-fourths of their sweat losses through drinking during exercise. Your goal is to fully restore fluid losses from one training session to the next, while keeping in mind that thirst is not a reliable indicator of fluid losses. Not only are you already dehydrated by the time you feel thirsty, the thirst mechanism will shut down before you have sufficiently replaced all your fluid losses.

Pay attention to what stimulates your desire to drink. You may prefer a sweet product or something a bit salty. The temperature of the drink may also affect the volume you consume. It makes sense that a cool drink would be more palatable, particularly in hot weather, but it may be difficult to drink large amounts of a very cold beverage.

How Much Fluid Do You Consume?

Some athletes may feel reluctant to weigh themselves before and after every training session. You may also not have a scale available every time you train or would prefer not to get overly focused on a weight number. What you can do is obtain pre- and post-exercise weights after specific types of training sessions. These weight checks will provide you with valuable data. For example, you may discover that you replace only 50 percent of your fluid needs during hard training sessions but meet 80 percent of your fluid requirements during less demanding exercise, when it may be easier to consume fluid. Once you have established the replenishment levels of your best drinking efforts, you can develop a system for rehydrating after exercise. You may want to determine what your typical fluid losses are for specific types of environmental conditions, both indoors and outdoors, and for both hot- and cold-weather training. You can also check the color of your urine to evaluate your hydration efforts.

Remember, you also keep sweating and urinating after training, so simply drinking what feels good after training is not enough. Typically, you need to consume 125 to 150 percent of fluid losses to compensate over the first 4 hours of recovery. Generally, 1 pound equates to 16 ounces of sweat losses (500 ml per 0.5 kg). While you should consume 20 to 24 ounces of fluid for every pound of weight loss over the few hours after training, it is best to spread this fluid intake over several hours, if you have the recovery time, so as to minimize urine production. However, if recovery time is short, stick to large amounts at one time.

On days when you know you are to train or compete in extreme conditions, check your weight before and after exercise carefully. During intense training times and in hot-weather training, you can perform a daily check on your hydration status. After urinating in the morning, check your weight. If your usual weight is down by more than 1 pound (0.5 kg), you may not be keeping up with your usual fluid requirements.

SODIUM AND IMMEDIATE RECOVERY

Sodium not only may stimulate your drive to drink but also can enhance the rehydration process very effectively. In most athletes, sweating results in large fluid losses and relatively small sodium losses. When you finish exercise, your blood volume and total body water are reduced, so your overall blood concentration, including the sodium content of your blood, is increased. When you consume large amounts of plain water after exercise, you dilute your blood before your full blood volume has been restored. This dilutional effect shuts down the thirst mechanism, and you will urinate to bring the concentration of the blood to a normal level. The end result is that you have produced a large amount of diluted urine before you are fully rehydrated.

You can offset this negative effect by consuming some sodium after exercise. One series of studies determined that rehydrating with drinks containing sodium produced significantly lower urine losses than low-sodium drinks, indicating that more of the fluid consumed was retained and thus better hydration occurred. Therefore, it is recommended that when your fluid losses are significant, replace sodium losses as well. It appears that some individuals may have greater sodium sweat losses than others, so consuming sodium after exercise may be prudent unless medically contraindicated. Some athletes may actually require up to several grams of sodium over the course of the day, especially when training in extreme conditions.

If your fluid losses exceed 1 to 2 pounds (0.5–1 kg) during exercise, you should make a focused effort to drink fluids on a schedule and incorporate fluids into your recovery nutrition strategies. Products that contain sodium can also be integrated into your food and fluid choices to facilitate rehydration. If your recovery time is short, and the next training session is to take place in several hours, it makes sense to actively include sodium in your fluid and food choices.

WHAT SHOULD YOU DRINK AFTER TRAINING?

Sports drinks are formulated for tolerable consumption during exercise, not after exercise. Post-exercise, a 150-pound (68 kg) athlete requires 75 grams of carbohydrates, which translates to 40 ounces (1,200 ml) of a sports drink. Sports drinks are relatively low in sodium, though higher-sodium formulas are available. You may consider adding 0.25 to 0.5 teaspoon (575–1,150 ml) of salt to your total fluid intake, as twice the amount of sodium as found in a sports drink is optimal for rehydration. However, consuming a sports drink rather than a recovery drink may not be your most effective fluid recovery strategy, though it is preferable to plain water when rehydration is important.

Caffeine shouldn't impair the rehydration process, as it is not a diuretic. In fact, caffeine-containing drinks add to your fluid intake. But you should avoid alcohol in the hours after training, as it will increase urine production.

Although the recovery process is a continual effort that takes place from one training session to the next, you can get off to a good start by paying close attention to what you consume immediately and within the 2 hours after exercise. Then follow these post-exercise nutrition practices with food and fluid choices that match your daily training requirements. Table 5.2 outlines the principles of immediate nutritional recovery.

Practical guidelines for post-exercise recovery include:

♦   Be organized. Many of your meals and snacks are likely to be consumed away from home. Prepare foods and fluids the night before for the next day's training as needed.

TABLE 5.2 NUTRITIONAL RECOVERY GUIDELINES

TRAINING PROGRAM	POST-TRAINING NUTRITIONAL STRATEGIES (WITHIN 30-60 MINUTES)	ONGOING RECOVERY STRATEGIES (3 HOURS POST-TRAINING UNTIL NEXT SESSION)
Prolonged exercise at moderate intensity, or shorter-duration intense exercise	• Consume 0.5–0.7 g carbohydrates per pound of weight (1.0–1.5 g/kg). • Choose high-glycemic carbohydrates • Consume 10–15 g high-quality proteins if there has been muscle damage. • Drink 20–24 oz. (600–720 ml) for every pound (0.5 kg) of weight lost. • Consume sodium-containing foods and fluids to replace exercise sodium losses and stimulate rehydration.	• Consume the same carbohydrate amount again in 2 hours and every 2–3 hours after until daily carbohydrate targets are reached. • Continue rehydrating to baseline weight. • Include sodium in meals after a workout with moderate to high sweat losses.
Example: 150 lb. (68 kg) athlete who trains at moderate intensity for over 90 minutes	• Consume 75 g carbohydrates, 10 g protein, 24 oz. fluid, and 250 mg sodium from liquid recovery supplement and granola bar.	• Consume 75 g carbohydrates and 20 g protein at next meal that includes grains, lean proteins, and antioxidant-rich fruits and vegetables.

- Plan food and fluid choices so that you can consume the optimal amounts of carbohydrate, protein, fluid, and sodium for your immediate recovery nutrition needs.
- Use the food list provided in Chapter 4 to consume enough carbohydrates—0.5 gram per pound (1.2 g/kg) of body weight.
- After moderate to hard training, be prepared to consume the same nutrient amounts again in 2 hours.
- If your appetite is suppressed after hard training, focus on liquid choices such as high-carbohydrate supplements, smoothies, yogurt drinks, or sports recovery drinks.
- Avoid foods with a low glycemic index or that are very high in fiber immediately after training. These foods may not result in as speedy a recovery and may not be as well tolerated after training.
- Don't consume excessive amounts of protein immediately after training. Animal foods and high-protein supplements are very concentrated proteins, and often only small portions or doses are required for your nutritional recovery mix.
- Fat does not play an important role in the immediate recovery nutrition mix. Consuming fat immediately after training could delay gastric emptying and crowd out more important nutrients such as carbohydrates and protein.
- After training, drink on a schedule rather than according to thirst.
- Check labels to ensure that the foods and fluids you consume after training contain some sodium.

IMMEDIATE POST-TRAINING FOOD AND FLUID CHOICES

Practice to determine what post-training food and fluid choices suit your preferences, tolerances, and schedule. Recovery products concentrated in carbohydrates, providing anywhere from 50 to 100 grams per 16-ounce (480 ml) serving, are available. Some of these products also provide up to 25 grams of protein per serving. Sports tubes that provide only protein are also available and can be consumed with a high-carbohydrate food or fluid. Aim for recovery products that have a higher sodium content. Some favorite food choices among endurance athletes are:

- Cereal, dairy or soy milk, and fruit. High-glycemic cereals are good choices.
- Bagel with peanut butter, jam, and orange juice
- Smoothie made with soy or dairy milk, yogurt, and frozen fruit
- Yogurt, granola, and fruit
- Energy bar and fruit
- Baked potato with yogurt topping
- Pancakes with syrup
- Pasta salad with low-fat cheese
- Turkey sandwich with pretzels

JACK CASE STUDY: NUTRIENT TIMING

Jack previously determined his energy requirements for a specific day of training (4,132 calories), and his breakdown of carbohydrates (740 g), protein (132 g), and fat (74 g), in Chapter 4. He determined that 540 grams of this carbohydrate target would come from real foods consumed before, after, and between training sessions.

Jack often trains early in the morning to complete two workouts daily, and that morning he would complete a 60-minute high-intensity swim. Jack leaves early in the morning for a swim and consumes 8 ounces of juice (30 g carbohydrate) and some water on the way to the pool. He consumes 24 ounces of a sports drink (45 g carbohydrate) during the 60-minute swim, drinking when set breaks are allowed.

Because Jack will go to work straight from the pool, he makes sure to pack an appropriate breakfast that matches his post-workout recovery prescription. At a weight of 165 lb. (75 kg), Jack requires 90 g carbohydrate (0.54 g/kg) and 10 to 15 g of protein within 30 minutes of training. He also has checked his weight before and after training and found that he needs to consume 8 to 16 ounces (120 to 240 ml) of fluid to rehydrate.

For his recovery breakfast Jack finds that he can easily mix 6 ounces (180 ml) of Greek-style yogurt with ¾ cup (180 ml) of low-fat granola and a large banana for 95 grams carbohydrate and 20 grams protein after the morning swim. He consumes some water with his recovery breakfast, and the sodium naturally contained in the yogurt and cereal supports his rehydration efforts. This breakfast gets Jack off to a good start for replenishing his fuel stores in preparation for his evening run workout. Jack also focuses on eating the right balance at lunch and for his afternoon snack, making sure that he consumes lean protein, wholesome carbohydrates, and appropriate doses of healthy fats in preparation for the 90-minute evening run.

Having eaten an easily digested carbohydrate snack 2 hours before his evening work-out, Jack starts the run with a placid stomach. He consumes one gel packet every 30 minutes during the run. A few drops in tempo allow for the gel intake with about 12 ounces of water intake per packet. He finishes the run workout down about 1.5 pounds (0.70 kg), indicating that his hydration plan during runs needs to step up before race day. Jack rehydrates after the run with a recovery smoothie that provides 50 grams carbohydrate, 10 grams protein, sodium, and of course fluid. He arrives home within an hour of completing his run and consumes a dinner providing whole-grain carbohydrates, lean proteins, and healthy fats.

NUTRITIONAL STRATEGIES FOR COMPETITION

Fine-tuning your food and fluid strategies before, during, and after training can also set the stage for competition day. Although the meals and snacks that you consume on race day are important, specific nutrition strategies in the days and hours leading up to competition can also benefit your performance. Many endurance athletes taper train-ing before an important event, and this period of relative rest presents an important opportunity to fuel up. Adjusting your pre-race meal to account for race day nerves and the hard effort ahead is also an important consideration. Having a specific plan for your nutritional strategies during endurance competition events—for example, the multiple heats that swimmers may need to complete over the course of a competition lasting sev-eral days—can give you that extra boost you need to do your best.

PRACTICAL USES OF SPORTS NUTRITION PRODUCTS

Endurance athletes can't avoid the intense marketing of various sports drinks, gels, wafers, blocks, chews, energy bars, recovery drinks, sports shakes, and high-energy drinks. While Appendix C presents a comparison chart of many of these products, a summary of some practical uses of these products is provided below. When you consume a wide variety of sports nutrition supplements over the course of a day or even a week, it is important to consider the other nutrients they provide, such as vitamins and minerals. Consider your intake in the context of your entire day's diet plan and be careful not to get too many vitamins and minerals through use of these products and supplements in combination.

Sports Drinks

Consume 16 to 24 ounces (480–720 ml) in the hour before exercise.

Consume 4 to 8 ounces (120–240 ml) every 15 to 20 minutes as your training session allows, or drink to match your sweat rate or minimize your sweat losses as much as possible.

Consume after exercise with high-carbohydrate foods and supplements.

Gels and Blocks

Consume one packet or one serving (20 g carbohydrate) in the 30 to 60 minutes prior to training and competition.

Consume during training with 16 ounces of water.

Consume as part of a recovery nutrition snack.

Energy Bars

Consume in the 30 to 60 minutes prior to training and competition.

‖ WEEK PRIOR TO COMPETITION: CARBOHYDRATE LOADING

When you have the luxury of tapering for an important competition such as a triathlon, marathon, cycling road race, or swim, you are presented with a prime opportunity to maximize your carbohydrate fuel stores. The combination of not dipping into your muscle glycogen as deeply as you would with regular training and maximizing your carbohydrate intake is known as "carbohydrate loading." Although this process traditionally takes place over the course of a week, some athletes adapt it to their needs by lengthening or shortening the carb-loading period. An athlete facing a short race or

Consume during training with fluid when a solid carbohydrate source is appropriate or desired.

Consume as part of a recovery snack after training.

Consume as part of a high-energy meal plan during heavy training cycles and for carbohydrate loading.

High-Energy Carbohydrate Drinks

Consume as part of a pre-training and pre-competition meal or snack.

Consume as part of immediate post-exercise recovery nutrition.

Consume as part of a high-energy meal plan.

High Carbohydrate Protein Drinks

Consume before and after resistance training for quality protein combined with carbohydrates.

Consume as part of a pre-training and pre-competition meal.

Consume as part of your immediate recovery nutrition plan.

Consume as part of a high-energy training meal plan.

Sports Shakes

Use as a pre-exercise snack for an easily digested carbohydrate and protein source.

Include in a carb-loading meal or competition morning meal for easily digested nutrients.

Drink as a recovery snack after training.

Include in a high-energy nutrition plan.

Use as a quick meal or snack for convenience.

competition may load carbohydrates over just a 24- to 48-hour period before competition, whereas an athlete preparing for an ultraendurance event, such as an Ironman triathlon or ultramarathon, may taper for several weeks and then load carbohydrates for the last week of his or her taper.

Why Carbohydrate-Load?

Research indicates that muscle glycogen stores return to normal with 24 hours of rest and a high-carbohydrate diet if there is no significant muscle damage. However, it may be ideal to rest and eat for an additional 24 hours to bring muscle glycogen levels from the normal full level of 100 to 120 millimoles per kilogram (mmol/kg) to the supercompensated level of 150 to 200 millimoles per kilogram. Carbohydrate loading will allow you to perform at your desired pace for a longer period of time and is especially useful for competitions where you anticipate that your time will be longer than 90 minutes. During longer race tapers designed for a longer event, focus on reaching a full recovery so that your muscles are rested and fueled for the big day.

The Traditional Carbohydrate-Loading Regimen

Sports dietitians currently recommend the "modified" carbohydrate-loading regimen because it is gentler than but just as effective as the old strategy, which contained a stringent "depletion" phase. Devised in the 1960s, this depletion phase started a week before competition and lasted 3 to 4 days. It involved depleting glycogen stores through a combination of hard training and a low-carbohydrate diet. This was followed by 3 to 4 days of combined rest and a high-carbohydrate diet to glycogen-load the muscle. Athletes often complained of feeling poor and training poorly during the depletion phase. This difficult strategy was phased out after research in the 1980s showed that it was unnecessary to achieve the high levels of muscle glycogen that the technique produced.

Follow the "Modified" Carbohydrate-Loading Regimen

A 3- to 4-day taper combined with a high-carbohydrate diet was found to be sufficient to achieve the same glycogen-loading levels. Below are a few guidelines to consider when carbohydrate loading:

- Gradually taper your training for 1 week prior to the event (longer if that is outlined in your training program). Eat your normal training diet that matches your intake with your training during days 7 to 4 of the 1-week taper countdown. Consume at least 3 grams of carbohydrates per pound (6.6 g/kg) of body weight.
- For the last few days of the week, taper your training further, or even rest completely on days 3 to 1 of the countdown. Consume a high-carbohydrate diet providing 4 to 5 grams of carbohydrates per pound (9–11 g/kg) of body weight.
- The carbohydrate amounts required for an athlete to glycogen-load can vary from the above recommendations. Ideally, on days 7 to 4 you will consume more total

carbohydrates than previously in your training, or in excess of what a particular training session normally requires, and on days 3 to 1 you will carb-load.

- Consider carbohydrate loading up to day 2 before the race so that you don't feel the need to get a high amount of carbohydrate the day before the race; you can simply rest and eat appropriately. This ensures that you don't overeat the day before the race and that you will wake up race morning looking forward to your planned pre-race meal.

- Your caloric needs may decrease during this time because of the marked decrease in training. You can lower both your protein and fat intake in the 72 hours before the race, as requirements for these nutrients are decreased.

- If you cannot taper for a full week, reduce your training for 3 days and load up on carbohydrates.

- Exercise lightly the day before the competition to relieve any muscle stiffness and to keep your muscles "sharp" for competition.

- Have a food plan laid out ahead of time that ensures that you consume enough carbohydrates to glycogen-load. Carbohydrate loading is not synonymous with "pigging out," nor is it a food free-for-all. You don't want high-fat foods to replace those precious carbohydrates.

- You may want to emphasize low-fiber and compact carbohydrate food sources to minimize gastrointestinal upset and to ensure that you consume the prescribed carbohydrate amounts.

- Be aware that for every gram of glycogen you store in your body, you also store up to 3 grams of water. This effect can result in a weight gain of several pounds. This extra fluid will help delay dehydration during the event.

- Pay close attention to what you eat the day and night before the competition and the day of the competition. Specific guidelines will be provided later in this chapter.

- Monitor urine color to determine if you are adequately hydrated. Pay attention to daily hydration needs, but keep in mind that you may not be creating as large a fluid deficit as you would during periods of heavier training.

- If you are competing in an event lasting longer than 6 hours, or if you are a heavy and salty sweater, be generous with the salt shaker and consume salty foods such as pretzels, tomato juice, and salty soups.

- Don't try any new or unusual foods or spicy items that may not agree with you in the days leading up to a race.

Having a sound menu plan in mind can take some of the stress off of carbohydrate loading. Table 5.3 provides a list of some high-carbohydrate, low-fiber foods that should be well tolerated and that provide 30 grams of carbohydrates per listed serving. Starches, breads, and cereals that are low in fiber are fairly concentrated sources. Fruit and fruit juices are also good sources of carbohydrates. Sports nutrition supplements such as energy bars, gels, concentrated carbohydrate drinks, and high-carbohydrate meal replacements may also fit nicely into your meal plan for their predictability and easy digestion.

The food lists in Chapter 4 provide an extended list of 30-gram carbohydrate servings. You have to consider how you will prepare and portion foods as you decrease your intake of proteins and fats during this carbohydrate-loading phase so as not to overeat calories and shut out the carbohydrates required for full replenishment of stored fuel. Many meals and snacks can be fat- and protein-free, with just enough consumed for satiety and fullness. Consuming between-meal snacks is another strategy for obtaining the recommended carbohydrate amounts. Using sports supplements and commercial products may make life simpler during carbohydrate loading. Table 5.4 provides a sample menu for a very high-carbohydrate-loading day at more than 600 grams of carbohydrates. If this level exceeds your carbohydrate needs, simply trim back some of the carbohydrate portions or one or more of the listed snacks.

TABLE 5.3 LOW-FIBER, HIGH-CARBOHYDRATE FOODS

30 GRAMS OF CARBO-HYDRATES PER SERVING	SERVING SIZE (OZ./C./TBSP.)	(G/ML)
Animal crackers	16 crackers	
Apple	1½ medium	
Apple juice	8 oz.	240 ml
Applesauce, sweetened	½ c.	120 ml
Bagel	2 oz.	60 g
Bread, white	2 slices	
Canned fruit	1 c.	240 ml
Carnation® Breakfast Essentials™ Drink	1 envelope	
Carrot juice	10 oz.	300 ml
Cold cereal, low-fiber	1.5 oz.	45 g
Cooked cereal	1 c.	240 ml
Cranberry juice cocktail	8 oz.	240 ml
Dinner rolls	2 rolls	
English muffin	1 muffin	
Fig bars	3 bars	
Graham crackers	6 crackers	
Granola bar	1 medium	
Grape juice	6 oz.	200 ml
Grapefruit	1 large	
Jam	2 tbsp.	40 ml
Jelly beans	25 small or 1 oz.	30 g
Milk, skim	20 oz.	500 ml
Muffin, low-fat, low-fiber	3 oz.	90 g
Pasta, cooked	1 c.	240 ml
Pita pocket	1½ rounds	
Potato, baked, no skin	1 medium	
Pretzels, white flour	1½ oz.	45 g
Raisins	4 tbsp.	80 ml
Rice, cooked, white	⅔ c.	200 ml
Rice cake, 4 inches diamete	4 cakes	
Saltines	8 crackers	
Sports drink	16 oz.	480 ml
Sports gel	1 packet	
Sweet potato, no skin	4 oz.	120 g
Tortillas, 6-inch, corn or flour	2 tortillas	
Waffles (toaster)	2 small	
Yogurt with fruit	1 c.	240 ml

48 HOURS BEFORE THE EVENT

This is your big day to load up on carbs, for several reasons. You are not likely to have much of any type of activity on this day, so it is truly a rest day, and you still have one more day of your taper after consuming a large dose of carbohydrates. This allows for plenty of digestion time after a few substantial high-carbohydrate meals. Good carbohydrate choices on this day include white rice, bread, bagels, low-fiber cereal, fruit, juice, a variety of sports nutrition supplements such as high-energy drinks and bars, and small amounts of very lean protein such as poultry or fish. Minimal oils should be used in food preparation. A large carb-loading meal with pasta, rice, or potatoes can be used as a base for this meal, but a 3-ounce portion of protein would also be fine. Stick with cooked, easy-to-digest vegetables; you should probably skip the salad. Drink plenty of fluids (but don't over-hydrate), and include fluid choices that also provide carbohydrates. You may need to eat five or six times on this day to take in the total grams of carbohydrates required. Carry high-carbohydrate snacks and fluids with you wherever you go so that you can continue to steadily fuel and hydrate your body. A light evening snack can top off your carbohydrate intake for the day.

TABLE 5.4 HIGH-CARBOHYDRATE, PRE-COMPETITION MENU

MENU	SERVING SIZE (OZ./C./TSP./TBSP.)	(G/ML)
BREAKFAST		
Orange juice	1 c.	240 ml
Cornflakes™ cereal	1 c.	240 ml
Banana	1 large	
Skim milk	1 c.	240 ml
Toast	2 slices	
Margarine	1 tsp.	8 ml
Jelly	4 tbsp.	80 ml
SNACK		
Yogurt with fruit	6 oz.	200 ml
Granola bar	1 medium	
LUNCH		
Lean turkey	3 oz.	90 g
White bread	2 slices	
Pretzels	¾ oz.	20 g
Pear	1 large	
Apple juice	16 oz.	480 ml
SNACK		
Energy bar	1 medium	
DINNER		
Cooked rice	2 c.	480 ml
Ground turkey	3 oz.	90 g
Cooked peas	1 c.	240 ml
Bread	2 slices	
SNACK		
Frozen yogurt	12 oz.	360 ml
Fig Newtons®	4	

Total: 654 g carbohydrates, 140 g protein, 38 g fat, 3,545 calories

THE DAY BEFORE THE EVENT

The day before the event, your nutritional focus should be on consuming adequate carbohydrates but also sticking to very simple and easy-to-digest foods. Only minimal amounts of fats and proteins are required the day before the event. Following a few strategies can contribute to a successful race day:

- Consume your large meal by 5:00 p.m. or even earlier if you expect a very early morning start. Since most races and events do start early in the morning, the last thing you want is to feel groggy and full from consuming a large dinner late in the evening before a race.

- Your pre-race meal on event morning is an essential component of your nutrition plan. It is important that you wake up that morning feeling hungry and ready to eat. The day before and especially the night before the event, you do not want to try any new and unusual foods that could result in gastrointestinal upset. Be especially careful to limit fiber-containing foods, gassy foods such as broccoli and beans, and alcohol.

- Practice having various meals the night before an important morning training session to see what works best for you. Make simple meals that can be ordered in most restaurants when traveling. Pasta dishes low in fat are a common favorite among athletes, but other choices also work well. Try rice-based dishes, baked potatoes, and white breads. Avoid salads and other raw vegetables and raw fruits the night before an important training session or race.

- Carry carbohydrate-containing foods and fluids to keep the fuel supply steady. Sports drinks and high-carbohydrate drinks that contain sodium provide a great way to hydrate the day before the race. Continue to go heavy on the salt as needed by salting your food and consuming salty items.

RACE MORNING

Depending on your race time, personal tolerances, and experience, you should consume a light to large meal 3 to 4 hours before competition. Many seasoned endurance athletes have identified this time period as optimal for pre-race eating, as you can achieve a good balance between optimal food consumption and adequate digestion time. Ideally you will greet the morning well hydrated and with muscle glycogen stored at peak levels by practicing proper nutrition techniques for several days before the race. The main focus of this pre-race meal should be to replenish your liver glycogen stores. This valuable fuel falls to low levels overnight, especially if you spend your night tossing and turning from pre-race nerves. With the right timing and portions, eating 3 to 4 hours before exercise will allow you to:

- Restore liver glycogen to normal levels. Liver stores are important for early start times, since they are low after an overnight fast.

- Store carbohydrates in the muscle as needed, if portions are large enough.
- Avoid hunger during longer events and competitions and leave your system feeling placid and comfortable during competition.
- Top off fluid levels and pre-hydrate before an event.

On the morning of competition, it is especially important to choose foods that you enjoy and tolerate and that also provide both a physiological and a psychological edge. For every hour you allow yourself to digest, consume just less than half a gram of carbohydrates for every pound of body weight.

For example, if you decide to eat a large meal 4 hours before a triathlon or swimming competition, you can consume 2 grams of carbohydrates per pound. For a 150-pound (68 kg) athlete, this translates to 300 grams of carbohydrates (and 1,200 calories).

It is probably easiest on your stomach if a good portion of this fairly substantial meal consists of dense, low-fiber foods and some liquid carbohydrate sources. You can obtain 300 grams of carbohydrates by consuming one large bagel topped with 2 tablespoons (40 ml) of jam, followed by a fruited yogurt and 32 ounces (960 ml) of a concentrated sports drink. The small amount of protein in the yogurt may help keep you full a bit longer. You can also add peanut butter or cream cheese to your bagel if a small amount of fat is well tolerated.

Some athletes can only tolerate smaller meals close to exercise, particularly competition. Every athlete needs to iron out individual tolerances in terms of foods, portions, and timing. Table 5.5 provides pre-competition meal suggestions.

In the hours leading up to the race, continue to hydrate with a sports drink. These drinks provide easy-to-digest carbohydrates and sodium as well as fluid. You may want to stop drinking, however, 30 minutes or more before the start of the race to allow your stomach to empty comfortably and to empty your bladder. Some athletes even like to top off their carbohydrate intake in the 90 minutes before the start of competition with an energy bar or gel. Practice this strategy during training to determine if it works well for you.

Meal timing and portioning are especially important the day of competition. Make sure that you have a well-thought-out and thoroughly rehearsed game plan for eating times and portions on the day of the event. Experiment with meal and snack timing in training, and try to mimic the schedule of an upcoming competition. For earlier start times, you may want to consider one moderate-sized meal several hours beforehand. If you do not want to rise as early as this strategy requires, however, a smaller meal can be consumed closer to the event.

TABLE 5.5 MEAL TIMING BEFORE TRAINING AND COMPETITION

TIMING	CARBOHYDRATE/FOOD RECOMMENDATIONS	SAMPLE CARBOHYDRATE AMOUNTS	SAMPLE FOODS	START TIMES
Night before	• High-carbohydrate meal • Low in fiber • Easy on fat • Optimal fluids	200–300 g carbohydrates for dinner and evening snack	Grains: pasta, rice, potatoes, bread, couscous Lean protein Cooked vegetables	Essential for early starts Helpful for any start time
3–4 hours prior	• Carbohydrates: 1.5–2 g/lb. (3–4 g/kg) of weight • Low-fat proteins in moderate amounts • Easily digested fat in low to moderate amounts • Low fiber • Optimal fluids	Example: A 150 lb. (68 kg) athlete would consume 225–300 g carbohydrates.	Grains: cereals, bread, crackers, milk, yogurt, fruit, juices, jelly, muffins, bagels, waffles, pasta, rice, potatoes Lean protein Limited fats	*For early-morning starts:* Eat at 4:00 a.m. for 7:00 a.m. start. *For mid-morning starts:* Eat at 7:00 a.m. for 10:00 a.m. start. *For mid-afternoon starts:* Eat at 10:00 a.m. for 2:00 p.m. start. *For evening starts:* Eat at 4:00 p.m. for a 7:00 p.m. start after adequate carbohydrate meals earlier in day.
2 hours prior	• Carbohydrates: Up to 1 g/lb. (2 g/kg) of weight • Minimal low-fat protein • Low fat and fiber • Plenty of fluids	Example: A 150 lb. (68 kg) athlete would consume 130–150 g carbohydrates.	Grains: cereals, bread, English muffin, bagel, crackers Milk, yogurt, smoothie, liquid meal supplements Fruits, juices, jam Sweet potato Energy bar	*For early-morning starts:* Eat at 5:00 a.m. for 7:00 a.m. start. *For mid-morning starts:* Eat at 8:00 a.m. for 10:00 a.m. start. *For mid-afternoon starts:* Eat at noon for 2:00 p.m. start after a large morning breakfast. *For late starts:* Eat at 6:00 p.m. for 8:00 p.m. start after adequate carbohydrate meals throughout the day.
1 hour prior	• Carbohydrates: 0.5 g/lb. (1 g/kg) of weight • Emphasize liquids: 50–100 g easy-to-digest carbohydrates in the form of liquid or gel, solid if tolerated • Limit or avoid protein • Limit fat and fiber	Example: A 150 lb. (68 kg) athlete would consume 65–70 g carbohydrates.	Concentrated carbohydrate drinks, sports drinks, gels, blocks, liquid shots, sports bars	*For early starts:* Eat at 6:00–7:00 a.m. for 8:00 a.m. start. *For mid-morning starts:* For 10:00 a.m. start, have snack/liquid at 9:00 a.m. in addition to 6:30–7:00 a.m. meal.
Immediately prior	• Carbohydrates	Example: A 150 lb. (68 kg) athlete would consume 20–30 g carbohydrates.	Sports drinks, gels, blocks, jelly beans, liquid carbohydrate, energy bars if exercise starts at moderate intensity for at least 30 minutes.	*For any start time*

Later start times may necessitate eating one large meal earlier in the day, followed by a series of snacks as the start of competition approaches. On competition day, you can enjoy sports nutrition supplements that are easily digested and well tolerated. Liquid meal replacements, high-carbohydrate energy drinks, and sports drinks and gels can be consumed leading up to the start time. Refer to Tables 5.4 and 5.5 for pre-competition meal and snack timing suggestions. For the 150-pound (68 kg) athlete, this translates to 300 grams of carbohydrates (and 1,200 calories).

During the competition or event, you should follow the race nutrition plan that you have developed, fine-tuned, and practiced, practiced, practiced during training.

ATHLETE PROFILE

Developing a Hydration Plan: Brad

Brad, an enthusiastic multisport athlete, has competed for several seasons in Olympic-distance triathlons, half-marathons, and mountain bike races. This season he wants to improve his racing and finishing times, so he enlisted a more structured training program and decided to seek the services of a sports dietitian.

The sports dietitian reviewed Brad's racing practices and determined that he needs to develop a strategic hydration and fueling plan for each race. Brad used the "Sweat Loss Worksheet" (see Appendix F) to estimate his sweat rate for the various disciplines in which he trains. He learned that his sweat rate is higher than he had realized and that he was consuming only about 50 percent of his hourly sweat rate when training. For early-morning training sessions and for training sessions lasting longer than 60 minutes, Brad was advised to consume a carbohydrate-electrolyte beverage or sports drink to offset low liver glycogen and muscle fuel depletion, respectively. The quality of his early-morning workouts has since improved, and Brad is now able to maintain his desired pace for longer evening and weekend workouts.

As the season progressed, Brad rechecked his sweat rate and found that it had increased as he acclimated to warmer weather. Having improved his hydration and fueling strategies, he was able to meet 80 percent of his sweat losses through practice. Brad also checked various race sites to determine what sports drinks and gels would be offered on the courses and trained with these products in the weeks leading up to the race. With the assistance of his sports dietitian, Brad determined how many grams of carbohydrate he requires per hour for various competitive events and matched this with his sweat rate and the volumes that he is able to consume per hour. He also has a plan for using carbohydrate gels and blocks as needed.

By race day, Brad felt that he was well prepared, with a fueling and hydration plan for each race that he followed as outlined. He packed needed nutritional items the night before, ensuring that he had the proper equipment to carry fluids and other items for each race and planned for transitions and aid stations specific to each race.

WEIGHT LOSS, MUSCLE BUILDING, AND CHANGING BODY COMPOSITION

Boosting Your Strength-to-Weight Ratio

Endurance athletes come in a variety of shapes and sizes. Some began participating in sports in grade school or high school when their bodies were developing and growing and their body composition was still in flux. Others started participating in their chosen sport well into their years as masters athletes. Some may be genetically blessed with a physique that is well suited to their sport and attain their body-composition goals easily, while others need to work hard to achieve these goals. Whichever category you fit into, you may find that focusing on body composition can improve your strength, fitness, and performance. Building muscle and strength and decreasing body fat also help you build a good foundation for optimal health as you age. This focus can be particularly helpful after age thirty-five, when loss of a small amount of muscle mass is a normal part of the aging process.

REACHING YOUR BODY-COMPOSITION GOAL

There are smart and sensible ways to attain a lean and strong body. However, some athletes resort to destructive methods of manipulating their body composition in an attempt to attain an overly idealized body that may not be realistic for their age, growth and development, level of training, body type, or genetic tendencies. It is easy to assume that dropping a few "extra" pounds will improve your performance and that intense training builds muscle strength. But athletic success is not always that simple. Examples abound of athletes at all levels who have restricted their diet or increased their training in an attempt to improve body composition, with the end result being a decrease in energy levels and performance. It is important to keep an open mind regarding your "best weight." Don't compromise your recovery and energy to build a few pounds of muscle or lose a few pounds of fat.

Optimal performance in endurance sports depends on a number of interrelated factors, including the ability to sustain power near your anaerobic threshold, a high VO_2max, efficient technique, a high power-to-weight ratio, and a low level of body fat. The last two factors mean that an endurance athlete carrying excess weight or lacking in muscle strength can be at greater risk of injury when performing the skills required for his or her sport. Of course, being overweight or ignoring the strength-training component of your program will also have adverse performance effects.

But less is not necessarily better. When striving to make body-composition changes, athletes need to realize that they will perform their best when they reach and maintain their own optimal body composition, not some idealized body composition that would require excessive training efforts and restrictive food strategies. Severe food restriction and excessive training can result in low energy levels and poor-quality training sessions, increase the risk of injury, and pose both short- and long-term health risks.

Reaching body-composition goals for optimal performance can go hand in hand with strength training or resistance training, a common element of endurance training programs. The high levels of muscle mass and strength that can be achieved with resistance training are important factors in athletic performance, whether it is on the road or in the pool. Optimal and effective methods for gaining muscle mass have long intrigued sports nutritionists and the industries that pay for heavy marketing and promotion of muscle-building products. However, the keys to maximizing strength include your genetic potential, an appropriate resistance training program, and specific muscle-building nutritional strategies supported by solid scientific research.

Clearly, many endurance athletes can benefit from building muscle and maintaining optimal levels of body fat. Let's take a look at some strategies for doing just that.

BUILDING MUSCLE

Muscle growth is the result of the balance between muscle protein synthesis and muscle protein breakdown. You build muscle when synthesis exceeds breakdown over a period of time. Research indicates that the interaction between exercise, particularly resistance exercise, and protein that you consume leads to the greatest stimulation of protein synthesis or muscle building. This interaction actually lasts at least 24 hours, and over time each resistance training session and the meals that follow it lead to the building of muscle protein. How well you build this muscle or protein depends on several factors, with the most important being:

- The timing of protein intake
- The amount of protein intake
- The type of protein consumed
- Other nutrients ingested with the protein

Besides protein-specific guidelines, several of the nutritional strategies for muscle building center not only on your daily training diet but also on the intake of certain nutrients timed specifically around your weight training sessions and in key amounts in your daily diet—all designed to optimize your muscle-building efforts. The keys to optimizing muscle-building efforts include:

- Attaining enough calories so that your body has the energy required to build muscle
- Consuming enough carbohydrates so that you meet the fuel demand for both resistance training and training for your endurance sport
- Having enough total protein in your daily diet
- Consuming fluids and carbohydrates during your workout

NUTRITIONAL REQUIREMENTS FOR BUILDING MUSCLE

Calories and Carbohydrates

When you strength train, you likely are also participating in regular training for your sport and could be burning significant amounts of stored body fuel from various types of exercise sessions. During weight training, the stored fuels of creatine phosphate and muscle glycogen serve as important energy sources. When combined with other components of your endurance training program, resistance training can provide a further drain on your body's carbohydrate fuel stores. Although you may typically think of increased protein intake in relation to strength training, one main goal should be to consume adequate energy to build muscle tissue.

One of the most important nutrition guidelines for effectively building muscle is to consume enough calories. Because of the increased energy it takes to build body tissue, falling short on your calorie requirements will impair your rate of muscle building. An additional 350 to 500 calories or more daily are needed to gain 1 pound (0.5 kg) of muscle mass per week. Further increases in muscle building require additional calories. Once you gain the muscle and strength that you desire for your sport and performance, it also takes an adequate amount of energy to maintain this increased weight. Keep in mind that these additional calories are the calories required above your energy needs for training and recovery in your endurance sport and for resistance training. The combination of your endurance training program and your weight training can have a significant impact on your energy needs.

Often the perception is that extra calories consumed to build muscle should be protein calories. Specific protein guidelines are reviewed below. However, although protein is required to build muscle tissue, it is only one of the ingredients needed for the tissue-building process. The amount of protein that you require as an endurance athlete should be adequate to cover your daily needs for muscle building; your protein needs may increase only slightly, if at all, when you are adding resistance training to your day. In fact, many of the extra calories needed for muscle building should come from carbohydrates in your diet. The most important factor in your protein intake is not amount, but timing.

Just keep in mind that when it comes to fueling exercise, carbohydrate is the master fuel, even for repeated high-intensity efforts. That makes muscle glycogen an important fuel source during weight training, and an intense session may deplete 30 percent of your muscle glycogen stores. When this type of training is combined with your endurance training, muscle glycogen stores can become significantly depleted in a day or over several days. Regardless of how quickly you deplete these stores, it is important that you replenish glycogen stores adequately after training, whether in the weight room at the gym, after a workout in the pool, or after a bike or run.

Protein

Although large amounts of protein are not necessary, protein is still important for the repair and growth of muscle fibers. Strength training causes the breakdown of muscle fibers, which respond by making bigger and stronger muscle fibers to protect against further stress. Protein is one of the main construction materials needed for this repair process to take place. Athletes who strength train do have higher protein requirements than sedentary individuals, but the amount of protein they consume for endurance training is likely more than adequate to put them in positive protein balance. Positive protein balance means that you consume enough protein to meet all the protein-requiring processes and functions in your body, including the synthesis of new muscle tissue.

If you do consume protein in excess of what is required for both your strength and endurance training, this extra protein is burned for energy, which is not a very efficient process, or simply stored as fat, which may not be desirable. More is not better, and eating twice as much protein as your body requires won't make your muscles twice as big. Strength training also makes your body more efficient at using the protein in your diet.

Real foods can easily be part of a well-balanced diet that meets your protein requirements for both weight training and endurance training. Stick with the high-quality sources of protein mentioned in Chapter 2, such as lean red meat, poultry, fish, skim milk dairy products, and soy products. You will also obtain protein from some plant foods, all of which contribute to your total protein intake. Fat in your diet should continue to round out your calories just as it would for your regular training diet.

TIMING YOUR NUTRITIONAL INTAKE

After weight training, your body synthesizes new muscle protein and replenishes muscle glycogen. Several studies have indicated that an athlete's nutritional intake in the hours before and after weight training can have a significant impact on his or her muscle-building efforts. Consuming the right amount of the right type of protein at the proper time around your weight training session is more effective in promoting muscle building than just increasing your overall daily protein intake. Carbohydrate can be added to protein recovery snacks for refueling and is likely to provide some support of protein resynthesis.

Protein Timing, Amount, and Type

The window for building protein begins just before resistance training and extends up to 24 hours after training. The preferred window for protein building is the 3 hours after training. Ongoing resistance training can reduce your sensitivity to protein feedings to under 16 hours, rather than 24, making it even more important to time your post-workout protein intake properly.

For this reason it is recommended to consume protein prior to and after your resistance training efforts as your training schedule and access to the proper food and supplements allow. Aim for 15 to 20 grams of protein in the meal or snack that you eat in the 1 hour before strength training, emphasizing high-quality sources such as low-fat dairy products, whey protein, and protein from animal foods, as the essential amino acids in these foods are the most potent stimulators of muscle protein synthesis. Recent research confirms that more is not better. One study found that the muscle-building response increased incrementally with up to 20 grams of protein. There was no difference in response when doses were increased to between 20 and 40 grams.

Combine your protein with 35 to 50 grams of carbohydrates. Go for the higher carbohydrate amount if your resistance training session is followed by an endurance workout in order to start replenishing muscle glycogen.

Again, include both carbohydrates and protein in the next snack or meal that you consume after weight training to continue to facilitate the recovery and muscle-building process. Aim for some recovery nutrition foods and fluids within the 1 to 2 hours after weight training. Carbohydrates and protein consumed after resistance training should also stimulate both muscle glycogen and protein synthesis. High-glycemic carbohydrates can be emphasized after resistance training, just as they can after your regular training sessions. Aim for 15 to 20 grams of protein and 50 grams or more of carbohydrates in your recovery snack or meal.

Often your nutritional choices before and after weight training will, out of necessity, depend on practical considerations. Keep snacks on hand to consume both before and after resistance training. Aim for convenience choices, such as low-fat shakes or smoothies. Pack protein-containing snacks such as yogurt with fruit, a peanut butter–and–honey sandwich, or low-fat cheese and crackers to take with you to the gym. A commercial sports supplement containing a mix of carbohydrates and protein is convenient and meets your nutritional requirements in the hour before and after weight training.

During Resistance Training

What you consume during resistance training may be beneficial to your recovery and the quality of your training sessions. Although adenosine triphosphate (ATP) and creatine phosphate in the muscle are your primary fuel sources during weight training sessions, muscle glycogen can become depleted to varying degrees between training sets, depending on the intensity and duration of your training. Between sets, your muscle will use the glycolysis energy pathway to regenerate ATP stores. Consuming a sports drink for the carbohydrates it provides can help you maintain muscle glycogen stores and provide energy during your workout. These drinks also provide fluid and assist you in maintaining adequate hydration levels. Of course, consuming plain water during resistance training is also recommended. As with any training session, start your workout well hydrated.

PROTEIN SUPPLEMENTS AND WEIGHT TRAINING

Athletes who become serious about strength training inevitably wonder whether they should take protein supplements. The number of choices can be bewildering—there are many products on the market containing protein from a variety of sources. These products can optimize muscle building, but again, the timing of the protein intake is the key. The protein in the supplements is not necessarily any better than the protein contained in foods; however, the supplements are convenient and may make your protein consumption at the right times easier to accomplish when you are not at home. The supplements can be consumed with moderate amounts of carbohydrate, so follow the recommendations described above for your diet on a day that includes strength training.

YOUR WEIGHT TRAINING DIET

The nutritional strategies for optimizing muscle building and increasing strength are complex and interrelated. Consuming adequate calories is a key to providing your body with the energy to build muscle in the hours after it has been damaged and broken down. Too, your daily protein needs must be met, and the timing of your protein intake is also important, particularly before and after training. Weight training, like your regular training for your sport, is a fuel-depleting exercise. Consuming carbohydrates with your protein both before and after training can facilitate energy for training and recovery after training, and consuming carbohydrates during training itself can also fuel your efforts.

WHAT FORM OF PROTEIN SUPPLEMENT SHOULD YOU CHOOSE?

Which of the protein sources used in these supplements is best? Basically, there are several sources that provide high-quality protein.

Whey protein is the component of milk that is separated out when making cheese and other dairy products. It is a high-quality protein that contains all the essential amino acids and is an especially rich source of the branched chain amino acids (BCAAs), which are especially important for muscle building—particularly leucine. Whey protein isolate is the highest form, at 90 percent protein, and is lactose-free. Whey protein is soluble and easy to digest and is often referred to as "fast" protein as it gets to the muscles quickly and is one of the most potent stimulators of protein building.

Casein, also found in milk, is a "slow" digesting protein. It helps prevent muscle protein breakdown, ultimately preserving muscle mass. Whey and casein work well together to prevent muscle breakdown. Because protein synthesis is dynamic, consuming milk sources of protein regularly at meals and snacks is recommended. Because casein provides benefits as a slow protein, do not use the hydrolyzed form, which is more rapidly broken down.

Soy protein is an excellent source of protein—especially soy protein isolate, which is 90 percent protein. It is a high-quality protein choice for vegetarians and is lactose-free. Soy protein concentrate is only 70 percent protein. Like whey protein, it is considered a "fast" protein and can promote increases in lean body mass. When soy protein has been compared with milk protein, studies have shown that the milk protein leads to greater gains in muscle mass. Soy protein, however, is still an effective protein for muscle mass increases.

Albumen, the high-quality protein found in eggs, is easily digested and high in the BCAAs, especially leucine. Egg protein is absorbed more slowly than whey and faster than casein. It supports muscle building and can be obtained from real food sources or is often incorporated into high-protein energy bars. Egg protein is obtained from egg whites and is considered the standard against which to compare other proteins—though real eggs may not be as convenient a protein source as supplements, depending on the timing and location of your training.

To gain muscle mass while following a strength training program, you need an additional 350 to 500 calories daily for a muscle gain of 1 pound (0.5 kg) per week. These additional calories can come mainly from carbohydrates and some protein. Here are some strategies for obtaining additional calories:

- Add a bit more protein to sandwiches and dinners.
- Top carbohydrate foods such as bagels with jams and honeys.
- Add another snack to your meal plan.
- Add a fruited yogurt, fruit smoothie, low-fat shake, or instant breakfast drink to your meal plan.
- Add a pasta or rice salad side to your lunch.
- Consider an additional high-calorie shake or meal replacement.
- Make oatmeal and soups with milk.
- Add wheat germ, sunflower seeds, and dried fruit to cereals.
- Choose higher-calorie juices such as apple, cranberry, nectars, and blends.
- Choose calorie-dense cereals such as muesli, granola, and Grape-Nuts®.
- Eat higher-calorie starchy vegetables such as peas, corn, and winter squash.

Table 6.1 summarizes the nutritional strategies for building muscle mass.

TABLE 6.1 NUTRITIONAL FACTORS IN DAILY DIET FOR MUSCLE BUILDING

NUTRIENT	ROLE OF NUTRIENT	
Carbohydrates	Fuel source during weight training. Required in diet to replenish glycogen stores for comprehensive training program that includes aerobic and anaerobic conditioning.	
Protein	Required for muscle building. Protein needs are easily met on a well-planned diet for a comprehensive training program that includes weight training and aerobic and anaerobic training for an endurance sport.	
Fat	Adequate amounts needed to maintain hormone levels, including testosterone. Healthy fats should be emphasized for cardiovascular health.	
Calories	Provide additional 350–500 calories or more in daily diet to build 1 lb. (0.5 kg) of muscle per week.	
ONE HOUR BEFORE WEIGHT TRAINING	**DURING TRAINING**	**AFTER TRAINING**
• Consume 15–20 g high-quality proteins from whey, dairy, soy, or animal sources. • Consume 25–50 g or more carbohydrates. • Pre-hydrate with 16–24 oz. (600–720 ml) fluid.	• Consume 16 oz. (600 ml) of carbohydrate electrolyte beverage, if desired. • Consume gel and water for carbohydrate and fluid sources, if desired	• Consume 15–20 g high-quality proteins from whey, dairy, soy, or animal sources. • Consume 25–50 g or more of carbohydrates if complete back-to-back endurance training. • Rehydrate with 20 oz. (600 ml) of fluid per lb. (0.5 kg) of weight lost during session.

JACK CASE STUDY: MUSCLE BUILDING

Jack typically competes at a low body fat level of 8 percent and usually gains a few pounds during the off-season. He mainly trains indoors during the early part of his training season as he lives in a colder winter climate. This indoor training also allows him to focus on resistance training and building strength in weaker areas to improve the coming season's performance and prevent injury. During indoor training time, Jack remains focused on muscle building and meeting his energy requirements for training, knowing that he will arrive at his "racing weight" and body fat level with increased training volume and intensity as the season progresses.

Jack often completes his endurance training and weight training sessions back to back, so he consumes a sports drink during the endurance session to offset muscle glycogen depletion, as muscle glycogen is also a fuel source during resistance training. He found a recovery supplement that can be purchased and consumed at his health club that provides 20 grams of whey protein and 50 grams of fast-acting carbohydrate. He added an energy bar to the mix to increase his carbohydrate intake to levels needed for recovery from the

CHOOSING A PROTEIN SOURCE

Like many other sports nutrition strategies and choices, use of protein supplements rather than real food before and after resistance training is a matter of what is most convenient for you. These products should be taken with a carbohydrate source such as juice. Often, only a small scoop of the protein supplement is needed to provide 15 to 20 grams, though higher doses may be encouraged on the label.

But the supplements can be expensive and do not necessarily offer any muscle-building advantage over real protein foods. High-quality protein can be obtained from milk and yogurt, tofu and other soy products, and poultry and lean meats. Practical protein and carbohydrate combinations for your pre– and post–weight training meals or snacks would include home-made smoothies that use a variety of quality protein ingredients such as soy milk, yogurt, and/or cow's milk. Fruit juice or fruit can be added for carbohydrates. A generous serving of yogurt with fruit can make a good protein-and-carbohydrate combination. Low-fat cheese is also a high-quality protein source that can be consumed with fruit or a granola bar.

endurance training session as well. Total intake is 28 grams protein, with 20 grams coming from high-quality whey protein in the liquid supplement, and 75 grams of carbohydrate.

Jack has built 3 pounds (1.4 kg) of muscle in the off-season and feels stronger for the upcoming training and racing season. His weight training will be adjusted to maintain this gain as he ramps up his endurance training.

WEIGHT LOSS

Many endurance athletes wish to lose weight for both health and performance reasons. For example, masters endurance athletes may originally have competed in sports whose optimal body composition requirements contrast with the optimal levels of muscle and fat required for swimming, cycling, running, or triathlon. Consequently, many endurance athletes desire to undergo significant body-composition changes in preparation for competition.

Losing body fat can improve performance. But it is important to achieve these levels through scientifically proven methods and safe and health-preserving strategies. To lose body fat and weight, you have to expend more calories than you consume, or you have to create a negative energy balance. A combination of the proper nutrition strategies with training is most likely to produce success than either one alone. Rapid weight loss can have serious health consequences and also lead to significant decreases in performance. Goals of a healthy weight-loss plan include:

- Achieving a modest energy deficit
- Maintaining lean body mass
- Gradually reducing body fat
- Consuming a high-quality diet rich in vitamins, minerals, and phytonutrients
- Avoiding any significant decrease in resting metabolic rate

LOSING FAT

There is no doubt that achieving optimal levels of body fat can improve performance for cycling, running, and triathlon. Athletes of all shapes and sizes compete in these sports. Each sport, including swimming, also requires some optimal level of lean body mass.

Body composition is what truly matters, and training and diet can profoundly influence the ratio of lean mass to fat mass for any endurance athlete and body type.

USING A SCALE

When endurance athletes monitor their weight and attempt to become leaner in hopes of improving their performance, their efforts to manipulate body composition often result in frequent weight checks on the scale. It is important that you keep the scale in perspective, however, as it provides only a rudimentary measure and tells you little about body fat levels or changes during the training season. There are other methods of estimating body fat that are much more useful for training purposes.

The scale obviously weighs all of you—muscle, fat, bone, water and fluid fluctuations, and body organs—and does not differentiate among these body tissues. For this reason, highly muscular athletes may weigh at the high end of their "ideal" weight. Conversely, thin, small-boned people weigh less. Your body weight is influenced by more than what you eat and how much you train. Many of the factors that affect your weight are determined by genetics and are often out of your control.

The best use of a scale is to monitor long-term changes over time as they coincide with monitored body-composition changes and to measure short-term changes related to your hydration status. As mentioned previously, weight loss after a hard training session provides feedback regarding your level of hydration. It is recommended that for every 1 pound (0.5 kg) of weight lost during exercise you rehydrate with 24 ounces (720 ml) of noncaffeinated fluid.

Long-term weight changes as measured by a scale can provide you with a crude indicator regarding changes in body composition over time or even help you determine whether you are keeping up with or exceeding your energy needs. Chronic unwanted weight loss can indicate that you are not meeting your caloric requirements, and perhaps that you are pushing yourself to an overtrained state. It is also important not to get overly focused on an idealized weight obtained from a height and weight chart, or on the weight and body fat levels of the top athletes in your endurance sport. Although certain body fat averages have been measured for specific sports, a number of interconnected factors other than body fat affect an athlete's performance. Athletes can be successful at varying degrees of reasonable body fat levels, with some competitors at the low end of the body fat range and others at the high end. Top athletes do not always fit the lean and muscular ideal for their sport, and a low body fat level does not guarantee success.

TECHNIQUES FOR MEASURING BODY FAT LEVELS

Regardless of the body fat measurement technique you employ, keep in mind that they all measure your body fat indirectly. When choosing a body fat measurement technique, consider the following guidelines:

- The technique and formula used to estimate your body fat should be valid for athletes in your sport, for your gender, and for your age range.
- A reliable technician should perform the technique.
- The same technique should be repeated over time to obtain long-term data and to measure progressive changes.
- The results should be interpreted by a knowledgeable expert who is aware of the limitations of the technique and can advise you appropriately.

Clearly, the measurement of body composition is far from an exact science. One commonly utilized technique, skinfold testing, has a standard error of 3 percent. This means that if an athlete tests at 15 percent body fat, his or her actual body fat level could range from 12 to 18 percent. Body fat assessments provide a possible range of body fat rather than an absolute number. When monitoring your body composition over time, it is very important that you not try to compare the results you obtain via different techniques and technicians. Table 6.2 provides a perspective on body fat measures for male and female endurance athletes in various endurance sports. But no individual athlete should feel pressured to

TABLE 6.2 BODY FAT LEVELS FOR HEALTH AND ENDURANCE SPORTS

RATING	BODY FAT LEVELS (%)
At risk (low levels)	Males: <5 Females: <9
Very low	Males: 6–10 Females: 10–15
Below average	Males: 11–14 Females: 16–19
Average	Males: 15–18 Females: 20–25
Above average	Males: 19–24 Females: 26–29
At risk (high levels)	Males: 25 or more Females: 30 or more

SPORT	AVERAGE MEASURED BODY FAT LEVELS (%)
Running	Males: 6–13 Females: 10–19
Cycling	Males: 8–10 Females: 12–18
Triathlon	Males: 5–11 Females: 7–17
Swimming	Males: 7–12 Females: 14–24

meet a certain body fat number: Each athlete is unique and performs best at a body fat level appropriate to his or her own genetic inheritance and training level, among other factors.

Body fat simply refers to the number of pounds of fat on your body, often expressed as a total percentage of body weight. It is a body tissue that does not contribute to performance and does have to be carried, particularly when cycling and running uphill. Lean mass is everything but body fat. It includes muscle, organs, and bones, and is more accurately referred to as fat-free mass.

It is important to choose one method of body-composition analysis that you can use over a few years. If you jump around regarding technique and tester, it can be confusing to compare data and monitor progress. Don't compare skinfold results with a handheld device or fall back on data from several years prior, particularly if you have more years of training stored in your body.

The body fat measurement techniques listed below are the ones most commonly used. They all contain some inherent range of error, and they all provide only an estimate of body composition rather than an exact figure derived from a direct measurement of body fat. Accuracy also can vary among technicians. If you decide to obtain a body-composition assessment, find an experienced technician who works with athletes regularly.

Hydrostatic Weighing

The hydrostatic method, a water-displacement technique, is often cited as the "gold standard" of body fat assessment, despite having a standard error of at least 2 percent. Hydrostatic weighing involves being weighed underwater after expelling as much air from your lungs as possible. Your body density is estimated from the difference between your weight on land and your weight under water. Your body fat is then extrapolated from this information.

Like all methods, hydrostatic weighing is not error-free. This method assumes a constant fat-free body density and may not be appropriate for all population groups. There is some potential error related to your hydration status and how much air is actually left in your lungs when you are weighed. In addition, the procedure for underwater weighing can be a bit uncomfortable. The method can be useful, however, and is offered at some sports medicine centers and universities. Health clubs may offer it as a special service several times throughout the year. This technique, when administered by a skilled technician over time, can help you to gauge body-composition changes.

Air Displacement

Also known as *body plethysmography*, this technique measures body density through air displacement rather than water displacement. Your body fat percentage is calculated based on standard equations. This technique provides body fat estimations similar to those of underwater weighing, though more data are needed on the results obtained from this method for competitive athletes. To complete the procedure, you sit in an enclosed capsule (a Bod Pod) while a computer measures the amount of air displaced.

This is an expensive system, but it is more convenient than underwater weighing. It is not yet widely available, though some universities and health clubs do offer it.

Bioelectrical Impedance Analysis (BIA)

Use of bioelectrical impedance analysis has markedly increased over the past ten years because it is relatively inexpensive, portable, and convenient. BIA is based on the conductive property of different tissues within the body. Because muscles contain a high percentage of water, they conduct current more quickly than fat stores. The BIA machine passes a small and undetectable current through the body and analyzes the resistance to the flow of the current. The slower the signal, the more body fat you have.

Although BIA is relatively quick and simple, it may overestimate body fat in lean individuals, and the results can be affected by hydration levels. If you are not well hydrated, you will appear to have a higher level of body fat than you actually have. You should be well hydrated for the test, but you should not drink fluids for 4 hours before the test so that you will have an empty bladder. It is also best not to exercise within 12 hours of the test. Alcohol and diuretics should be avoided prior to this procedure as well.

Many individuals are now purchasing a home scale (Tanita brand) that measures body fat with this technique. To use the scale effectively, take the readings at the same time of day each time, be well hydrated, and have an empty bladder. Avoid early-morning readings when you are most likely to be dehydrated.

Skinfold Calipers

The skinfold caliper technique is the most widely used and the most inexpensive and convenient method of measuring body fat. For this procedure, a technician uses calipers to indirectly measure the double thickness of subcutaneous fat underneath the skin. Several standard skinfold sites have been identified on the body: abdomen, arm, thigh, hip area, and back of shoulder. They must be accurately marked, and the skinfold is then pinched and gently pulled away from the body. The sum of several skinfolds (anywhere from three to seven sites) is plugged into a formula that is then used to estimate total body fat.

This technique has several disadvantages. It requires a skilled technician, and it assumes that subcutaneous fat is proportional to total body fat. Moreover, the formulas for skinfold measurements are based on body-composition measurements from underwater weighing. The formulas used for skinfold measurements should be appropriate for athletes and their sport. When formulas for the general population are used, body fat is often underestimated in athletes. Skinfold measurements may also underestimate body fat in very lean athletes.

However, when kept in perspective, this technique can be useful. Besides calculating the body fat percentage, you can use it to obtain a number that is the sum of all the skinfolds measured. This absolute number is not formula-dependent and can be monitored over time. For example, a twenty-year-old male cross-country runner may have a three-site skinfold sum of 40 millimeters and an estimated body fat of 11 percent. A follow-up measurement several months later may show an increase in body weight along with a decrease in the total skinfold sum to 36 millimeters. These results would indicate a probable loss in body fat and an increase in muscle mass. This trend can be monitored every several months and over a year's time to provide useful feedback regarding training and diet.

Tape-measure readings can also be combined with skinfold assessment, with measurements taken at thigh, arm, and abdominal sites. The more skinfold measurement sites required by the formula, the better—you should never compare body fat estimations made over time using different formulas.

CHANGING BODY COMPOSITION

Because body composition is the result of genetics as well as training and diet, some athletes may naturally have a body composition considered optimal for their sport, while others have to struggle to stay within a preferred range. Extreme effort to maintain a set body composition may not be worth the energy it takes, as it may compromise the quality of your diet and training. It is also important to keep a healthy perspective on body fat. Aim for an appropriate range rather than a specific number. Body fat levels may change over the course of a season—and over the course of your life—depending on the phase of your training, your age, and the stage of your competitive career.

If you are considering trying to improve your body fat composition, have it assessed by a skilled technician. An optimal goal for weight can be determined, but it is important to be realistic regarding how much body fat you want to lose and how quickly you should try to reach your goal. This may require some professional advice and some realism on the athlete's part.

First, consider your genetics. Experts suggest that genetics strongly influences the amount of fat your body stores. If you have a history of struggling with body fat and can say the same of your family members, consider a moderate and gentle weight-loss goal. Next, look at your lifestyle. Food choices are heavily influenced by your schedule, commitments, environment, and stress levels. It is important for your weight-loss and body fat goals to be reasonable, as you have to meet the energy demands not only of training but of life in general—and work or school—as well.

Dieting Pitfalls

Dieting certainly presents several pitfalls for the endurance athlete. An athlete who is glycogen-depleted, electrolyte-depleted, low on protein, and dehydrated from dieting will not perform at his or her best and likely will perform poorly. Rigid dieting and too much calorie restriction can deplete body fuel stores. Intense weight-loss efforts can also result in hormonal imbalances, iron-deficiency anemia, compromised bone health, and loss of muscular strength and power. Severe dieting can make you crabby, tired, and obsessive. Dieting just isn't fun.

Food is fuel for your hardworking body, and your body does not respond positively when fuel runs low. A low fuel gauge sends out a slew of appetite-triggering brain chemicals that drive you to eat. What many dieters perceive as a lack of willpower is really the body's drive for self-preservation. Restricting foods can lead to overeating and even binge eating, thwarting weight-loss efforts. Besides playing games with the body, dieting wreaks havoc with the mind. Restrictive eating can lead to feelings of deprivation and a preoccupation with food.

Besides triggering overeating, drastic calorie reduction can break down body protein stores for energy. This muscle loss not only hinders your strength and power but also negatively impacts your metabolism.

The most important factor that determines your resting metabolic rate (RMR) is the amount of fat-free mass (muscle, bone, body organs) that you have. Because these are calorie-burning tissues, the more fat-free mass you have, the higher your metabolism.

Your total body weight or body mass also affects your resting metabolic rate. The higher your body mass, the more calories your body needs for basic maintenance.

Starting as early as age thirty, you lose some muscle mass every year. Resistance training twice weekly can help maintain this muscle mass and prevent a loss in resting metabolic rate. Muscle is what keeps your furnace burning.

Dieting can also slow down your resting metabolic rate. When you restrict calories, your body becomes more efficient at using less energy. The more severe your calorie drop from your normal intake, the greater the decrease in your resting metabolic rate. Resting metabolic rate will return to normal once a more normal calorie intake is resumed. One way to avoid a big drop in RMR is to drop your calorie requirements by only 15 percent of your maintenance requirements. For example, if you require 2,500 calories for a particular type of training day, a 15 percent decrease in calories would be a deficit of 375 calories, for a total caloric intake of 2,125 calories.

How Do I Determine a Goal Weight?

First, have a body-composition analysis and keep in mind the inherent degree of error with each technique. Consult Table 6.2 for the classifications for good health and for the ranges often seen for your gender and in your chosen sport. Of course, the body fat values provided are a range; optimal levels for endurance athletes can vary. Some endurance athletes can safely reach the lower end of the ranges in an appropriate time frame, while others have to compete at higher levels because it is not possible to get down that low without adversely affecting performance. It is recommended that women not strive for body fat levels in the single digits, as this is unhealthy.

When considering your weight and athletic history, put your high-school weight—and if you are an older endurance athlete, even your college weight—where it belongs: in the past. Your weight and body-composition goals should reflect where you are as an adult endurance athlete, including muscle mass developed for your sport through training. Losing unwanted muscle through dieting is even harder than decreasing body fat. Chances are that you do need this muscle for your sport. Don't try to attain a weight or body fat number that has been unreachable or difficult to reach in the past. Instead, set a more realistic goal. If you have reached this number in a healthy manner, you can then reevaluate if that lower number fits into your lifestyle and training plan, and if it is even required for improved performance. It is also expected that optimal body fat levels would increase as you reach your forties, fifties, and later. Keep in mind that the same body fat can look different on different people, so choosing an ideal based on someone else's appearance (let alone performance) is not the best strategy.

When you have obtained your baseline body fat, your technician can calculate what weight you would need to reach for your new body goal. This calculation assumes that your current level of muscle mass remains the same. Because both fat mass and lean body mass can change over time, your weight goal can be recalculated with subsequent body fat checks.

Training and Weight-Loss Dangers

Many weight-loss diets, particularly those that are designed for weight loss of greater than 1 to 2 pounds (0.5 to 1 kg) weekly, often do not provide enough energy and carbohydrates for endurance workouts and high-intensity workouts. That's why it is recommended that you only reduce calories by 10 to 20 percent so that adequate carbohydrates for training and recovery are part of your meal plan. Too low of an intake can result in inadequate replenishment of glycogen stores, use of muscle for fuel stores, and decreased energy. Muscle loss also results in lowered RMR.

Because of the potential pitfalls of cutting too far back on calories and the subsequent decrease in performance, it is recommended that you focus on weight-loss goals early in the season—preferably before and in the early months of base training. This should minimize any negative impact that dieting or calorie restriction can have on your training and recovery. Calorie restriction in the build phase of training and in the weeks leading to a race could have a greater negative impact on your training than trying to lose body fat earlier in the season.

Endurance athletes wanting to lose weight may wonder where they should cut back on calories. Fad diets would have you convinced that carbohydrates should be drastically reduced in the diet. But as an endurance athlete you need the carbohydrates in your diet to match that particular training cycle. Keep in mind that your body prefers to convert carbohydrates into glycogen—the all-important fuel. Protein is important to preserve muscle mass, and it can also be used for energy production, though this is not preferable. Protein in your diet stimulates thermogenesis or heat production. It is also the nutrient that promotes the highest level of satiety or fullness.

A good place to cut calories is from fat. Dietary fat is more likely to be converted to fat than any other nutrient. Fat burning is most likely to occur when the total amount of calories that you require exceeds the amount of calories burned. The fats that you do eat should mainly be monounsaturated fats, omega-3 fatty acids, and omega-6 fats high in essential fats.

Alcohol can also encourage fat storage and should be limited. Because alcohol is not stored in the body it must be burned and converted to energy. Excess calories from alcohol are ultimately converted to fat. Also, many alcoholic drinks contain sugars, making them high-calorie beverages.

Balanced weight-loss plans should include the following:

• Reduced total fat at about 20 to 25 percent of total calories
• 2–3 grams of carbohydrate per pound (4–7 g/kg) for base training
• 0.8 gram of protein per pound weight (1.6 g/kg) to preserve lean body mass and promote fullness

Overall, you will slightly decrease fat and carbohydrate intake and possibly increase protein intake. Alcohol intake should be kept to a minimum.

Calorie Requirements and Weight Loss

Your calorie target is the number of calories that you consume each day to create a calorie deficit that will get you to your weight- and fat-loss goal in a reasonable amount of time. Chapter 4 provides guidelines for estimating your caloric requirements based on your weight, estimated RMR, daily activity, and that day's energy training demand. Because your training requirements can vary daily, your weight-loss calorie level can also vary from day to day. The key is to cut back enough for some weight and fat loss, but not too much!

Depending on how much weight you need to lose and your energy requirements for that day's training, a reasonable calorie deficit is 350 to 500 calories daily, or a weight loss of 0.5 to 1 pound weekly (0.25 to 0.5 kg). Athletes with more weight to lose can cut back 750 to 1,000 calories earlier in the season on higher-volume training days for a weight loss of 1.5 to 2 pounds (0.7–1 kg) weekly. Just keep in mind that the body reacts to smaller deficits by burning more fat and to larger deficits by loss of lean tissue and glycogen depletion and a decrease in RMR. Larger deficits should be followed on training days that require more calories. For example, if your energy requirements for a particular training day are 3,800 calories, a deficit of 750 calories would still allow for 3,050 calories to be consumed. On a lighter training day when only 2,700 calories are required for weight maintenance, you would consume 1,950 calories—a level that could be too low and result in hunger and subsequent overeating. Think of a reasonable calorie deficit as ranging from 10 to 20 percent of your energy requirements for that day. On a 2,700-calorie day this would be a deficit of 270 to 540 calories, with the midpoint at 405 calories.

HEALTHY WEIGHT-LOSS GUIDELINES

A healthy weight for an athlete is about how you feel and perform, not just about how you perceive how you look or what the scale is telling you. It can be difficult in our society to keep a healthy perspective on weight. The ideal has become more muscular and leaner than ever, while as a whole the population is gaining weight. Often the ideal portrayed in the media is unhealthy and unrealistic and can only be attained through excessive exercise and overly restrictive eating.

Healthy weight loss starts with setting a realistic goal and avoiding quick, unbalanced, and extreme weight-loss approaches. Try to accomplish your goal in a reasonable amount of time and during the off-season for your sport. Let's take a look at some sensible weight-loss guidelines.

Set a realistic body-composition and weight-loss goal. It is very likely that your training program emphasizes both muscle building and maintaining a low level of body fat. Often, real body-composition changes do not result in drastic body weight changes, as the scale measures all body tissue, not just fat. Elicit the advice of a qualified professional who can assess your body-composition results and recommend changes in body composition that are appropriate for your age, gender, growth and development, current training program, and sport.

Set a realistic calorie deficit. Keep in mind that when you attempt to lose body fat, you have to restrict calories; however, when you desire to build muscle, you need to consume adequate calories. It is important to find a balance between your body-composition and strength-development goals. Females should not exceed a weight loss of 1 pound (about 0.5 kg) weekly, and males, 2 pounds (about 1 kg) weekly, especially during heavy training periods. Losing 1 pound (0.5 kg) weekly requires a deficit of 500 calories daily. Greater weight loss requires even more restriction. Losing 2 pounds (1 kg) weekly requires a daily 1,000-calorie deficit, clearly calling for some intense calorie-cutting and calorie-burning efforts that are not always appropriate during periods of growth and/or heavy training cycles.

Remember that trimming no more than 200 to 300 calories daily may be the safest and most effective long-term weight-loss approach. This mild reduction should have no metabolism-lowering effects and will not precipitate feelings of hunger and deprivation. However, if you are stepping up your muscle-building efforts, your best results may be obtained by following the proper training program and the nutrition program that is optimal for building muscle mass.

Consume enough energy or calories so that you stay above a threshold that is considered too low and would result in a lowering of resting metabolic rate. Your calorie intake should not go below your RMR and daily activity calories. You should avoid very low calorie intake on harder training days.

Have your energy intake spread over the day to avoid energy lows and hunger. Planning regular meals and snacks should keep you on an even keel all day.

Reduce carbohydrates as part of your energy cutbacks, but keep enough to fuel muscle. Daily carbohydrate intake should also fluctuate over the course of a week according to daily fuel needs.

Train for some sessions without fuel support. Early or light recovery sessions can be completed first thing in the morning before eating or without a sports drink.

Consume carbohydrates before, during, and after key training sessions. Fuel is required to keep up the pace during high-intensity sessions.

Consume adequate protein to maintain lean mass and control hunger.

Leave room for social eating and treats. Make sensible choices when eating out and consume favorites in smaller amounts and perhaps with less frequency.

Keep a food journal to assess your current eating habits. Write down your food intake, the times of your meals and snacks, and your portion sizes for 1 week. Record your training sessions as well, noting the duration and intensity of training in conjunction with your food intake. You can also record your moods, thoughts, and feelings to determine some of your eating triggers, such as stress or fatigue. It may be helpful to note your energy levels and recovery during and after various types of training sessions.

Assess your intake. Make sure that you are following the principles of post-exercise recovery nutrition. Monitor your hunger and fullness patterns. Do you often wait until you are ravenous before eating? Do you get overfull at meals? Do you eat for comfort or in reaction to stress fairly often? Do you have significant drops in your energy levels during the day?

You may be surprised at how much you actually consume during the day. Writing down your food intake can help you stay on track while you are trying to lose weight and, more important, can help you improve the quality of your diet and nutritional strategies, as it makes you accountable and conscious of your food choices.

Have a healthy strategy or plan for reducing your caloric intake and improving your diet. There are a number of effective ways to reduce your caloric intake and improve your diet. It is important that you eat well after exercising, practicing the recovery nutrition guidelines supplied in Chapters 4 and 5, and that you time your meals and snacks appropriately before training. If you eat out frequently or consume too much fast food, you may have a large amount of hidden fat in your diet.

Other techniques for reducing fat intake are choosing leaner meats, switching to low-fat dairy products, minimizing added fats and those used in cooking, and decreasing the frequency of sweets. You can also cut back on high-calorie fluids. Alcohol is an obvious choice, as are sodas and perhaps juices. Pay attention to portions when you eat out or grab items on the run. A bagel or muffin can easily provide more than 300 calories.

Plan ahead. Preparing meals ahead of time can help you avoid fatty restaurant foods. Learning how to shop for quick, low-fat, nutritious foods can be extremely helpful in improving your diet and changing your body composition. You can also pack healthy snacks such as fresh fruits and vegetables. Programming your food environment for success or learning how to manage the environment in which you make your food choices will go a long way toward supporting you in reaching your weight-loss goals.

Eat breakfast and add some protein. Don't skip breakfast, as people who do so are more likely to overeat later in the day. Chronic breakfast skippers are much more likely to struggle with weight management. Studies also show that when you consume up to 30 grams of protein at breakfast, you have a better handle on hunger throughout the day and at later meals.

Eat balanced meals at the right times. Having real meals will leave you feeling satisfied. Make sure that you consume meals throughout the day, and don't set yourself up for periods of intense hunger. Besides having a complete breakfast, have a full lunch, and don't consume all your calories in the evening. Your body works best on a steady supply of fuel throughout the day. As you can see from the nutrition guidelines outlined for pre-training eating, recovery nutrition, and nutrition strategies designed to optimize muscle building, eating small, frequent meals is ideal and effective.

Have some protein, fiber, and fat with your meals and snacks. These foods will keep you feeling full longer and help prevent the hunger that leads to an unplanned trip to the vending machine. Choose lean proteins and small amounts of healthy fats. Choose fiber-rich versions of all foods such as raw fruits and vegetables and whole grains. Look at your food journal to determine what times of day you get hungry. Add a bit more protein to the preceding meal or snack if hunger sets in quickly at specific times.

MONITORING PROGRESS

One of the more important components of your weight management plan is monitoring progress. Following are some important components of monitoring progress:

Step 1: Have accountability. This may involve accountability to a sports dietitian, yourself, or a program. Often this involves not just checking weight but also checking up on your food intake. You can keep a food journal electronically, in a notebook that you carry with you, or through many of the online programs that are now available.

Step 2: Check weight, but keep it in perspective. Regular weigh-ins are helpful, but how often you need to check weight varies from person to person. Keep in mind that daily weight checks are not useful other than to monitor fluid shifts and levels of body fuel. If you do check your weight daily for any period of time, it might be useful to have an objective and informed person help you check the data and provide a perspective. For example, you might see transient weight gains after hard workouts from shifts in fluid, muscle by-products, and inflammation. Becoming familiar with your own patterns of weight fluctuation helps to soften any emotional impact that weight checks can trigger.

Step 3: Check body composition at appropriate intervals. Body-composition changes take more time to register. Depending on the rate of your weight loss, checks should occur every 4 to 12 weeks, with longer intervals for slower weight loss.

Step 4: Review your food journal to look at current eating patterns, portions, and ongoing problem areas.

Step 5: Plan nonfood rewards. Reward yourself for consistency and progress.

Tune in to hunger and fullness. Paying attention to your body's physiological signals is one of the best ways to gauge when to start eating and when to stop. Of course, you must plan your eating around your training and your schedule for work or school, but becoming aware of hunger and fullness can also provide valuable direction regarding your food intake and portions. You can also use the 20-minute rule: stop eating before you are completely satisfied, then wait 20 minutes to see whether you feel full. Usually, this amount of time allows your body to stop giving you hunger cues.

Reduce your intake of energy-dense liquids. Watch out for liquid calories from fruit juices, alcohol, lattes, and other high-sugar drinks. Chew rather than drink your calories.

Choose low-glycemic carbohydrate foods. This can help improve hunger management, increase feelings of fullness, and help delay or soften hunger between meals. You can also make your meals lower in GI by consuming protein with higher-glycemic carbohydrates.

Do a portion check at meals. Review recommended portions in your meal plan and check portions regularly to make sure that you are staying on track. Watch out for larger or jumbo sizes when eating out. It isn't a bargain if it is more than you require.

Enjoy the meal and have some treats. Food is not only fuel but also a source of enjoyment. This means sitting down and enjoying your meals whenever possible, eating slowly and savoring the food, and making sure that favorites are regularly included in your diet.

Have a plan for various social eating situations. Social eating can be one of the biggest challenges. Try to get familiar with the menu ahead of time and plot your strategy. Control portions and don't be hesitant to leave food on the plate.

ATHLETE PROFILE

Weight Loss: *Angie*

Angie wanted to take her cycling to a higher level. She had enlisted the assistance of a coach and was part of a women's racing team. While she planned to race in time trials and criteriums, some of her upcoming races would require climbing. For performance and health reasons, Angie felt that weight loss was a primary goal.

Angie met with a sports dietitian in order to develop a weight-loss plan early in the season, several months before her first race. The sports dietitian assessed her usual food intake, reviewed her training program, and measured her body composition. It was calculated that Angie needed to lose 15 pounds to reach a body fat of 15 percent, a typical level for a competitive female road cyclist.

Angie often trained early in the morning, followed by a long workday. She typically ordered lunch from a fast-food or area restaurant close to work. She often ordered in dinner as well after the end of a long day.

Angie's energy requirements for various types of workouts were estimated by the sports dietitian. Then Angie was provided with specific meal plans that included a calorie deficit to promote a weight loss and body fat loss of about 1 pound weekly, and which provided adequate carbohydrate and protein for recovery. Angie was given sample menus that outlined the timing of meals and snacks around her training sessions.

Because Angie ate out frequently, it was recommended that she frequent restaurants that provide nutrition information and stick with specific calorie amounts at each meal. It was also recommended that she prepare more meals at home. Simple recipes were provided, including those that could be prepared on the weekend and reheated during the week.

Angie began keeping a daily food journal and tracking her meal plan targets so that she could determine where she was overeating calories or consuming sources of hidden fat. The food journal increased her awareness of her eating habits, encouraging her to plan ahead and to double-check portions.

Angie lost 0.5 to 1 pound weekly and was more than halfway to her goal weight by the time her first race arrived.

ERGOGENIC AIDS
Separating Fact from Fiction

AT A GLANCE
KEY POINTS

Be discerning about supplement use and aware of scientific backing and safety data.

Supplements can be cross-contaminated with illegal or unsafe substances.

Only a limited number of ergogenic aids are backed by sound scientific data.

Smart nutrient strategies can provide a better performance boost than ergogenic aids.

The term ergogenic *literally means "work-producing,"* etymologically speaking, but in modern parlance it refers to the numerous supplements and other substances said to enhance athletic performance. Nutritional ergogenic aids can be nutrients, metabolic by-products of nutrients, or other substances commonly found in foods. When put into supplement form they exist in concentrated amounts. Advertisers of these products claim they can provide performance benefits by increasing muscle size and strength, promoting fat burning, or improving speed. Several ergogenic aids, such as carnitine, are touted as aids to "enhance fat burning," and creatine is reputed to enhance muscle building when taken during a strength training program.

Apparently many consumers have believed the promises behind the ads, as sales of these products have become a serious and lucrative business. All sports nutrition product sales, including sports nutrition supplements, increased 9.5 percent, from $20.8 billion in 2009 to $22.7 billion in 2010. This value includes sales for sports and energy drinks and shots, sports nutrition supplements such as energy bars and gels, weight-loss pills, and weight-loss meal-replacement supplements. Just sports nutrition supplements alone reached sales of $3.2 billion in 2010, according to the *Nutrition Business Journal.* Chapters

4, 5, and 6 outline practical uses for sports nutrition products such as sports drinks, gels, bars, and high-carbohydrate and meal-replacement supplements that are backed by both research and the practical experience of athletes. Using these products knowledgeably and appropriately carries minimal risk and provides some clear performance benefits that support your training and competition goals. However, some sports drinks and recovery drinks may contain ingredients that are not necessary or not even proven to be safe for athletes to consume, especially young and developing athletes.

IS THE SUPPLEMENT LEGAL, EFFECTIVE, SAFE, AND UNCONTAMINATED?

The marketing surrounding ergogenic aids is effective, but it is important for you to verify that any product you ingest in the quest for top performance is legal, effective, safe, and uncontaminated. Unfortunately, many of these products are backed solely by strong and enticing claims, anecdotal hearsay, high-profile athlete and coach testimonials, and referenced "research" that has not been published in full in a reputable scientific journal. In reality, many of these supplements have not been thoroughly and appropriately tested. Moreover, many of the supplements that have been tested independently of the manufacturers who supply them don't live up to their performance claims. Despite this lack of evidence that ergogenic aids can do what their manufacturers claim they can, or even that they are safe to take, it can be tempting to top off all your hard work and optimal training diet with an easily ingested supplement that promises a quick and effective performance boost.

With new products coming out monthly, athletes need to be discerning when evaluating nutritional ergogenic aids or performance enhancers. It is important that you learn to make knowledgeable choices about these products. Keep these tips in mind before you use them:

- Understand how the ergogenic aid purportedly functions.
- Know both sides of the story of current research supporting or opposing the supplement.
- Be aware of any safety concerns surrounding the product.
- Know whether the product is a legal supplement for athletes to take.
- Be aware that a supplement can cause you to test positive through cross-contamination.

Chances are you may try a supplement because it is widely talked about among other athletes you train with or compete against, or because it is surrounded by enticing marketing claims for building muscle, burning fat, or increasing energy output. But these supplements are never going to be an effective substitute for a solid training program and an optimal performance diet.

Another important consideration when evaluating the safety of these supplements is the age of an athlete. The American Academy of Pediatrics does not recommend high-performance supplements in the diet of child athletes. These supplements are also routinely tested on adults (if at all) and not on young and growing bodies or athletes of high-school age. Studies of collegiate athletes are limited, as are long-term safety data. What safety information is available does not usually address safety issues in high-school athletes. Some supplements are also banned by the National Collegiate Athletic Association (NCAA).

REGULATION OF ERGOGENIC AIDS

Athletes are bombarded with claims of the magical effects of nutritional ergogenic aids on performance. Advertising and claims surrounding these products have increased exponentially since the Dietary Supplement Health and Education Act (DSHEA) was passed in 1994. DSHEA significantly changed how all dietary supplements—such as vitamins, minerals, herbs, amino acids, metabolites, and even hormones—are tested, marketed, labeled, and manufactured. Unlike regulation of makers of a drug or food additive, supplement manufacturers are not required to prove that a dietary supplement works. Under DSHEA, manufacturers are merely responsible for making sure that their products are safe.

The government does not review these products before they are put on the market, but the Food and Drug Administration (FDA) can take action against any unsafe dietary supplement products. The FDA cannot evaluate the thousands of products on the market, and it makes selective use of its time and resources. It usually responds only to products that have caused significant adverse health effects on a large scale.

The labels on these products often include a loosely defined "nutrition support claim." These claims may relate to the "structure and function" of the body and "general well-being." Although a certain set of conditions must be met to make these claims, they do not require prior FDA approval. Manufacturers must be able to substantiate that the claim is "truthful and not misleading," but they cannot promise to prevent or cure a disease.

The FDA assumes that the discerning consumer realizes that it is up to each company to decide how to prepare and package its supplements and that these manufacturing practices may affect the products' purity, safety, potency, and overall quality. According to the FDA, consumers can contact the manufacturer and request product safety information and research support, which would preferably not be only in-house data. They can also question whether the firm has a quality-control system in place and whether any adverse event reports have resulted from use of a particular product.

GOOD MANUFACTURING PRACTICES

In 2003, the FDA began developing Good Manufacturing Processes (GMPs) in coordination with the supplement industry. Two websites, www.nsf.org and www.consumerlab.com, currently list products that have been evaluated for appropriate quality control. Both of these sites also test products for banned substances and can certify that products do not contain substances banned for athletes. Some supplement companies have their own GMPs in place and may be regulated under the National Nutritional Foods Association (see www.nnfa.org).

Consumers should also review the "Supplement Facts" labels on the packages of dietary supplements. Unlike serving sizes for conventional foods, the dosage on labels is not standardized—which means it's important to remember that the amounts that are recommended may be higher than needed or safe. The label will provide the following information:

- Statement of identity
- Net quantity of ingredients
- A structure and function claim statement
- Directions for use
- Supplement facts
- Other ingredients, listed in descending order of predominance by common name or proprietary blend
- Name and address of packer, manufacturer, or distributor

Unfortunately, even if companies are accused and fined regarding false claims on dietary supplements, they may not be deterred from promoting new products. Fines often may be rendered insignificant by a large volume of sales generated while claims are being investigated.

EVALUATING ERGOGENIC AIDS: SAFETY, EFFECTIVENESS, AND LEGAL ISSUES

Before taking an ergogenic aid, it is essential to understand how to evaluate its safety and effectiveness objectively and to make sure it is legal in sports training and competition. The first question should be, Is this product effective? Does solid research back up the company's claims? Valid scientific testing of a nutritional ergogenic aid costs time, money, and resources. Tests of a supplement's effect on athletic performance should be conducted with well-trained athletes and can be specific to the type of sport, such as cycling or running. For these and other reasons, much of the supplement industry forgoes testing and relies heavily on testimonials, anecdotes, and untested scientific theories rather than valid research to promote its products. But a theory is not proof. A theory is a hypothesis or intriguing idea that requires testing. What the manufacturer calls a "scientific breakthrough" may be a new and interesting idea with little or no basis in fact.

DOES IT HAVE SCIENTIFIC BACKING?

Conducting a scientific trial remains the best way to examine the effectiveness of ergogenic aids in performance. Testing should mimic real athletic performance conditions as much as possible. Researchers should also control for age, level of training, and nutritional status. Various dosages, supplementation periods, types of exercise, and performance testing may need to be incorporated.

Studies should control for the placebo effect as much as possible by incorporating a double-blind design. In this approach, different groups of subjects receive the substance being tested or a placebo. To minimize bias, the test subjects, and the researchers in direct contact with the subjects, do not know which product is being administered when and to whom. In addition to a placebo trial, there may be a control group who receives no treatment. These are only some of the features needed in a well-designed testing strategy.

But even with a well-designed study, a large change in performance is required for the outcome to be considered statistically significant. In many cases, the changes produced by nutritional supplementation are small. Although a 1 to 3 percent change may not be statistically significant from the scientist's perspective, it may be useful in elite competition. In addition, researchers report only the overall performance effect within a group. The positive results of individuals within the group may be diluted by the negative or neutral responses of other subjects. Not all subjects respond in the same way to a particular substance.

Companies may state that they are in the process of conducting research, or that their research is "in-house" or has simply never been published in reputable peer-reviewed journals. The value of this research is difficult to assess. Unfortunately, even well-designed studies can be quoted out of context. Research findings are extrapolated to produce inappropriate conclusions. And good preliminary studies require verification through additional sound research. Furthermore, consumers may be impressed by an ergogenic aid because the company has patented its product. Yet patents are not granted based on the effectiveness of the product, but rather on its distinguishable differences. Patents can be obtained with a theoretical model rather than objective double-blind research.

Specific nutritional ergogenic aids can benefit athletes under certain conditions. However, the supplement industry is an extremely profitable business that relies on unsupported theories and testimonials to market products. Ergogenic aid theories may even be extrapolated from clinical research on disease states or nutrient deficiencies. To say that a product will then produce a performance improvement is not a scientific breakthrough but a leap of faith. Even with proven ergogenic aids, it is important to keep their role in perspective. Although they may produce small performance improvements, ergogenic aids are no substitute for proper training, nutrition, and psychological preparation.

Unfortunately, the amount and quality of the research behind a product are not apparent to the average consumer. Often this information needs to be obtained from an informed sports dietitian and other sports-related health professionals to help the athlete make an informed decision about a supplement.

IS IT SAFE?

The next question to consider in determining whether you should use an ergogenic aid is, "Is this product safe?" As previously mentioned, supplement manufacturers are not required to prove a product's safety. Negative effects from a product may be acute, mild, or temporary, but they can also be serious and chronic. Some dietary supplements may be toxic or decrease the absorption of other nutrients, especially in high doses. Surprisingly, independent testing has found that many supplements do not even contain the ingredients marked on the label. Products are often watered down or contain unlisted ingredients that may be harmful or illegal. It is hoped that this concern will be resolved when all companies comply with adopted GMPs. You can also check ConsumerLab.com, an independent tester of health and nutrition products, including "sports and energy products." It publishes results of its tests for identity, strength, and purity. For example, creatine products were tested and the results reported in 2010. The message is, buyer beware.

IS IT LEGAL? DOES IT CONTAIN UNWANTED AND BANNED INGREDIENTS?

As a competitive athlete, particularly if you may be drug-tested both in and out of competition, you do not want to inadvertently take a dietary supplement that contains a banned substance. Therefore, the third question to ask is, Is this product legal for my sport? The past decade has seen a significant increase in the number of positive test results for illegal substances at the elite and professional levels that are claimed to be due to contaminated or mislabeled dietary supplements. All athletic governing bodies have some regulation regarding the use of ergogenic aids. (Products banned by the NCAA, for example, are listed at www.ncaa.org.) Even if you avoid illegal products such as ephedra or androstenodione, checking labels does not guarantee 100 percent that you will avoid banned products. Cross-contamination can occur in the manufacturing process, and the purity of these supplements is often questioned. In fact, some professional teams have resorted to batch-testing any supplement that their athletes utilize to prevent an inadvertent doping positive due to cross-contamination. The World Anti-Doping Agency provides a complete list of banned substances at www.wada-ama.org/en/.

COMMON ERGOGENIC AIDS

This section will review some popular nutritional ergogenic aids for scientific validity as determined by quality research. It will also look at some of the safety concerns and practical issues regarding the use of these supplements. Not surprisingly, sports physiologists and sports nutritionists do not overwhelmingly support the majority of these supplements. They would prefer that athletes train and eat properly, two strategies that very effectively improve performance! Many professionals are especially concerned about young athletes taking supplements that have not been proven safe for them, as supplement testing is usually done on adults.

Ergogenic aids marketed to endurance athletes are often designed to increase muscle mass and strength and decrease body fat. Some are also reported to improve performance by increasing power output during exercise. Table 7.1 summarizes several ergogenic aids that are discussed in more detail here.

ERGOGENIC AIDS THAT AFFECT BODY COMPOSITION

Creatine

Creatine is one of the best-researched ergogenic aids on the market, making it possible for sports nutritionists to provide clear and confident recommendations regarding this sports nutrition supplement.

What Does It Do? Creatine is often advertised as a steroid alternative, but its use is really more comparable to glycogen loading. Just as carbohydrate ingestion maximizes the glycogen content of the muscle, "creatine loading" can increase muscle creatine stores. Your normal intake of creatine is about 2 grams daily (perhaps less for vegetarians), and it is also synthesized in the liver and kidneys. Creatine is an essential fuel of the adenosine triphosphate–creatine phosphate (ATP-CP) system. Loading the muscle with creatine is designed to increase ATP resynthesis. This power system typically stores enough fuel to last 6 to 8 seconds. Creatine can also buffer lactic acid and transport ATP to be utilized for muscle contraction.

What Is the Evidence? Muscle biopsies have confirmed that rapid loading can be achieved with 25 to 30 grams of creatine daily, taken in five or six 5-gram doses per day for 5 or 6 days. A more gentle loading protocol is 3 grams daily over 28 days. Unlike carbohydrates, creatine appears to remain trapped in the muscle for 4 to 5 weeks after a loading phase without ongoing supplementation. About 30 percent of individuals who creatine-load appear to be "non-responders"—that is, they do not adequately load creatine into the muscle. To counter this problem, experts recommend consuming creatine with carbohydrates. Ingesting 75 to 100 grams of carbohydrates along with the creatine has been demonstrated to enhance creatine accumulation in the muscle. In addition, a 2- to 5-pound (1–2 kg)

TABLE 7.1   SUMMARY OF ERGOGENIC AIDS

SUPPLEMENT	CLAIMS	SCIENTIFIC DATA	SAFETY
Amino acids	Facilitate muscle building and exercise recovery	Not supported by well-designed research	Can upset balance of amino acid metabolism when taken in large doses
Beta-alanine	Increases carnosine content of the muscle which acts as a buffer and antioxidant	Sound theory with data emerging	May cause skin tingling with no damage, only discomfort; more long-term data needed
Bicarbonate	Buffers acid build-up in cells due to high-intensity training	Studies show modest effect in exercise performance for short, high-intensity exercise	Safe in recommended doses when taken with water; possible gastrointestinal side effects
Caffeine	Promotes endurance; may improve power output for shorter distances	Good data support claims for endurance exercise Limited data on power sports indicate need for more research	Can be used safely in moderate doses High doses not required for ergogenic effect
Carnitine	Metabolic fat burner	Not supported by well-designed research	L-carnitine form only may be consumed in doses of 1–2 g daily for 6 months
Chromium	Builds muscle and burns fat	Not supported by well-designed research	Should not exceed 200 mcg daily
Creatine	Supports training for increased muscle mass	Well supported by scientific data	Can be used by adults when following scientific protocols
Glutamine	Supports the immune system Promotes protein synthesis	May benefit athletes with a true glutamine deficiency; more data required	Often incorporated in sports nutrition supplements Too much could upset amino acid balance
HMB	Builds muscle strength Inhibits breakdown of muscle and protein	Limited human data supporting claims; several studies found no benefits	Doses at 3 g taken for 6–8 weeks appear safe
MCT oil	Provides fuel during training and spares muscle glycogen; Enhances fat burning	Tested mainly for endurance exercise; not supported by well-designed research	May cause mild gastrointestinal symptoms
Prohormones	Promote muscle building	Increase muscle mass and strength	Banned by USADA and IOC; long-term safety concerns and possible adverse health effects
Protein supplements	Facilitate muscle building	When consumed before and after resistance training in the proper dose and with the proper timing, can facilitate building of muscle tissue	Can consume 15–20 g high-quality protein in conjunction with carbohydrates before and after weight training Can consume protein from real foods; supplements not required Exceeding recommded dose provides no additional benefits
Pyruvate	Improves endurance; promotes muscle building and fat loss	Not tested on athletes; not supported by research	Not much safety data
Quercetin	Antioxidant, anti-inflammatory, increased oxygen capacity	Trivial to small effect on human endurance capacity; limited data showing reduced stress	Safe in 1,000 mg doses for up to 12 weeks
Ribose	Improves muscle recovery, energy, and endurance Rebuilds ATP	Published research is limited; current data far from conclusive	Not enough safety data
Weight-loss supplements	Promote body fat loss and weight loss	Many ingredients not supported by well-designed research; risks may outweigh benefits	Risks of supplements may be serious; some ingredients may be banned

weight gain is associated with creatine loading. Scientists believe this to be water gain, however, as urine output decreases during the loading phase.

We know that creatine ingestion can load the muscle, but how does it affect performance? Creatine loading appears to increase the rate of creatine resynthesis during recovery (20 seconds–5 minutes) from bouts of high-intensity exercise (6–30 seconds). Creatine loading delays fatigue during activity that includes repeated, all-out surges of energy interspersed with rest periods.

After completion of one loading phase of creatine, you can maintain these higher creatine levels with a low daily dose of 3 grams for at least 60 days. Creatine loading may only be necessary once or twice yearly due to the cyclical nature of your training and the muscles' ability to hold creatine for several weeks.

Do I Need It? Creatine could potentially assist team sport players such as hockey players or soccer players, but it is unlikely to provide any performance benefit for most endurance training sessions and competitions. Of course, many endurance athletes incorporate resistance training into their programs, and creatine loading does appear to allow more repetitions to be performed and consequently to increase one's strength.

Are There Side Effects? Though it is not documented in the scientific literature, anecdotal reports abound that creatine loading is associated with muscle cramping and GI upset. If you decide to load with creatine, make sure that you consume plenty of water to help prevent any side effects. Taking more than 30 grams of creatine daily over a 5-day period offers no additional benefits for loading. As is often the case with nutritional supplements, more is not better. In fact, there are some concerns that taking creatine in high doses or taking it over a long period of time can lead to liver and kidney damage. People with kidney disease should not take creatine.

Creatine is currently legal. However, there have been concerns about cross-contamination of creatine products in past years, as athletes ingesting this supplement have tested positive for banned prohormone products. No creatine studies have been done with high-school athletes or athletes who are still growing and developing. Many high schools and colleges likely have their own policy regarding creatine supplementation in their athletes. The NCAA does not allow use of creatine (see the sidebar "The NCAA and Nutritional Supplements").

Beta-Hydroxy-Beta-Methylbutarate (HMB)

What Does It Do? Beta-hydroxy-beta-methylbutarate, or HMB, is primarily marketed to strength and power athletes and is one of the fastest-selling supplements on the market. Endurance athletes who weight-train and want to facilitate muscle recovery may be interested in this supplement because it is promoted to decrease protein breakdown, and in doing so to enhance muscle size and development, decrease exercise-induced muscle damage, and promote fat loss. HMB is not actually a nutrient but a metabolic by-product made naturally by the human body in small amounts when the amino acid leucine is metabolized. You produce only about 0.2 to 0.4 gram of HMB daily. The form used in supplements was first developed by scientists and then patented in the early 1990s by the company that produces HMB, which has sponsored much of the research on its effects.

What Is the Evidence? Initial HMB research was conducted mainly with animals, but its effects on humans have also been studied. Some researchers found greater muscle mass gains and fewer markers of muscle damage in subjects taking the supplement; however, these studies have not always controlled for diet and training load, both of which can have a significant impact on muscle gain in conjunction with weight training. Several studies found no ergogenic benefit from HMB supplementation in regard to muscle mass and both anaerobic and aerobic exercise performance.

Although a study of HMB use in runners did find that the supplement helped to prevent exercise-induced muscle damage, other studies have not produced similar findings. A recent review of existing studies of HMB supplementation suggested that this supplement may provide a small improvement in muscle size and strength when combined with resistance training. Further research is needed, however, particularly on trained athletes.

Further published data on this supplement are needed. A daily dose of 3 grams divided into three 1-gram doses appears to be safe when taken for a 6- to 8-week period. Higher doses have not resulted in greater effectiveness.

Do I Need It? Likely you can accomplish more with the nutritional guidelines outlined in Chapter 6 for muscle building than with HMB supplementation. If there is any benefit, it is more likely to be in the early phases of a new resistance training program. However, once an athlete adapts to a higher workload of resistance training, HMB would not be expected to provide any additional benefit.

Are There Side Effects? HMB supplementation at the recommended dosage appears to be associated with minimal side effects. Long-term data are lacking.

Amino Acids

What Do They Do? The marketing of amino acid supplements is heavily targeted to athletes who benefit from building muscle mass. Supporters of amino acid supplementation claim that the protein used in these products is more readily digested and absorbed than the protein found in foods. This statement simply is false. Your body is well equipped to handle protein from whole foods by secreting a number of enzymes that help you to absorb amino acids. This absorption process occurs at a high level of effectiveness.

What Is the Evidence? The amino acids arginine, lysine, and ornithine are often sold individually or in combination as "legal anabolic compounds" and "recovery agents." Advertisements claim that these products can promote the release of growth hormone and thus increase lean body mass and decrease body fat. These claims surfaced after two studies found that infusing these amino acids directly into the bloodstream stimulated the release of human growth hormone, which is involved in building muscle tissue. The effects of oral supplementation of amino acids on human growth hormone are questionable, however. Several well-controlled studies have verified that oral supplementation does not have the same effect as intravenous infusion. Other studies have been criticized for their design. One study that provided a large oral dose of arginine and ornithine found a slight increase in growth hormone release. However, this increase was most likely stimulated by the resistance training itself rather than the amino acid intake. High oral dosages of these supplements are also associated with gastrointestinal problems.

Arginine, lysine, and ornithine are available individually or in mixtures in powder or tablet form. Several research studies have used 2- to 3-gram dosages; a dosage of 6 grams may cause gastrointestinal distress. High doses of certain amino acids may also inhibit absorption of other amino acids. Moreover, the dosages used in several studies can easily be obtained by consuming high-protein foods. The use of any amino acid supplement, either alone or in combination with others, is unlikely to be beneficial and is not recommended.

Do I Need Them? As explained in Chapter 6, timing your consumption of a high-quality protein source before and after weight training is the most effective strategy to facilitate muscle building and recovery. High-quality protein supplements that provide the branched chain amino acids and foods high in these amino acids can be used appropriately. Full muscle recovery also entails following specific nutritional guidelines to obtain enough calories and protein in your daily training diet. Protein metabolism is very complex. It is affected by a variety of factors, including amino acid concentration in the blood, competition with other available amino acids, and the presence of other nutrients.

Are There Side Effects? Amino acid mixtures could potentially lead to nutritional imbalances, as an excess of one amino acid may negatively affect the absorption of another. Amino acid supplement dosing may also be misleading. A bottle listing up to 500 milligrams in a capsule actually contains less than 1 gram of amino acids, whereas only 1 ounce of chicken contains 7,000 milligrams, or 7 grams, of amino acids in the form of whole protein. Clearly, amino acid supplements cannot meet the dosing found in a compact source of natural protein such as chicken or a manufactured supplement such as whey protein. Using expensive amino acid supplements simply is not necessary and could actually be harmful.

Glutamine

What Does It Do? Glutamine is an amino acid synthesized in the muscle tissue. It is the most abundant amino acid in the body and is used as a fuel source by the cells of the immune system. Impaired glutamine status has been associated with the overtrained state in athletes, and overtrained athletes are thought to be more susceptible to upper respiratory tract infections as well as other kinds of infections. Blood glutamine levels fall during endurance exercise and remain lowered during the recovery phase for several hours after exercise. Glutamine depletion is thought to become cumulative if recovery between sessions is inadequate, and overtrained athletes do sometimes have low blood glutamine levels. However, adequate daily carbohydrate consumption may be the most effective means of preventing glutamine depletion.

Does It Work? The theory behind glutamine supplementation is that it could help prevent the immune system problems suffered by overtrained athletes. Research data do not consistently support this theory. What is more likely is that glutamine supplementation benefits those athletes with a true deficiency and that it is not a general cure for immune system problems.

Another theory regarding glutamine supplementation is that it promotes protein synthesis and helps maintain a positive protein balance in the muscle by preventing protein breakdown during periods of heavy training. Limited data have not shown glutamine to improve muscle gains in comparison with a placebo.

Glutamine may also stimulate the synthesis of muscle glycogen. Obviously, glutamine performs some very important functions in the body. However, more research on glutamine supplementation in athletes is needed.

Do I Need It? There is no conclusive evidence that glutamine supplementation lowers the incidence of illness when an athlete's diet contains adequate protein, or that it decreases protein breakdown following resistance training.

Is It Safe? A dose of less than 0.1 gram of glutamine per pound (0.3 g/kg) of body weight is safely absorbed and does not appear to cause any harm when taken for several weeks. Higher doses for up to 5 days also seem safe.

Chromium

What Does It Do? Chromium is a trace mineral that is often marketed as a legal alternative to anabolic steroids and human growth hormone. Scientists have long known that chromium enhances the effects of insulin, which regulates glucose metabolism. Adults with impaired glucose regulation have been measured to have positive responses with chromium supplementation. Insulin also promotes the uptake of amino acids into muscle cells and regulates protein metabolism. Because of this protein-building function, some researchers have theorized that chromium intake should lead to an increase in muscle mass.

Proponents of chromium supplementation for athletes maintain that many athletes are chromium-deficient and that a supplement would improve their protein synthesis. Other proponents believe that high chromium doses could stimulate muscle building. It has not been firmly established that athletes are in fact chromium-deficient; however, the North American diet is high in refined grains, which may trigger a higher release of insulin and require more chromium in the diet than is normally consumed.

What Is the Evidence? Studies of chromium supplementation have produced mixed, but mostly negative, results. The more recent and better-designed studies monitored and controlled for exercise training and carefully measured body composition. These studies found no significant gains in muscle mass with chromium supplementation. Earlier studies, which showed some positive results, were not as carefully controlled. Several studies have shown that even higher doses do not lead to significant gains in muscle mass.

Do I Need It? There is inadequate evidence to support the use of chromium for muscle building.

Is It Safe? More information is needed about the safety of chromium supplementation, especially at dosages beyond 200 micrograms. Because chromium is a mineral, large chronic doses are unwise. Minerals often compete with one another for absorption, and one study found that iron status was compromised with chromium supplementation.

Clearly, adequate chromium intake from whole foods is important. Especially good sources are whole-grain breads and cereals, mushrooms, asparagus, apples, raisins, cocoa, peanuts, peanut butter, and prunes. Various sports nutrition supplements such as recovery drinks and bars often include chromium as well, as do many regular multivitamin and mineral supplements. Try not to exceed 200 micrograms daily from supplemental sources. Most diets likely do not exceed 50 micrograms of chromium daily.

Overall, chromium's ability to build muscle mass in athletes appears highly doubtful. Supplementation in safe doses is only appropriate to correct a deficiency and compensate for an inadequate diet.

Prohormones

Prohormones are widely sold in dietary supplements and are currently banned by the World Anti-Doping Agency (WADA), an international independent organization created in 1999. WADA developed and implements the World Anti-Doping Code, which harmonizes anti-doping policies in all sports and countries (www.wada-ama.org). The U.S. Anti-Doping Agency (USADA) was created in 2000 and is the independent anti-doping agency for Olympic-related sports in the United States (www.usantidoping.org). Like WADA, USADA bans prohormones.

What Do They Do? These products include the "andro" and the "nor" prohormones. Andro products, namely androstenedione, are testosterone precursors that transform into this hormone in the body and are promoted as muscle builders. Other androgenic products are androstenediol and dehydroepiandrosterone (DHEA). Nor products are precursors to the steroid nortestosterone (nandrolone), which is similar in structure to testosterone. Available nor prohormones are 19-norandrostenediol and 19-norandrostenedione. These nor products break down into the same metabolites used to detect nandrolone usage. Andro prohormones may lead to an elevated testosterone-to-epitestosterone ratio.

What Is the Evidence? Despite all the sales and the hype, scientists continue to debate if these substances that lead to testosterone production are even effective at building muscle mass and strength. Studies have demonstrated that use of prohormones does not increase serum testosterone levels or produce any significant changes in lean body mass, muscle strength, or performance when compared with a placebo.

Do I Need Them? Prohormones are on the banned list and pose a high risk to legal supplement contamination.

Are There Side Effects? Prohormones are easily purchased in the United States and over the Internet because they are classified as dietary supplements. Often these supplements are geared toward building muscle, enhancing recovery, and "maintaining hormone levels." Since the late 1990s, a rash of elite athletes have tested positive for the steroid nandrolone. Many of these athletes have claimed that it occurred through the inadvertent ingestion of the dietary supplements that contain nor hormones. Although athletes can read labels carefully to avoid these banned products, it is becoming clear that this may not be enough. A study conducted at the Olympic Laboratory at the University of California at Los Angeles checked urine tests after supplementation with androstenedione and 19-norandrostenedione. As expected, the 19-nor produced nandrolone metabolites exceeding IOC limits. But the results of the andro supplementation were especially of concern. This test actually produced nandrolone metabolites in the urine! Twenty of twenty-four positive urine samples exceeded doping limits. Based on these findings, researchers tested several andro supplements. Seven of eight tested capsules contained varying amounts of 19-nor. Researchers speculated that the supplements had been contaminated with 19-nor in the manufacturing process. Many supplement companies use the same equipment to blend, encapsulate, and bottle both prohormone and nonprohormone products.

Some of these prohormones may carry unwanted side effects. One study that supplemented with andro did not find higher testosterone levels or increased muscle strength but a rise in blood estrogen and a reduction in the good HDL cholesterol in male subjects. These side effects could result in potentially serious health effects. A second study tested andro combined with an herbal product designed to decrease estrogen production. The estrogenic profile was not reduced from the herbal supplements despite claims to the contrary by the manufacturer.

No athlete engaging in competition should take prohormones, because they are illegal. Read labels carefully to ensure that they are not contained in any of the products you purchase, and be aware that cross-contamination is a real concern. Banned substances may turn up in supplements even if they are not listed as ingredients.

Weight-Loss Supplements

What Do They Do? Weight-loss supplements are typically marketed via strong claims purporting that they can speed up metabolism, burn fat, and decrease appetite. Although the ingredients found in some weight-loss supplements are legal (and ineffective), other weight-loss supplements contain banned substances and may be dangerous to use.

What Is the Evidence? Weight-loss supplement ingredients can include bitter orange, chitosan, ephedrine or related stimulants, hydrocitric acid, hoodia, pyruvate, and chromium. The amount of evidence for each weight-loss ingredient varies, and for many the evidence is not very strong.

Do I Need Them? It is recommended that you avoid these supplements due to limited scientific support and safety concerns.

What Are the Side Effects? Until 2004, the most widely purchased weight-loss supplement was ephedra. Because it had a high incidence of reported side effects, the FDA banned it, and it is not currently available in the United States. Ephedra, also called ephedrine or Ma Huang, stimulates the central nervous system and improves appetite control. However, because it is a stimulant, reported side effects include nervousness, headache, heart palpitations, dizziness, insomnia, and anxiety. Ephedra was banned in sports before it was banned by the FDA, and its use is easily detected in drug tests.

Another weight-loss supplement on the WADA monitoring list, which has products not on the prohibited list for patterns of misuse, is phenylpropanolamine (PPA), also known as norephedrine. This product claims to suppress appetite and stimulate metabolism. However, it can also increase the risk of a bleeding stroke, and its safety risks far outweigh its effectiveness. The FDA warned consumers to stop use of a product containing PPA, caffeine, an herb called yohimbine, and diiodothyronine, a form of thyroid hormone. The FDA received multiple reports of liver injury or liver failure with use of the product over a 2-week to 3-month period.

Many weight-loss supplements are currently marketed as being "ephedra-free." However, these supplements may also contain banned products that are sources of synephrine or pseudoephedrine, including citrus aurantium, or bitter orange. Synephrine is banned by the NCAA and is on the WADA monitoring list, and pseudoephedrine is banned by WADA. Many other ingredients in weight-loss supplements lack solid research backing. Other weight-loss supplement ingredients to avoid are caffeine, cola nut, ginseng, and willow bark. Many of these supplements contain high amounts of caffeine, and they are often strong stimulants. Like ephedra, they can produce potentially dangerous side effects.

ERGOGENIC AIDS THAT AFFECT EXERCISE PERFORMANCE

Carnitine

What Does It Do? Often promoted as a "metabolic fat burner," carnitine is a non-essential nutrient formed in the liver from two amino acids. Your skeletal muscles contain at least 90 percent of the carnitine in your body. Carnitine is of interest to athletes because it carries fat into the cells to be burned for energy during exercise. If carnitine supplementation did increase fat burning and decrease your body's reliance on glycogen and blood glucose, it could enhance performance. Carnitine is found in large quantities in meat and dairy products, however, so a carnitine deficiency is unlikely.

What Is the Evidence? Carnitine is unlikely to be an effective ergogenic aid, as carnitine supplementation does not appear to increase muscle carnitine levels (as measured by muscle biopsies). Glycogen sparing with carnitine supplementation was also not found in the studies conducted on its use. Only one study found a slight increase in muscle carnitine content after supplementation with 2 grams daily. Other studies found no improvements in exercise performance with carnitine supplementation. Two studies that did find a positive performance effect have been criticized for their methodology and design.

Do I Need It? Few studies conducted on carnitine have included athlete subjects, and the effect on body fat has not been widely studied in athletic populations. For these reasons and the very limited evidence in any population, carnitine is not recommended.

Are There Side Effects? Carnitine supplementation appears to be safe if you consume the L-carnitine form of the nutrient only. DL-carnitine can be toxic, as it depletes L-carnitine and may lead to a deficiency. Two to 4 grams daily can be consumed for 1 month, though 1- to 2-gram doses have been taken for 6 months.

Pyruvate

What Does It Do? Pyruvate is commonly sold as DHAP, which is a combination of pyruvate and dihydroxyacetone. Manufacturers claim that it can improve endurance exercise, promote fat loss, and increase muscle mass.

What Is the Evidence? Studies that have tested pyruvate on endurance performance need
to be put in perspective. These studies, using a small number of untrained subjects exercising at moderate intensity, may not have much relevance to endurance athletes. In addition, several of the study protocols used 25 grams of pyruvate combined with 75 grams of
dihydroxyacetone. Many commercial preparations contain much smaller doses. However,
these studies did measure an increase in endurance with the supplement.

Pyruvate does not appear to have much validity as a fat burner. One often-quoted
study restricted participants to a 1,000-calorie diet daily and no activity—a result not
applicable to an athlete participating in endurance sports.

Several more recent studies have evaluated aerobic exercise performance, mainly in
cycling, with pyruvate supplementation. No positive effects were found.

Do I Need It? There is not adequate scientific support to recommend pyruvates as a fat
burner for athletes.

Are There Side Effects? Large doses over 5 grams may cause abdominal discomfort and
bloating.

Caffeine

What Does It Do? One of the oldest known drugs, caffeine belongs to a group of compounds called methyl-xanthines. Caffeine is found naturally in coffee beans, tea leaves,
cocoa beans, and cola nuts, and caffeine-containing foods are a normal part of the North
American diet, from coffee, tea, and chocolate to soft drinks. Many of these products
provide 30 to 100 milligrams per serving.

But does it enhance performance for endurance athletes? Although it appears that
caffeine does provide some muscle glycogen–sparing effects, this appears to be limited
to the first 15 to 20 minutes of exercise. Researchers are not certain exactly how caffeine
produces this effect. The classic explanation is that caffeine elevates free fatty acids in the
blood, which exercising muscles use for energy while conserving muscle glycogen. Caffeine may also impact the enzyme that breaks down glycogen. Besides sparing glycogen,

caffeine stimulates the central nervous system (increasing alertness), stimulates blood circulation and heart function, and releases epinephrine, all of which could enhance a variety of performance-related functions. Caffeine also stimulates calcium release from the muscle, which stimulates muscular contraction, and could have other direct performance effects on the muscles.

What Is the Evidence? Recent evidence has added to our perspective on caffeine. While the mechanisms by which caffeine are still unclear, it likely changes the athlete's perception of fatigue through effects on the brain.

Caffeine can enhance performance over a wide range of exercise protocols. These include not only endurance events lasting 90 minutes or longer and ultraendurance events lasting over 4 hours but also high-intensity exercise lasting 1 to 5 minutes and prolonged high-intensity exercise lasting 20 to 60 minutes. Many recent, well-designed studies of elite athletes have found that caffeine can effectively enhance performance when consumed in relatively low amounts. Doses as low as 1.5 to 2 milligrams per pound (3–5 mg/kg) of weight are effective. The optimal dose appears to be 2.25 to 2.7 milligrams per pound (5–6 mg/kg). Consuming higher amounts provides no additional performance benefits and may result in rapid heart rate, nervousness, and gastrointestinal discomfort. Most studies have had subjects ingest caffeine 1 hour prior to exercise.

There is also evidence that small doses of caffeine—0.5 to 1.4 milligrams per pound (1–3 mg/kg)—can aid performance if taken before competition, at various times during competition, or toward the end of an exercise session or race when an endurance athlete can become fatigued.

Are There Side Effects? Not all athletes react to caffeine in the same way. Some individuals may have a performance response to caffeine while others may not. Caffeine's diuretic effect has long been debated, but it appears that it is essentially insignificant. Studies indicate that caffeine does not increase urine output during exercise. Athletes who wish to use caffeine as an ergogenic aid in competition should experiment while training to determine their personal tolerance to caffeine during exercise and their own performance response. At higher levels caffeine has the potential to increase heart rate, affect fine motor control and technique, or interfere with sleep. It is best to work with the lowest effective dose possible to achieve a performance enhancement.

On January 1, 2004, caffeine was removed from the WADA prohibited-drug list and was placed on the monitoring list. Previously caffeine intake was not to exceed a threshold dose checked with a urine test.

Medium Chain Triglycerides

What Are They? Medium chain triglycerides, or MCT oils, have been promoted to athletes for several years. Because of their shorter molecular chain size (compared with long chain triglycerides), MCTs empty from the stomach more quickly and are more easily absorbed into the bloodstream. In fact, they are absorbed as quickly as glucose and transported to the liver, where they are metabolized and rapidly burned for energy. Their ergogenic benefit supposedly results from their ability to provide quick fuel during exercise and spare muscle glycogen during extended training.

What Is the Evidence? Of the several studies conducted with MCT oil, one found a performance improvement while the others did not. One study determined that the amount of MCT oil that can be tolerated within the gastrointestinal tract might be limited. GI symptoms ranging from mild to severe can result. Consuming carbohydrates prior to exercise (as recommended in this book) could also negate the effects of MCT supplementation. MCT oil is promoted as a metabolism enhancer and fat burner. However, these claims are not supported by research.

Do I Need Them? Overall, this supplement is not recommended to athletes as there is inadequate evidence that use of MCTs before and during exercise spares muscle glycogen.

Are There Side Effects? At intakes of greater than 30 grams daily, there is a high risk of gastrointestinal symptoms that can be severe enough to impair performance.

Glycerol

What Is It? Glycerol is a colorless liquid alcohol found naturally in fats and is produced from the breakdown of fat. It is available as a glycerine solution or as part of hyperhydration supplements for athletes. Its use is thought to facilitate hyperhydration before training and competition because it holds and attracts water like a sponge. If taken properly and with the correct amount of fluid, glycerol can hold about 36 ounces of fluid in the body. It may be useful for offsetting sweat loss in environments where the possibility of dehydration is extreme.

What Is the Evidence? Study results are still mixed on glycerol hyperhydration. Several studies have suggested that hyperhydration derived from glycerol ingestion can help an athlete maintain a low heart rate and body core temperature during exercise in the heat. Other studies, however, found that it exerted no beneficial physiological effect during endurance exercise.

Do I Need It? Glycerol hyperhydration supplements have been targeted to endurance athletes because of their fluid needs in long-distance events. It may be appropriate for situations in which dehydration and excessive heat conditions are likely to occur. It may also be useful for rehydration in situations where quick recovery from fluid losses is required.

Are There Side Effects? When diluted and mixed properly, glycerol appears to be relatively safe to use. Dosages used in research have been limited to about 0.45 to 0.7 gram per pound (1–1.5 g/kg) of body weight, with each gram of solution diluted with 0.75 to 1 ounce (25–35 ml) of water. Glycerol solutions should be consumed 1 to 2.5 hours before exercise, but athletes experimenting with glycerol must be very careful. Some physiologists recommend that it only be used under medical supervision. Some athletes taking glycerol have reported headache, bloating, nausea, vomiting, or dizziness. Pregnant women or individuals with high blood pressure, diabetes, or kidney disease should not use glycerol because of its potential negative side effects.

Do not exceed the recommended amounts of glycerol, and experiment first with this product in training before attempting to use it in competition. You will experience some weight gain with glycerol use, and you will still need to consume adequate amounts of fluid while competing.

Ribose

What Does It Do? Ribose is hyped as a supplement that can improve muscle recovery, boost energy, enhance endurance, support cardiovascular fitness, and rebuild ATP. A sugar formed from the conversion of glucose, it is considered the starting substance for ATP production and is part of the metabolic pathway that results in ATP resynthesis. It has been suggested that ribose supplementation could enhance recovery of the muscle ATP content.

What Is the Evidence? Published research on the effect of ribose on athletic performance is limited. Ribose did benefit one group of men who suffered from cardiac ischemia,

THE NCAA AND NUTRITIONAL SUPPLEMENTS

Collegiate athletes competing in the sports of swimming, cycling, cross-country track, and triathlon need to be aware of the National Collegiate Athletic Association's (NCAA) policy on supplements. The NCAA's current policy regarding sports nutrition supplements states that it is not permissible for an institution to provide any substance to student athletes unless it is a non-muscle-building product and is included in one of the four classes of permissible supplements. Permissible supplements include vitamins and minerals, energy bars, calorie-replacement drinks, and electrolyte-replacement drinks. A listing of nonpermissible supplements includes amino acids, chrysin, chondroitin, creatine and creatine-containing compounds, ginseng, glucosamine, glycerol, HMB, L-carnitine, melatonin, Pos-2, protein powders, and tribulus. However, a supplement that contains protein is permissible if it does not obtain more than 30 percent of its calories from protein and falls under one of the four permissible categories.

The NCAA is concerned about the lack of quality control in the production and manufacture of nutritional supplements. Supplements geared toward muscle building have been found to be contaminated with substances currently on the NCAA banned drug list. In one study funded by the International Olympic Committee, approximately 15 percent of 600 over-the-counter supplements were found to contain nonlabeled ingredients that could result in a positive doping test. The NCAA promotes the superiority of a well-balanced diet over nutritional supplements and is concerned about the long-term safety of some of these products.

Currently, student athletes wishing to take muscle-building supplements must obtain them on their own. Athletes should seek out sound nutrition advice from qualified sports nutritionists and information on the scientific data behind these products, rather than depending on advertising claims and professional athlete endorsements. It is not worth risking eligibility to take products that may offer no real benefit. It is much safer—and more effective—to follow healthy nutritional strategies. Be sure to consume adequate calories and protein, eat a variety of nutritious foods, and strive for optimal nutrient timing to reach your performance goals.

The NCAA encourages students to refer to the Resource Exchange Center (REC), which is sponsored by the National Center for Drug Free Sport, at www.drugfreesport .com/rec, for more information.

but study results on these subjects are not applicable to athletes. Three other published studies measured its effects on repeated high-intensity exercise in trained male athletes. Ribose supplementation did not affect power output. Another study that combined the ribose supplements with creatine and glutamine found no improvement in muscular strength and endurance or in body composition. Many studies looking at the ergogenic effects of ribose have been presented at conferences, but not published in full for further evaluation.

Do I Need It? Adequate data do not exist to support use of this expensive supplement for sprint training.

Are There Side Effects? Ribose has not been used for long periods of time, though daily doses of up to 20 grams appear to be tolerated. Higher doses may result in gastrointestinal side effects. Manufacturer labels often recommend taking 3 grams prior to and 3 grams after exercise. The patent holder recommends that ribose be consumed with carbohydrates on an empty stomach. Current data are too limited to safely recommend a cycling or maintenance dose.

Sodium Bicarbonate

How Does It Work? Sodium bicarbonate, commonly known as baking soda, is an alkaline salt thought to buffer the acid buildup in the muscle cells caused by training that stresses the anaerobic glycolysis (or lactic acid) energy system. During exercise that stresses the lactic acid system, acid accumulation inhibits muscle contraction and is associated with fatigue. The majority of both laboratory and field studies show that bicarbonate supplementation, or "soda loading," improves performance in high-intensity tasks, both continuous and intermittent, that last from 1 to 7 minutes. This effect appears to be moderate. Only two studies, however, have found that bicarbonate enhances endurance exercise lasting 1 hour. Overall, this supplement should not be of great benefit to an endurance athlete because its effect is more applicable to short, high-intensity tasks.

What Is the Evidence? A review of 29 studies of bicarbonate loading and exercise performance concluded that it has a modest positive effect upon performance. Benefits are seen in prolonged, intermittent sprint protocols, and prolonged high-intensity events, and perhaps for interval-based training sessions.

Do I Need It? The best scientifically supported use of bicarbonate loading is for events of 1 to 7 minutes at high intensity, and some evidence for use during prolonged, intermittent sprint protocols, so the benefit to endurance athletes is likely to be limited in training. It is not recommended for use in competition.

Are There Side Effects? Sodium bicarbonate appears to be safe when taken in the recommended dose of 140 milligrams per pound (0.3 g/kg) of body weight. For a 150-pound

ERGOGENIC AID CHECKLIST: EVALUATING DIETARY SUPPLEMENTS

Before taking any supplement or ergogenic aid, make sure that you understand what is behind the claims. Can you derive the same benefit by adjusting your food intake? Try to find out if there are any negative effects. Consider the costs of taking a supplement that may have limited scientific backing.

Following is a list of important considerations regarding dietary supplements and ergogenic aids:

1. What are the claims around the supplement? If it sounds too good to be true, then it probably is.
2. How does the product work? Verify that the supplement benefits some aspect of your endurance training program. If you take a supplement, how long will you take it for? How will you know that the supplement is providing a benefit?
3. What is the scientific evidence? Is the product backed by scientific claims published in peer-reviewed scientific journals? Often, unpublished in-house research is cited in marketing materials and advertisements. "Clinical Trials" could have been completed at the manufacturer's own lab with no objective evaluation of the data such as "placebo-controlled" or a "double-blind" design.
   - Beware of testimonials that manufacturers often use to entice you to purchase a product—often by a famous athlete or coach. A testimonial is anecdotal evidence that highlights one person's experience rather than well-designed research.
   - Beware of extrapolated data that may have been found in one population group (often in the clinical setting) and then applied to a different population (the athlete). For

continues

ERGOGENIC AID CHECKLIST: EVALUATING DIETARY SUPPLEMENTS *continued*

example, a supplement that benefits a group with heart disease does not necessarily improve athletic performance in an athlete.

4. Check the ingredient list. All ingredients should be listed. For example, a whey protein product may also contain creatine and other "muscle-building" ingredients, proven or unproven. Don't be fooled by claims of a "proprietary" blend of ingredients or a "patent," as these terms do not connote effectiveness of a product.

5. Is it safe? Do any of the ingredients have unwanted side effects, such as increasing heart rate and raising blood pressure? Does the supplement interact with other products or medication that you are taking? Supplement manufacturers do not have to disclose possible side effects as drug manufacturers do.

6. Is it legal? Does it contain substances banned by athletic organizations? Consult the governing bodies for the sports in which you plan to participate.

7. Is it worth the money? Some supplement protocols can reach high monthly dollar amounts. Often, you can obtain similar nutrients and benefits from food sources.

8. Who is the manufacturer? Does the company produce other reputable products? Does it have a history of producing safe and reliable products?

(68 kg) athlete this translates to a dose of 5 teaspoons of baking soda, which provides 21,000 milligrams, or 21 grams, of bicarbonate. Baking soda should be consumed with plenty of water, about 1 to 2 quarts (1–2 L), when taken 1 to 2 hours prior to exercise. This fluid may or may not mitigate reported side effects in some individuals, which include nausea, bloating, abdominal pain, and diarrhea. Experimenting with this supplement in training can help you determine whether you are prone to these unwanted side effects and whether it seems to provide any benefit for you.

Beta-Alanine

What Does It Do? Chronic supplementation with the amino acid beta-alanine increases the muscle content of an important compound called carnosine, which acts as an antioxidant. Carnosine also has the ability to buffer the acidity in the muscle produced by high intensity activity.

What Is the Evidence? Supplementation with 5–6 g daily of beta-alanine increases muscle carnosine content by approximately 60 percent after 4 weeks, and by approximately 80 percent after 10 weeks. After beta-alanine supplementation is stopped, it may take up to 15 weeks for muscle carnosine to fall to original levels. The theory around use of beta-alanine as an ergogenic aid is sound, but evidence is still emerging. Beta-alanine has the potential to increase the capacity to train hard by reducing the damage associated with high levels of muscle acidity and may be a good alternative strategy to bicarbonate loading.

Do I Need It? Beta-alanine supplementation would potentially improve performance in high-intensity sustained events lasting 1–7 minutes, such as track cycling, swimming, and middle-distance running. It may also be useful during interval or resistance training sessions or during high-intensity efforts within or at the end of a prolonged event, such as a cycling road race. Beta-alanine products can be expensive.

Are There Side Effects? Beta-alanine supplements are associated with skin tingling in some individuals. Symptoms can range from mild to very painful but do not cause any damage other than discomfort. Symptoms can be lessened by using small, multiple doses or sustained release products. The long-term effects of beta-alanine supplements have not been investigated.

Quercetin

What Does It Do? Quercetin is a flavonoid found in a variety of foods, such as apple skins, berries, black tea, and some leafy green vegetables. It is believed to be an antioxidant and an anti-inflammatory, offering potential immune benefits to athletes. The effects of quercetin on the enhancement of exercise performance by increasing oxygen capacity have also been studied.

What Is the Evidence? Despite much potential, quercetin has not produced striking results in human clinical trials as was predicted from animal studies. Some human studies have shown a modest effect at lowering inflammation while others have shown no effect. Trials combining quercetin with omega-3 fats and epicallocatechin 3-gallate (EGCG) have produced the most promising results with reduced markers of inflammation, oxidative stress, and immune disruption. A recent meta-analysis or review of existing data on the effects of quercetin ingestion on endurance capacity had researchers conclude that while quercetin provides a statistically significant benefit in human endurance capacity (VO_2max and endurance exercise performance), the effect was trivial to small.

Do I Need It? Current data is not strong enough to support the regular use of quercetin supplementation.

Are There Side Effects? Quercetin study doses were often 1,000 mg, divided into two doses. Supplementation usually lasts 1–3 weeks but may last several weeks longer with no significant side effects reported for use up to 12 weeks.

Choosing an Ergogenic Aid: *Jack*

Jack wanted to use supplements appropriately during the training and racing season, as he felt that this could give him a competitive edge. He received advice from a sports dietitian as to which supplements have sound scientific backing and when they can be used appropriately to derive a performance improvement.

Early in base training when Jack was trying to increase muscle strength, he did a creatine load at a 30-gram daily dose (divided into six doses) for 5 days to prepare for 8 weeks of training that included three resistance training sessions weekly. After the loading phase, he consumed a 3-gram daily dose during the 8-week training cycle. He was able to complete these demanding training sessions at the desired level and build muscle and strength to prepare him for the next training cycle.

As Jack entered more intense training sessions, including longer-distance bike rides and runs, he decided to experiment with caffeine use in training in preparation for use during races. Jack normally consumed a strong 16-ounce (500 ml) cup of coffee in the morning and decided to stick with this strategy rather than add more caffeine to his pre-workout or pre-race meal. With his weight at 165 pounds (75 kg), Jack's optimal caffeine dose was 225 milligrams 1 hour before the race. He did not want to increase his pre-exercise caffeine and possibly experience gastrointestinal side effects or jitteriness on race morning. He decided, however, that caffeine intake on the run might be a useful strategy, as he was competing in a half-Ironman and could take this supplement for the last leg to combat brain or central nervous system fatigue. Jack experimented with a caffeine-containing gel and aimed for about 100 milligrams of caffeine over the run, which would provide 0.6 milligrams per pound (1.5 g/kg), the test dose supported by research. He found that in training he tolerated this product well and to good effect. He employed this strategy during the run leg of the half-Ironman and found that the caffeine helped him to maintain mental focus and concentration in the last hour of a very long race. Jack had a PR finish for his half-Ironman and qualified for age-group Nationals.

PART III
SPORT-SPECIFIC
NUTRITIONAL GUIDELINES

*Putting Your Sports Nutrition Plan
into Action*

Though all endurance sports share similarities, they are not exactly alike. Each one presents a unique set of challenges and demands. Triathletes, cyclists, runners, and swimmers must function differently to achieve the top levels of their sport. Nutritional considerations must take this into account. The principles presented in Part II apply to all endurance sports, but athletes can greatly benefit from nutritional fine-tuning for their specific type of sport. Part III shows endurance athletes how to do just that.

Triathletes can adjust their nutrition race plan specifically for short-course and long-course racing. Cyclists can modify their nutrition plan for road, criterium, or mountain bike racing. Runners can adapt their training, taper, and competition nutrition plans for 10K races or longer distances, such as the marathon. Endurance sports such as swimming, which impose large training demands for races measured in minutes, also have their own unique nutritional considerations.

NUTRITION FOR TRIATHLON
(AND OTHER MULTISPORT EVENTS)

Since being introduced as a medal sport at the Sydney Olympic Games in 2000, triathlon competition has received a great boost in exposure. In the past two decades there has been a rapid increase in both amateur and professional race participation. Membership in the sport's governing body, USA Triathlon (USAT), increased to 135,000 in 2010, up from 21,000 in 2000. USAT sanctioned 3,115 races and clinics in 2009.

Many triathlon fans "discovered" the sport while flipping through television channels and came across weekend coverage of the inspiring and grueling Hawaiian Ironman® Triathlon World Championship. While triathletes can participate in Ironman and half-Ironman races around the world, race events designed to attract first-timers wanting to participate in the sport at a recreational level have increased exponentially. These new events, particularly the sprint-distance and the women-only races, have greatly fueled the sport's growth. Triathletes can also take their act off-road with events such as the XTERRA® series. These events draw endurance athletes who have participated in one of the three triathlon disciplines and who are looking for some cross-training, variety, and new

8

AT A GLANCE
KEY POINTS

Meal timing is essential for optimal fueling during training and recovery.

Prioritize recovery nutrition between two-a-day sessions.

Address weight loss early in the season to avoid energy depletion during hard training.

The longer or harder the session, the more essential the need for replenishment.

How you fuel for the long-course can make or break your race.

Practice effective nutrition intake on the bike and run.

TYPES OF EVENTS

Triathlon

Sprint Distance (short): 0.5-mile swim, 12.4-mile cycle, 3.1-mile run
There are "super-sprint" options for the newbies or super-speedsters in the sport.

Olympic Distance (intermediate): 0.93-mile swim, 24.8-mile cycle, 6.2-mile run
XTERRA races are often held at this intermediate distance or at shorter distances.

Half-Ironman (long): 1.2-mile swim, 56-mile cycle, 13.1-mile run
The growing Ironman 70.3 race series (70.3 designates the sum of the course miles completed) offers over fifty races around the world. Long-course triathletes can choose from this race series or take part in independent races at or near this distance.

Ironman (ultra): 2.4-mile swim, 112-mile cycle, 26.2-mile run
With more than twenty-five races to choose from around the world, triathlon competitors craving the ultradistance in triathlon events have more options than ever. Despite the challenge of this race distance, it is not unusual for the full Ironman races to fill up within twenty-four hours after registration opens.

Duathlon
Duathlon races combine the sports of cycling and running, typically in a run-bike-run sequence. Distances can vary and include:

challenges in their exercise and competition programs. Some single-sport endurance athletes participate in events as part of a relay team.

Triathlons also have a broad age appeal. USAT statistics show that most triathlon participants are between the ages of thirty and forty-four, but there are many younger athletes competing at the shorter distances as well as older competitors embracing the triathlon lifestyle beyond their middle years. Although triathlon competition is essentially an individual sport where competitors attempt to set their own best time, triathletes often train together and there is a real sense of community within the sport.

Although certain physiological characteristics seem essential for competitors at the elite level, people of all shapes and sizes are embracing the sport at the recreational level. Elite competitors have a high VO_2max, low body fat, high anaerobic threshold, and econ-

- 2-mile run, 10-mile cycle, 2-mile run (Formula One® race)
- 5K run, 30K cycle, 5K run
- 10K run, 40K cycle, 5K run (international or short-course race)
- 10K run, 60K cycle, 10K run (Powerman® or long-course race)

Aquathlon

Aquathlons combine the sports of running and swimming, and races are generally completed in less than 45 minutes. The races follow the run-swim-run format, and distances generally include a 1.5K run and a 1,000-meter swim followed by another 1.5K run.

Winter Triathlon

Winter triathlons are not just regular triathlons held between the months of November and March; rather, the winter triathlon is a separate sport that combines running, mountain biking, and cross-country skiing.

Adventure Racing

Adventure racing includes a variety of race distances such as sprint, one-day, and expedition-style races. Race sections include a variety of components, trekking, mountain biking, paddling, and rappelling among them.

omy of movement. Many other factors influence competitive success, but at the age-group level, anyone who is willing to train can participate. Athletes can choose from a variety of races and distances, and special nutritional considerations are appropriate to each.

TRAINING NUTRITION

Whatever the distance a multisport athlete is racing, the proper training diet is essential to a successful and enjoyable racing experience. Because of the diverse nature of their sport, many triathletes complete training for two disciplines daily. Though some schedule two training sessions back to back, others schedule two separate training sessions with a recovery period in between—training, for example, for one sport in the morning and for another in the afternoon or evening. For those who schedule two workouts, weekends are often reserved for long back-to-back training sessions. Sessions are mainly aerobic with some interval workouts, and strength and conditioning in the off-season.

Depending on the race distance, triathletes may train anywhere from 8 hours weekly (for the sprint distance) to 25 hours weekly (for the ultradistance). Clearly, the nutritional demands of multisport training vary depending on the type and distance of the course. Race nutrition demands can also vary depending on the level of the competitor. Racing itself can last over 1 hour for a sprint first-timer, from 2 to 4 hours for Olympic-distance competitors, from 4 to 8 hours for a half-Ironman, and from 8 hours to just under the 17-hour cutoff for the Ironman distance. Despite spreading the work out among various muscle groups, any race distance can challenge muscle fuel stores and blood glucose levels. Multisport athletes are also often challenged by the environmental conditions in which they compete. Their races often take place in hot and humid conditions, challenging fluid and electrolyte stores. Long-course racing presents its own unique set of challenges, as competitors must fuel and hydrate for several hours within the constraints of their own stomach and intestinal tolerances.

Because of the nature of their training, multisport athletes need to match energy intake, and particularly their intake of carbohydrates, to their training sessions and training cycles. They must also know how to adjust protein and fat intake levels for optimal training. It is important for the multisport athlete to understand sensible meal and snack timing as well in order to ensure a steady cycle of fueling before training and refueling afterward, particularly when there is a short recovery period between training sessions.

Optimal daily hydration remains important for multisport athletes, but with multisport training and competition it is crucial for an athlete to become familiar with his or her own sweat rate for each training discipline and to develop techniques for rehydrating and refueling during training. And although it is important for any multisport athlete to meet his or her fueling needs during training, this aspect of nutrition can make or break the efforts of the long-course triathlete.

NUTRIENT REQUIREMENTS

Triathletes often plan their race season well in advance. This type of planning allows triathletes plenty of time to map out their training program and look at weight and body-composition goals.

Multisport athletes, particularly long-course triathletes, have training days that demand a very high energy intake. Energy needs can vary throughout the week depending on the level of training for the day. For example, say an intermediate-course male triathlete who weighs 165 pounds (75 kg) completes an easy 45-minute swim one morning and an easy 45-minute evening spin on the bike. His energy needs for the day would amount to approximately 3,000 to 3,300 calories. For this same athlete, a weekend endurance ride lasting 3 to 4 hours would require an intake ranging from 3,800 to 4,450 calories. The same athlete would require more calories if he were training for a long-course distance. Two hours of moderate training would require him to take in 3,600 calories, while a long bike ride of 5 hours or more would demand an intake of more than 5,000 calories for the day.

Refer to Table 4.4 to appreciate the peaks and valleys of an athlete's carbohydrate requirements as training builds and progresses and then decreases during recovery weeks. Carbohydrates are an important fuel for the triathlete during any period of training. Although fuel demands can be low during the preparation phase of training, long-course triathletes often require hefty doses of carbohydrates even early in the season owing to the volume of their training. Fat intake may need to be higher for long-course competitors on high-volume days that include more than 4 hours of training. Protein requirements build steadily as training increases in both duration and intensity; both long workouts and shorter speed workouts have high carbohydrate demands.

CHANGING BODY COMPOSITION

Without exception, elite competitors in triathlon events exhibit low levels of body fat. Although this is not the case with competitors at the recreational level, some age-groupers may also want to improve body composition over the course of the season. (Refer to the weight-management guidelines outlined in Chapter 6.) Triathletes wanting to lose weight should start as early in the season as possible, since weight loss is more easily tolerated during the preparation cycle. As you approach the build phase of your training, the rate of weight loss should slow down because the fuel demands of your training program will increase and adequate recovery is essential. It is important to have realistic weight and body-composition goals and to monitor your changes in body composition throughout the season. Weight-loss efforts are not advised during the last build to an important race or during a race taper.

Regardless of your competition focus, meeting your energy needs is essential for recovery. Attempts to lose weight quickly may result in fatigue and lackluster training.

Keep in mind that optimal body fat levels are not the same for all individuals—an "ideal" weight that results in hormonal imbalance, loss of muscle and power, and compromised immune function will not make you a better triathlete. Lean and successful triathletes achieve their low body fat levels through an intense training program and proper fueling.

TIMING MEALS AND SNACKS

As a triathlete, you may faithfully keep up a vigorous schedule of training twice a day all year-round. Although multiple training sessions are essential for refining your swimming, cycling, and running skills and accelerating your conditioning, they also present a nutritional timing challenge. It may sometimes seem that your life is one continuous cycle of training, eating, and recovery.

It can be a challenge to determine how to time meals and snacks around multisport training schedules. You don't want to train with an empty or half-empty tank, or one that is too full prior to exercise. But figuring out just the right amount of fuel to consume for training more than once daily—and when to consume it—can be tricky. Depending on when you have swimming, cycling, running, or resistance training in your training schedule, it may be difficult or even impossible to eat several hours prior to exercising.

Even if you find that your gastrointestinal (GI) system can adapt fairly well to eating close to exercise, as many triathletes do, clearly you must think ahead to the day's schedule in planning your food choices. Three factors will most likely affect those choices: whether you are going for a swim, bike ride, or run; how hard you expect to train; and the timing of your training sessions. Generally, the higher the intensity, the lighter the pre-exercise meal, or the longer the time interval between eating and training. Running will likely present the greatest digestive challenge, with swimming next in line and cycling the most gentle on your GI system. And although large meals before exercise could make you drowsy and lethargic and possibly cause digestive distress, your real challenge lies in determining the size of the meal and the meal choices that work best for you before particular types of exercise sessions.

In general, a moderate snack providing 1 gram of carbohydrates per pound (2 g/kg) of body weight can be consumed 2 hours prior to training. This snack can include some easily digested solid food, such as a granola bar and yogurt, along with fluids. If you need to eat within an hour of exercise, try an easily digested energy bar, piece of fruit, carbohydrate gel, 24 ounces (720 ml) of a sports drink, or another high-carbohydrate sports nutrition supplement to boost energy levels. Your training schedule may dictate that you have a full meal during the recovery part of your day. Plan ahead, and be sure to include enough meals and snacks to supply the energy you need to train at your best.

Early-Morning Sessions

Early-morning training sessions are not uncommon for the serious triathlete. Often this early session is a swim, but it could easily include a run or bike ride. If your early-morning schedule does not leave much time for digestion before exercising, make sure that you consume a high-carbohydrate dinner, or perhaps even a high-carb evening snack, the night before. You want to start the training session with full muscle glycogen stores and minimize as much as possible the effects of the liver glycogen breakdown that occurs overnight. You can also experiment with small, low-fiber snacks beforehand to determine tolerances. Well-tolerated early-morning noshes may include an energy bar, half a bagel or English muffin, a small yogurt, a glass of juice, or a piece of fruit. These carbohydrate choices can boost your early-morning blood glucose levels and help keep them steady during training. Aim for 50 to 75 grams of carbohydrates before exercise. Of course, you should also drink plenty of water in the morning. If your early-morning training session is a long workout, consider consuming a sports drink while you train. This strategy is easy on your GI system and ensures a steady supply of blood glucose. It can also help you compensate for eating just a small amount of food before the exercise session and can be a useful fueling strategy even during a short workout.

During Training

Anytime that your schedule or personal food tolerances preclude adequate food intake prior to training, think about what you can consume while exercising. Sports drinks, bars, and gels provide glucose for your exercising muscles and can offset muscle glycogen losses that occur later during exercise. Proper refueling during exercise prevents your body from entering a greatly depleted state and will ultimately speed your recovery. Try to consume 30 to 75 grams of carbohydrates, or 0.5 gram of carbohydrates per pound of body weight (1 g/kg) per hour for workouts lasting longer than 75 minutes or during high-intensity interval sessions. For very long workouts, some triathletes may require up to 90 grams of carbohydrates per hour. If you decide to consume only water during very low-intensity workouts, keep in mind that muscle glycogen and blood glucose stores will eventually drop to low levels as training time progresses. Consider your training goals for that day and that week. Consuming carbohydrates during training sessions is especially important if another training session will quickly follow with limited recovery time in between. If your training schedule is not as demanding, then you may have more recovery time. But consecutive training sessions are not uncommon for multisport training. Hydration is important during any workout and during any part of your training cycle, and sports drinks provide the right balance of carbohydrates and fluid, as well as electrolytes, to stave off the depletion that can occur during heavy training.

RECOVERY NUTRITION

Because you are in a constant cycle of training and recovery, it is very important that you pay close attention to recovery nutrition. If you go into your second workout dehydrated or low on energy, you may not have a high-quality training session. In fact, you may end up digging yourself into an even bigger hole of energy depletion that will affect your training for the next day. Improper refueling can start a downward spiral of poor training and low energy. Follow the recovery nutrition guidelines provided in Chapter 5. Make sure that you plan to have foods on hand that will provide anywhere from 50 to 100 grams of carbohydrates, or at least 0.5 gram of carbohydrates per pound (1 g/kg) of body weight, and up to 20 grams of protein. Check your weight loss from the training session to see how much fluid you lost in sweat, and drink to rehydrate. You should drink about 16 to 20 ounces for every pound of body weight lost. Consume foods and fluids containing sodium after training in hot, humid weather to replace sodium losses and to enhance rehydration efforts.

The food choices that suit you best after exercise depend to a large extent upon your training schedule for the day. If your next training session is within 2 hours, a between-workouts snack is likely your best option. Aim for easily digested choices. You can try real-food options such as a banana smoothie and toast with jam after a hard session, knowing these foods will sit well until the next training session. At other times, a recovery drink that can be mixed quickly after training or ahead of time may be the most convenient choice. However, if your next training session is several hours away, you should consider having an actual meal. This will not only allow you to fill up on carbohydrates but also provide you with the opportunity to round out your protein and fat intake. Some triathletes practice both nutrition strategies after an arduous training block. They make certain that a good recovery snack is readily available immediately after training and follow this snack shortly afterward with a well-balanced meal.

PLANNING AHEAD

As a triathlete you need to plan ahead to have the proper meals and snacks available. Pack recovery foods and sports drinks the night before. Know what deli carries your favorite healthy lunch that provides just the right balance of protein, carbohydrates, and fat. And make sure that you have the right afternoon snack available when hunger strikes—and to prevent hunger during an early-evening workout.

The meal plan in Table 8.1 reflects the food and training schedule of a half-Ironman competitor. It provides about 3,940 calories, including 660 grams of carbohydrates, 132 grams of protein, and 97 grams of fat. This plan is for a full day of training with 2 to 3 hours of total training time. Short-course athletes could pare down the portions at meals, as they likely would train less and have lower energy, carbohydrate, protein, and fat requirements, but the meal timing and types of food choices would remain the same.

If you train both in the morning and over the lunch hour, the timing will be tighter. After a strenuous morning workout, have recovery foods available in the form of a quick snack, followed by a large breakfast. If it is feasible, your recovery meal can be a good-sized breakfast. You may want to follow with a mid-morning snack so that hunger does not set in during your lunchtime training session. If needed, consume a sports drink during the lunchtime training session. Lunch should follow as your recovery meal. Depending on the intensity of training, you may be hungry for an afternoon snack or an early dinner. The meals and snacks following your last training session of the day are your opportunity to refuel for the next day. Make sure that you continue to recover for the next 12 to 24 hours or up until the time when your next training session presents itself.

Evening training could receive a good fuel boost from an afternoon snack. Later training sessions often take place 5 hours or more after your last good meal. Dinner can

TABLE 8.1 MEAL PLAN OUTLINE

EARLY-MORNING SNACK

12 oz. (360 ml) apple juice

16 oz. (480 ml) water

Morning workout: 60–90 minutes

32–40 oz. (960–1200 ml) sports drink

RECOVERY BREAKFAST

8 oz. (240 ml) yogurt with fruit

½ c. (120 ml) granola

1 banana

LUNCH

5 oz. (150 g) turkey

1 oz. (30 g) low-fat cheese

2 slices bread

1 pear

1 c. (240 ml) pasta salad with vegetables

3 tsp. (20 ml) olive oil

PRE-EXERCISE SNACK

1 energy bar

8 oz. (240 ml) cranberry juice

1 apple

2 tbsp. (40 ml) peanut butter

Afternoon workout: 60–90 minutes

32–40 oz. (960–1200 ml) sports drink

DINNER

5 oz. (150 g) fish

1.5 c. (360 ml) cooked brown rice

1 c. (240 ml) broccoli

3 tsp. (20 ml) sesame seed oil

EVENING SNACK

1 c. (240 ml) frozen yogurt

1 c. (240 ml) strawberries

follow an evening training session as a recovery meal, and depending on the intensity of your training, you may even be hungry for an evening snack.

SPORT-SPECIFIC GUIDELINES

SWIM WORKOUTS

Triathletes frequently experiment with nutritional strategies around cycling and running workouts; you should view your swim workouts in the same way. Even though you will not rehydrate and refuel during the swim in an actual race, the proper nutritional strategies for any workout enhance the quality of your training and recovery. What you eat and drink, and how much you eat and drink before, during, and after swimming, depend on the timing of your swim workout and other details of that day's training schedule.

Before an early-morning swim, aim for some liquid carbohydrate sources such as juice or a sports drink. A light solid food such as toast or a banana could also be tolerated. Experiment with easily digested foods and fluids to give your early-morning blood glucose levels a needed boost. For afternoon and evening swims, experiment with a light afternoon snack providing at least 50 grams of carbohydrates. Swims late in the evening present a logistical challenge. Some triathletes do well with a small dinner 3 hours beforehand and a sizable recovery snack after swimming. Another option is a late-afternoon snack and a moderately sized post-swim dinner for refueling. You can aim for both solid and liquid carbohydrate choices, with moderate portions of lean proteins.

When your swim training exceeds 60 minutes, or is scheduled back to back with another workout, consider refueling during the swim session. Although sweat rates in the pool can be significantly lower than during land training, hydration is still a focus. And even a relatively short swim of 45 minutes can start the fuel-depletion process. These problems are only compounded by another workout in quick succession. Hydrating with a sports drink can offset glycogen depletion from the swim and help prepare you for the workout directly following your swim. Keep a sports drink at the end of your lane to rehydrate and refuel. Check your weight before and after training to gauge fluid loss during a swim workout.

Very long swim workouts may require a gel shot for a needed carbohydrate boost. Most sports drinks provide 13 to 19 grams of carbohydrates per 8-ounce (240 ml) serving. Sixteen ounces (480 ml) of a sports drink should provide 26 to 38 grams of carbohydrates, and a gel shot can provide another 25 to 30 grams and may be appropriate during harder workouts and for large athletes. Experiment to determine the mix that works best for you. You can replenish after the swim with a sports drink and/or gel if your next workout is in 15 minutes; otherwise, just refuel with a good meal or snack.

BIKE WORKOUTS

Regardless of the distance for which you train, your cycling sessions are likely to be the longest workouts of your training program. The cycling leg of a race also presents the most opportune and convenient time to rehydrate and refuel. Practicing your on-bike nutrition is thus essential for race preparation. The longer the ride, the more important this key skill becomes, as fuel, fluid, and electrolyte stores can easily become depleted if you neglect this part of your nutrition plan.

Your GI system is relatively stable during a cycling workout, allowing you to consume a greater volume of fluid during the bike ride than during the run. In addition, your fluid bottle is more accessible on the bike. Check your sweat rate for cycling training sessions. Aim to match this sweat rate with your fluid intake. It can be difficult at first to consume more than 1.5 quarts (about 1.5 L) per hour on the bike, but it becomes easier with practice. At the very least, minimize dehydration on the bike, and avoid drinking in excess of your sweat rate. This is only likely to occur in athletes with low sweat rates, however. Optimizing your fluid intake on the bike with your favorite sports drink results in a higher carbohydrate intake, which allows you to better meet your fueling needs, and a higher sodium intake, which better replaces sodium sweat losses.

Some practice tips may be helpful. First, use a larger fluid bottle if necessary, especially if your sweat rate indicates that you need at least 40 ounces (1,200 ml) of fluid per hour to prevent or minimize dehydration. Second, practice drinking while on the bike to increase your ability to handle the bottle easily during the race. Third, set a watch alarm to remind you to gulp every 15 minutes. Sports drinks work on the bike for any triathlon distance. Short-course athletes can pack their own fluids for the race, whereas long-course athletes should anticipate taking advantage of the drinks offered on the course. In fact, they should train with this product to be fully prepared for race day. Depending on the volume of fluid that you consume, sports drinks can nicely meet your fueling needs, particularly for the shorter events. But you may need to add gels and other carbohydrate sources for long-course racing. More information on race nutrition strategies is provided later in this chapter.

RUNNING

Hydrating and fueling during runs can be challenging. First, running jostles your stomach, and drinking may not always be comfortable. Second, it is not as convenient to carry fluids with you on a run as it is during a bike ride. Just as you can train your stomach to take in greater volumes of fluid during bike workouts, however, you can also practice during the run. The race course does offer fluid stations. To mimic this setup, you can run a loop with a safe place to stash your fluids. Track workouts allow you to hydrate conveniently, though high-intensity training runs can still pose an intake challenge. At the very least, train with a hydration belt.

RACE COURSE–SPECIFIC GUIDELINES

Many of the hydration and fueling strategies that you practice in training are an all-important rehearsal for race day. Still, there are some nutritional considerations unique to each race distance in the days leading up to the race, on race morning, and during the race.

SPRINT DISTANCE

This race distance may be short, but arriving at the starting line prepared still requires savvy nutritional planning. Focus on a diet ample in carbohydrates 24 to 48 hours prior to the race, and make sure your intake matches the energy needs of your training taper. Drink plenty of fluids to hydrate well, and have an early high-carbohydrate dinner the night before the race. Stick with easily tolerated foods and fluids for a couple of days before the race. Time your pre-race meal on race morning according to personal preferences and tolerances, with plenty of fluids and easily digested foods. Though race starts are likely early, pre-race eating 2 to 3 hours before the start time works best. In the 48 hours leading up to the race, make sure that you stay optimally hydrated. Drink fluids to stay hydrated before the race start—a sports drink is an excellent choice—and time bathroom breaks appropriately. (See Table 8.2 for a summary of nutrition guidelines for sprint- and Olympic-distance triathlons.)

Enjoy the swim, have a good transition, and consume a sports drink on the bike leg of the competition. With typical race times ranging from under 1 hour to just under 2

TABLE *8.2* RACE NUTRITION FOR SPRINT- AND OLYMPIC-DISTANCE TRIATHLONS	
SPRINT DISTANCE	**OLYMPIC DISTANCE**
Consume adequate carbohydrates during race taper.	Taper and consume adequate carbohydrates in the 48 hours before race.
Consume carbohydrates in excess of requirements 24 hours before race.	Hydrate optimally in the 48 hours before race. Monitor urine color.
Consume a high-carbohydrate meal 2–3 hours before race.	Increase salt intake 48 hours prior to race if you are a salty sweater and if race will take place in hot and humid conditions.
Hydrate with sports drink in the hours leading up to race.	Consume high-carbohydrate meal providing 1 g of carbohydrates per lb. (about 2 g/kg) of body weight for 2–3 hours before the start of race.
Drink 20–32 oz. or an amount to minimize sweat losses of fluid, preferably a sports drink, during bike leg.	Consume fluids from sports drink in the hours leading up to race. Top off pre-race meal with a carbohydrate gel, if tolerated.
Stop at aid stations for fluid during run to prevent further dehydration.	Drink sports drink on the bike to minimize sweat losses. Amounts needed can range from 24 to 40 oz. per hour.
	Stop at aid stations on run and consume sports drink provided to prevent further dehydration.

hours, it is important for some sprint-distance triathletes to play it right nutritionally on the bike. Cycling presents the opportune time to drink and maintain blood glucose levels. By race day you should be a pro at on-bike drinking due to plenty of practice. Pack two bottles of your favorite sports drink on the bike and drink as you are able for the quick run to the finish. Make sure that you have practiced drinking the particular sports drink available on the course during your runs.

OLYMPIC DISTANCE

Although top competitors may complete this race at about the 2-hour mark, for many age-groupers an Olympic-distance triathlon is a test of both technique and endurance, with 4-hour finishes commonly listed in race results.

Eat according to your energy needs as determined by the reduced training outlined in your taper for 24 to 48 hours and emphasize high-carbohydrate foods. Consume 3 to 4 grams of carbohydrates for every pound (6.5–9 g/kg) of body weight 2 days before the race, and close to the same amount the day before the race. Be aware that you may gain a bit of weight when carb loading over 2 days.

Time and size your meals appropriately for your start time, consuming 1 to 2 grams of carbohydrates per pound (2.5–4 g/kg) of body weight 3 to 4 hours prior to the race (see Table 5.1). You may wish to time your pre-race meal closer to the start time and decrease your carbohydrate intake accordingly. Practice the pre-race fluid tips outlined in Chapter

5 so that you start the race well hydrated. Hydrate to maintain fluid balance during the taper, and take care not to overhydrate. Large volumes of very clear urine may indicate that you are overhydrating. Include sodium in your pre-race foods, especially if you are a salty sweater and susceptible to muscle cramping.

When you start the bike portion of the race, begin fueling up with a sports drink. Some competitors may prefer gels and water for their carbohydrate-and-fluid combination. If you are racing in hot, humid conditions, make sure that the sports nutrition products you use contain adequate amounts of sodium. Sports drinks are more likely to contain adequate sodium than gels and other products. You can also increase your regular sodium intake for 48 hours before the race to prevent sodium depletion. Age-groupers who have longer finish times are at greater risk of sodium depletion than elite athletes who complete the course quickly. Ingesting low-sodium fluids such as plain water over several hours can dilute the blood and reduce your sodium to below-normal levels. Pack a relatively high-sodium sports drink for the bike leg of the race if needed.

Focus on maintaining an adequate fluid intake during the run. Chances are that your efforts on the bike have not replaced 100 percent of your fluid, carbohydrate, and electrolyte losses. Drinking during the run is not as easy as during cycling, but you can practice and acquire this technique in training. The sports drink available on the race course should provide better hydration than a gel-and-water combination.

OFF-ROAD

Most off-road races are similar to the Olympic-distance event in terms of length, but finish times are longer owing to the necessity of navigating the terrain on the mountain bike and while running on trails. Both present unique nutritional challenges. Carb-load in the 48 hours before the race, and have a good pre-race meal as you would for an intermediate-course race. Start the race well hydrated, and consume adequate sodium in the days leading up to the race. By the time race day arrives, you should have had plenty of miles of practice fueling on the bike. A sports drink is essential for completing an off-road race, and both fueling and hydration are essential if you plan to be on the course for more than 3 hours. During the race, a back-mounted hydration pack is a good off-road race option because it leaves your hands free to navigate the off-road bike terrain. But packing water bottles is also helpful, and with relatively long bike times, a gel shot can provide a handy carbohydrate boost. A gel flask mounted on your bike presents another practical fueling option.

LONG COURSE

The impact of optimal nutrition when competing in a half-Ironman or Ironman triathlon cannot be overestimated. Having a good fluid-and-food day can make or break your race. Long-course triathletes often search diligently for the perfect food and fluid choices, and many top competitors have developed their own distinct rehydration and refueling choices and strategies. Half-Ironman competition is challenging, and Ironman competition is grueling, so it is imperative that you begin the race with glycogen-loaded muscles, adequate liver glycogen stores, optimal hydration and topped-up fluid levels, and a placid and satisfied GI system.

HALF-IRONMAN RACING

Although many age-group competitors can expect to be on the course for more than 5 hours, most athletes tackle this race at a slightly higher intensity than the rate at which they would approach an Ironman, at the upper end of their aerobic zone. You may compete at more of a "tempo" speed, or at a higher heart rate, during some sections of the race, particularly if the race is the most important one of the season for you.

Because of the higher intensity sustained during this type of race, you may wish to temper your nutritional strategies to determine the proper balance of taking in adequate fuel and maintaining a placid GI system. You should hydrate, fuel, and replace electrolytes with a sports drink, choosing one high in sodium if you have high salt needs. Gels can also be added to the mix. But when you exercise at higher intensities, the more concentrated carbohydrate sources do not empty from your stomach as quickly as they do during less intense exercise. Be careful with any solid items, if you choose to use them at all. Drink to match or minimize sweat losses in both the biking portion and the running portion of the race. You may not start the run with the same level of dehydration as in an Ironman, but the higher running speed can affect your stomach tolerances. Read below on strategies for Ironman racing nutrition to develop your own personalized plan for race day. Tapering and eating to carbo-load for the race is recommended 2 to 3 days prior, as are all the steps in the days leading to and the morning of the race. You may fuel on the lower end of recommended amounts for half-Ironman racing in contrast to Ironman racing.

IRONMAN RACING

One study indicated that male Ironman competitors burn more than 10,000 calories of fuel during the race, and female competitors more than 8,000 calories. Energy intakes during the race, however, were less than half the amount of calories burned. It is not expected that fuel intake match fuel burned. The logistical constraints of the race make it difficult to refuel, and the GI system does not always tolerate adequate refueling during the race.

Eating for the Taper

Regular Ironman training can take up to 25 hours weekly and necessitates a high calorie intake with the proper balance of carbohydrates, fats, and proteins. However, Ironman competitors also have a welcome training taper prior to competition. The taper allows the body to fully recover before the race and gives the athlete an opportunity to refuel and carbohydrate-load. Ironman triathletes may actually cut their training down by a full 50 percent during the taper, and this reduction decreases their calorie and carbohydrate requirements.

Even with carbohydrate loading, your calorie and carbohydrate requirements may dip below training levels during the taper. When you load carbohydrates, you rest your muscles and burn minimal amounts of glycogen. You then eat to exceed your carbohydrate requirements in order to bring your glycogen levels to above normal. Your typical training diet should be more than adequate to accomplish this pre-race loading. In fact, continuing your normal caloric intake can lead to unwanted weight gain, as you may be training for only 1 to 2 hours daily.

During the carbohydrate-loading phase of your program, your portions may be smaller than on training days. But do consume a high percentage of your calories from carbohydrates. Of course, it is the total grams of carbohydrates that matter most, rather than percentages. If you are training for up to 2 hours daily, consume anywhere from 3 to 4.5 grams of carbohydrates for every pound (6.5–10 g/kg) that you weigh. For a 165-pound (75 kg) triathlete this translates to at least 500 grams daily, a significant amount that requires knowledge and planning. Gauge your hunger and fullness carefully. If you are too hungry or become hungry quickly, you are not eating enough to fuel up your body. However, feelings of uncomfortable fullness are not appropriate either. High levels of carb loading may be better tolerated 2 days before the race than the day before—you do not want to wake up on race morning feeling bloated and too full.

At the very least, your normal diet will fill up your muscle glycogen stores during a taper; at worst, you will gain some weight. A bit of weight gain may be inevitable, as the glycogen you store in your body will hold water in your muscles. This fluid gain does not have any detrimental effect upon performance and can be valuable during competition.

Another important focus of your pre-race nutrition plan should be staying optimally hydrated. Fluid intake is especially important if you are racing in a location where heat and humidity can reach extreme levels. You need several quarts or liters of fluids daily regardless of the training level for the day. During training, average sweat losses can range from 1 to 3 quarts (about 1–3 L) per hour. If possible, weigh yourself before and after training during your taper phase and consume 24 ounces (720 ml) of hydrating fluid for every pound of weight lost. A large volume of pale urine is an adequate indicator of hydration. Pay close attention to your sodium requirements during this time as well. Have recovery drinks containing sodium, add sodium to the foods you eat for several hours after training, and include plenty of sodium in your carb-loading diet.

Chances are you will be traveling when you compete in an Ironman. Pack some favorite foods, such as sports nutrition supplements and other portable items, including cereals, dried fruit, and granola bars, to take with you. You can also call ahead to your destination or surf the Internet to determine what types of restaurants and menus are offered near where you are staying.

The 48-hour period before a race is a critical time for true carbohydrate loading to ensure optimal fuel stores. Even if you simply eat "normally" during the bulk of the taper, increase your carbohydrate intake 2 days before the race. Aim for 4 to 5 grams of carbohydrates per pound of body weight. During this 48-hour carb-loading phase, the types of carbohydrates you choose are as important as the amounts you consume. Placing less emphasis on high-fiber foods can keep your GI system settled and help you "race light." Try to rely on carbohydrate-containing fluids and low-fiber foods. Concentrated low-fiber carbohydrate sources include jam, honey, soft drinks, energy bars, refined pastas, breads, cereals, sports drinks, and concentrated sports nutrition supplements. You don't want to encounter any digestive surprises in the 48 hours prior to Ironman competition. Limit hard-to-digest foods, excess fat and spices, and any unusual or new items. Stick with bland, simple, plain foods, and request special preparation as needed. Your meals may not be a culinary delight in the 48 hours prior to racing, but at least they won't talk back to you during the race. During this period, you may also need to streamline your protein and fat intake to make room for the carbohydrates.

Hyponatremia, or low blood sodium levels, whether mild, moderate, or severe, has been an increasingly serious problem at Ironman competitions. Certain individuals may be more susceptible to excess sodium losses than others, but what you consume before an Ironman can make a difference. Before the race, you may want to consume some high-sodium foods and salt your food at mealtime. Levels of sodium loss due to sweating and regulation of blood sodium levels are unique to each individual, but it would be prudent to start any long-course race with blood sodium levels at the high end of normal. Although you need to drink fluids steadily during the pre-race period, don't overdrink, since overhydration can dilute the sodium levels of your blood.

The Night Before

The night before an Ironman, easily digested, tried-and-true foods low in fiber are your best option. Many athletes like potatoes, rice, refined breads, and pasta with a mild sauce. You may want to limit salads and other raw vegetables, which are harder to digest. Have a reasonable amount of easily digested protein with the night-before meal. A late-evening snack can provide a little carbohydrate insurance, but it is probably best to consume a larger meal by early evening. Remember, you want to wake up hungry the morning of the race so that you can enjoy and easily down your pre-race meal despite race day nerves.

RACE MORNING

Race morning is another time for following sensible strategies regarding your food and fluid intake, so plan your breakfast in advance. This pre-race meal allows your body to refill its liver glycogen stores after the overnight fast that occurs when you sleep. Top off fluid levels enough to carry you through the swim and the first transition (T1) leading to the biking portion of the race. Some competitors find that small amounts of easily digested protein can also be tolerated the morning of the race. Experiment with your favorite choices on training days that mimic the timing of the race, and don't try anything new on race day. Table 8.3 summarizes some pre-race nutrition strategies for the Ironman.

During the Race

Despite all your heroic efforts to prepare nutritionally prior to an Ironman, consuming adequate calories and carbohydrates during the Ironman itself is essential to completing

TABLE 8.3 LONG-DISTANCE RACE NUTRITION

TIMING	IRONMAN® RACE NUTRITION STRATEGIES	HALF-IRONMAN RACE NUTRITION STRATEGIES*
3–7 days prior to race	• Consume a high-carbohydrate training diet. Decrease protein and fat portions slightly during taper in training. • Maintain a carbohydrate intake of 3–3.5 g/lb. (6.5–8 g/kg) of body weight. • Increase sodium intake. • Hydrate optimally during training and rehydrate after training. Monitor the color of your urine to assess hydration status.	• Start carbo-loading 3 days prior to race.
48 hours prior to race	• Carbo-load with 4–5 g/lb. (9–11 g/kg) of body weight. • Emphasize concentrated sources of carbohydrates low in fiber. • Consume salt and salty foods. • Optimally hydrate.	• Continue carbo-loading 48 hours before the race.
Night before	• Finish pre-race meal early, by 5:00–6:00 p.m. • Keep pre-race meal simple and somewhat bland. • Keep fat intake low and choose very low-fat protein foods in small amounts.	• Do the same as for Ironman.
Race morning	• Consume breakfast containing easily digested carbohydrates in the amount of 1–1.5 g/lb. (2–3 g/kg) of body weight 3 hours before race start. • Hydrate with a sports drink in the hours leading to start. • Top off carbohydrate intake with a gel or energy bar about 90 minutes prior to start.	• Do the same as for Ironman.
T1 and bike	• Have a predetermined fueling plan for the bike and practice on your long rides. • Consume a sports drink for fluid, sodium, and carbohydrates in amounts required to minimize dehydration. Work within gastric tolerances regarding volume. • Add a gel, banana, energy bar, or concentrated carbohydrate drink to your sports drink intake per hour as needed for fuel.	• Race on liquids and semisolids only to minimize the risk of overfeeding. • Concentrated carbohydrate sources are not well tolerated at higher racing intensities and increase risk of gut problems during the race. Stick with carbohydrates mainly from sports drinks and add gels and blocks as tolerated during training. • Avoid protein and consume slightly fewer calories per hour (50–75 calories fewer) than during an Ironman.
T2 and run	• Have a predetermined fueling plan for the run and practice in training. • Vary fluid intake with a sports drink and cola. Add a gel as tolerated and needed. • Maintain adequate sodium intake with a high-sodium sports drink and electrolyte tablets or mixes, if needed.	• A more intense race pace than that of an Ironman can lead to GI problems. • A sports drink or tested gel plus water combination is best, with amounts tested out at race pace. This plan is expected to be slightly dialed down from an Ironman plan.
Post-race	• Consume easily digested carbohydrates and small amounts of protein, if tolerated. • Consume sodium-containing foods and fluids for several hours after the race. • Eat and drink at regular intervals.	• Do the same as for Ironman.

*Half-Ironman modifications: Half-Ironman races are less than half the duration of an Ironman race for each triathlete. While a half-IM is still mainly an aerobic race, triathletes have moments of hitting the upper limits of anaerobic threshold, pushing you to a predominance of carbohydrate fuel. This carries an increased risk of bonking, greater sweat losses, and a higher risk of gut issues—all of which require the proper balance of carbohydrate, fluid, and electrolytes for gut tolerances. More concentrated race nutrition formulas tolerated in the IM likely are not well tolerated in the half-IM.

the race and performing at your best. Optimal eating and drinking fuel you to the finish after months of preparation, whereas inadequate nutritional intake can leave you feeling depleted and disappointed. As an Ironman competitor, you need to translate the nutrition guidelines for eating and drinking during exercise into combinations and amounts of sports drinks, sodium sources, gels, bars, and other foods that work for your individual preferences and tolerances and that maintain your energy levels toward the finish.

As in pre-race preparation, the most important nutrients during a race remain fluids, carbohydrates, and sodium. The basic sweat rate of 1 to 3 quarts (about 1–3 L) per hour can vary with heat, humidity, exercise intensity, acclimatization, and fitness levels. The more pronounced the factors, the greater your fluid losses. Studies indicate that the rate at which fluid empties from the stomach exhibits a great deal of individual variability, but in general, it ranges from 24 to 40 ounces per hour. Aim to consume this amount of fluid during your race, and practice maintaining this intake during training. Seasoned competitors have learned to tolerate greater volumes.

Estimated sodium losses from sweating range from 115 to 700 milligrams per hour, but they can reach as high as 2,000 milligrams per hour in nonacclimated athletes or salty sweaters. Check the labels of your favorite sports drinks to determine sodium content, and choose those that match your typical level of sodium loss. If you are prone to muscle cramps, it may be because you have very salty sweat. You can add small amounts of salt to a sports drink if needed. One-quarter of a teaspoon of salt contains 550 milligrams of sodium. Salt tablets generally contain several hundred milligrams of sodium per tablet. All salt or electrolyte tablets should be consumed with at least 8 ounces of water.

Of course, you need carbohydrates to maintain blood glucose levels and provide fuel for your muscles as glycogen stores are burned for energy. Try to replace carbohydrates at a rate of 0.5 gram, or 2 calories per pound of body weight, per hour. This translates to about 60 to 100 grams of carbohydrates, or 250 to 400 calories per hour. This sounds like a lot of calories, but Ironman competitors expend several thousand calories in a race. Generally, 32 ounces of a sports drink provides 55 to 75 grams of carbohydrates. Check the labels of any items you may consume during a race, such as energy bars or gels, to determine their carbohydrate content.

TRANSITION I (TI) AND ON-THE-BIKE NUTRITION

After a swim in choppy waters or saltwater, your stomach may feel a bit unsettled. You may swallow some water during the swim and even feel a bit nauseated. But the bike leg is your opportunity to consume adequate fuel and set yourself up for the run. It is also the longest leg of the long-course triathlon. Try not to wait more than 30 minutes on the bike before you start consuming fluids.

Once you and your stomach are settled on the bike leg, it is time to get down to business. Start consuming fluids as soon as you can tolerate them. Fuller stomachs empty faster to quickly replace sweat losses, so drink enough to produce that effect. Sports drinks can provide a perfect balance of fluid and carbohydrates and varying amounts of sodium. Plain water can wash down the taste of sweet gels and beverages in hot and humid conditions. Try out your favorite sports drinks and gels (and the brand available on the race course) during long training sessions on your bike that are near race pace. The more efficient you become at drinking on the bike, the less energy you will expend doing so. You may want to slow down slightly when you refuel, but the more you practice, the better you can maintain your pace.

Despite the fact that biking keeps your GI system relatively stable, most triathletes prefer to consume the majority of their calories from fluids. Gels are also well tolerated. Many top competitors have come up with their own fluid-replacement formulas so that they can have something a bit more concentrated than a sports drink while on the bike, perhaps even adding a bit of protein at times as well. Of course, anyone who consumes these personalized products has experimented with them in training. As far as solids are concerned, they are generally kept to a minimum, but they can provide a nice chew in the middle of all that drinking. Make sure that you limit solids to well-proven, tolerable foods. Some good options are fruit bars, cut-up sports bars, and bananas. Only your stomach knows for sure what works best.

Pack more gels, bars, and other treats than you think you will need. This allows you to have choices and satisfy cravings. Tape gel packets to your bike for easy handling or plant them ahead of time in a pack or the pockets of a cycling jersey. Experiment with various carrying systems. You may want to try a bladder hydration system or seat-mounted and/ or aerobar-mounted bottle carriers in addition to the traditional frame-mounted water bottles. Pack your turnaround bag with fluids and foods, and allow yourself enough choices that you can select an item that appeals to you at the time.

Practice keeping up with your fluid requirements. Once you become dehydrated, it can be difficult to empty fluids adequately from your stomach. As you attempt to catch up with your fluid losses and drink more, your stomach will become uncomfortable and bloated. Despite your intake of fluids, you may experience the symptoms of fluid and carbohydrate depletion. It can be hard to differentiate among the symptoms to know whether you require more fluid or more carbohydrates. If you don't need to urinate, then you are not drinking enough or emptying your stomach adequately.

TRANSITION 2 (T2) AND THE RUN

Maintaining proper hydration and carbohydrate intake can be a challenge during the run portion of a triathlon. Running is harder on your GI system than cycling and more likely to result in nausea and bloating. Moreover, by the time the running leg rolls around, you have been exercising for several hours and your fluids and glycogen stores may already be running low. If you do try to drink, you may feel fluid jostling around in your stomach. Nevertheless, it is important that you stop or slow down at aid stations and make a point of drinking fluids. Most competitors choose to stay away from solids and stick with water, sports drinks, gels, and cola during the run. Because the risks of hyponatremia can increase as the race progresses, many competitors also bring along salt or electrolyte tablets or continue to hydrate with a high-sodium sports drink.

There are a variety of steps you can take to set yourself up for good GI tolerance during the run. The plan that is best for you depends upon individual tolerances. Some competitors find that it is best not to consume anything for the last 15 to 30 minutes on the bike and to keep their intake very light for the first few miles of the run. Other competitors successfully down a whole bottle of sports drink in T2. Knowing how you will fare best during this transition takes practice and experimentation in training.

Alternating among gels, sports drinks, water, and cola can support your carbohydrate and fluid needs during the run. Alternating cola with water helps dilute the higher carbohydrate concentration of the former. The caffeine in the cola may also stimulate your central nervous system and improve your focus during the race. Slow down when you approach aid stations. If you try to gulp fluid from the cups provided while keeping up your running pace, you may not actually get much of it down—most of the drink will spill out. Taking the time to drink should improve your overall performance.

If you consume gels during the run, make sure that you take them with plenty of fluid. Also, look for some flavor variety in your gels and drinks to avoid the taste boredom that can occur during a long race. Switching to a different flavor may be just the change you need to increase your intake. Keep in mind that some gels—and cola—are not as high in sodium as sports drinks. Often competitors make a point of consuming salt tablets during the run, but make sure that you do not take excessive amounts of them and that you have no medical contraindication for taking these tablets. Also, like gels, salt tablets should be consumed with plenty of fluid. When a race is held in a hot climate, triathletes who arrive from cooler environments and have not had time to acclimatize are at greater risk of hyponatremia. Slower triathletes are also at risk of developing this condition, as longer race times provide more opportunity for sodium losses that are not adequately replaced.

Unfortunately, it can be difficult to discern whether your stomach is emptying properly. The symptoms of inadequate emptying of fluids from the stomach and of inadequate carbohydrate consumption and absorption are similar. If you are not producing adequate amounts of urine, however, the chances are greater that the fluids are not emptying properly. Once you become dehydrated, your risk of GI upset increases significantly. Dehydration will delay emptying, and attempts to rehydrate at that point will upset your stomach further. It is best not to stop drinking altogether, so try sipping fluids a little at a time. If you overfill and vomit, regroup and slowly continue to sip fluids. Your body needs the fluids, but try not to give it more than it can handle at this point.

It can be equally difficult to discern whether you are suffering from low blood sugar during a race. If you feel mentally sharp, you probably have adequate glucose available to fuel your brain; if you feel irritable or spacy, however, you may be experiencing low blood glucose levels. If symptoms of hypoglycemia occur, try a gel or soda and see if symptoms improve. Experienced triathletes know that every Ironman is different and that one key to success is learning how to listen to the body and how to provide what it needs during the race.

ADVENTURE RACING

Adventure racing is the ultimate multisport experience and offers new and fun challenges to cyclists, runners, hikers, and water sports enthusiasts. Races may include a variety of sports, such as mountain biking, trekking, mountaineering, race navigation or orienteering, and rafting, canoeing, or kayaking. Longer races may include horseback riding, whitewater swimming, and even caving. Some races have special tests that focus on team-building and problem-solving skills. Racers know ahead of time what disciplines their race will include, but not the duration and succession of these disciplines, which, of course, are part of the adventure of adventure racing.

Because of the variety of race distances and types of challenges in adventure racing, there are several categories in which teams and individuals can compete. The longer races often allow or even require a support crew of one or two people to transport the team's gear to transition areas along the race course. In "unsupported" races, in contrast, race personnel transport the gear. Typically adventure races have no official rest times, and the competitors must make their own decisions about when to stop, rest, or even catch short periods of sleep. The shorter races normally have a single transition area for all competitors, so that support team assistance is not required. Many races are designed to have a coed team, though this factor varies among race categories.

Training programs for adventure racing are determined by the makeup and distance of the adventure race in which an athlete will be competing. All adventure racing requires a good endurance and strength base and the necessary skills for various sporting disciplines. Most adventure racers train for 10 to 12 hours or more weekly, depending on the goal in mind—that is, whether it is finishing or winning.

Adventure racers training for endurance generally build an endurance base at 60 to 70 percent of maximum heart rate and train for more than an hour at this intensity. Generally these workouts include cycling and/or running. Their endurance training also consists of long, hard workouts of back-to-back sports, such as hiking followed by canoeing, topped off with a bike or run. These sessions work out all areas of the body and help simulate an adventure race. To further simulate race conditions, athletes should practice carrying a pack in training and bring foods and fluids with them as they work out.

Preparing for an adventure race requires a focus on the proper training nutrition strategies. Because your training can vary with your next scheduled race and the makeup of your race, your training nutrition plan may need to be adjusted throughout the season. Some of the nutritional fundamentals that you can follow for any training program are described here:

Post-exercise recovery nutrition. Endurance training requires that you begin the recovery process shortly after exercise. After training sessions lasting longer than 90 minutes, focus on consuming 0.5 gram of carbohydrates for every pound (1 g/kg) of body weight, and add 10 to 20 grams of protein to the mix. Consume 24 ounces of fluid for every pound of weight lost during exercise. Include sodium in your post-exercise intake, particularly after training in the heat and humidity.

Daily recovery nutrition. Recovery nutrition continues for the next 24 hours or until the next training session. Refer to Chapter 4 to ensure that your carbohydrate intake matches that day's training and recovery requirements. Round out meals with adequate amounts of protein and fat. If you plan to train twice in one day, make sure that several meals and snacks are consumed every 2 to 3 hours between training sessions.

Hydrate and fuel during training. Train yourself to drink during exercise so that it will be easy for you to use various hydration strategies during the race. Focus on consuming optimal amounts of fluids, carbohydrates, and electrolytes.

Here are some other tips for staying hydrated and well fueled in adventure racing:

- Practice consuming 4 to 8 ounces of fluid every 15 to 20 minutes. Experiment to determine your favorite brands of sports drinks so that you can consume a variety of flavors while racing. Aim for 30 to 60 grams of carbohydrates per hour, and up to 75 to 100 grams per hour for ultraendurance sessions.
- Experiment with a variety of carbohydrate sources such as gels and bars. You will need these foods during longer training sessions and competitions and may benefit from them even during short races.
- During adventure racing, you may want to consume a variety of foods to relieve any taste boredom, particularly in the longer races. Experiment with pretzels, granola bars, sugary candy, dried fruit, gorp, Pop-Tarts®, panini, beef jerky, and anything that appeals to you and is well tolerated. Heavier foods can be consumed on days when your training efforts will be relatively low in intensity.
- You may be allowed to bring along foods such as instant soup and powdered mashed potatoes when you compete. Experiment with different items during training to discover what works for you.
- Train with high-sodium products if you anticipate racing in hot and humid conditions, and particularly if you are a salty sweater. Experiment with sports drinks that are relatively high in sodium, as well as sodium tablets, if needed.

Practice nutrition guidelines for resistance training. Since strength training is an important part of preparation for adventure racing, it is important that you practice the nutrition principles outlined in Chapter 6. If your goal is to build muscle mass, you may be able to take in 350 to 400 extra calories daily above your current training requirements. In addition, time your protein intake properly before and after training. During training you can also consume a sports drink to provide carbohydrates to your muscles and enhance the quality of your exercise sessions. Practice good recovery nutrition techniques after intense strength training sessions, particularly when they occur back to back with an endurance training session.

Practice eating while exercising when training for any length race and with equipment and strategies specific to your race profile and length. This is especially crucial for expedition racing, where racers must eat well and stay well hydrated day after day to be successful. Learning to eat comfortably at low exercise intensities and at transition areas is essential. Purposely run, hike, or bike at a slow, steady pace after eating to give your system a chance to digest this fuel. This will train your system to make the most of refueling opportunities and allow you to determine your tolerances and learn new strategies for staying fed and hydrated during racing. If you practice, you will know what portions and foods to consume at varying intensities. Generally, gels and liquid products work best during high-intensity efforts, while solid foods are a welcome change at relatively low intensities. Many adventure racers, particularly those competing in the longer distances, can train their stomachs to tolerate a higher level of fullness during exercise than other endurance athletes usually can manage.

Refer to the sport-specific nutrition fueling and hydration guidelines provided in Chapters 9 and 10. For each discipline in your training program, there are specific techniques that are best for fueling and hydrating. Practice these techniques and become accustomed to using various types of support equipment, such as a back-mounted hydration system, a hydration belt, and a pack. Seal electrolyte tablets in plastic to keep them dry, and pack solid food items efficiently for easy access. Some of the logistical challenges of staying hydrated during adventure racing can be solved with practice. Here are some methods to try:

- Keep a bladder hydration system in your backpack for readily available fluid. Have the bite valve accessible.
- Learn to carry and drink fluid when running. Rigging a system in which a straw for drinking is available right at your mouth can be helpful.
- Have a drinking system that works with the personal flotation device (PFD) that you wear when paddling. One team actually sewed their drinking system onto the top of their PFDs so that they could easily hydrate when on the water.

COMPETITION NUTRITION

When racing, always start out with a fueling and hydration plan that matches the duration, intensity, and profile of your race. The longer the race, the more detailed and complex your nutrition plan needs to be.

Race foods and fluids can be divided into several categories: sports nutrition supplements, processed foods, real foods, and cooked (or meal) foods for the transition

RACE FOODS AND FLUIDS

Sports Nutrition Supplements

Sports drinks
Gels
Energy bars
High-energy carbohydrate drinks
Liquid meal replacements
Electrolyte tablets

Processed Foods

Pop-Tarts®
Gummy bears
Sour Patch Kids®
Potato chips
Snickers® candy bar
Pretzels
Starbursts®
Fruit Roll-Ups®
M & Ms®
Twinkies®
Chocolate

Real Foods

Sandwiches (peanut butter, honey, jam)
Dried fruit
Nuts and seeds
Trail mix
Jerky
String cheese

Transition Area Foods

Pasta or ravioli
Rice
Oatmeal
Soup
Sandwiches
Bagels
Yogurt
Soy milk
Chocolate milk

area. How far you move through all the race food categories depends upon your race distance. For shorter races, the sports nutrition supplements on the market should be adequate. A list of these foods and fluids is provided in the sidebar "Race Foods and Fluids."

SPRINT RACE

Pre-race. When preparing for a race lasting 4 to 8 hours, make it a priority to rest for 24 to 48 hours before the starting time and consume the carbohydrate amounts recommended for carb loading as outlined in Chapter 5. Hydrate steadily, and consume plenty of sodium from foods and fluids in the days leading up to the race. For very early start times, plan for simple solid and liquid foods to refill your liver glycogen stores before the race.

During the race. Although relatively short adventure racing competitions may be called "sprints," they can still require up to a full 8 hours of race time. Races of this length include much steady-state activity along with periods requiring the competitors to move into higher gear. Nutrition plans for sprints should be based on the level of exercise intensity that is expected and your tolerance level for various food items. Sprint racers should be familiar with their sweat rate in specific race and weather conditions, and sports drinks should be their fluid and fuel staple. By race time, they should have developed drinking techniques and strategies for each race discipline. For races lasting 2 to 4 hours, gels can also contribute some important carbohydrate fuel. In the longer sprint races—that is, those lasting over 4 hours—you can also use more solid items, like gummy bears, Fruit Roll-Ups, and energy bars. Any solid items should be consumed with ample amounts of water. Find the mix of semisolid and solid items that works best for you by experimenting during training. Caffeine-containing gels and cola can also provide a needed brain and endurance boost for racers hitting the 8-hour mark.

After the race. Some weight loss from fluid depletion is expected during even a sprint race, but competitors should rehydrate steadily with sodium-containing fluids to minimize this as much as possible. Recovery nutrition emphasizing carbohydrates (with some protein) is recommended. Food sources containing sodium should also be included.

ATHLETE PROFILE

Racing Without a Nutrition Plan: Maddie

Maddie was excited and nervous about completing her first half-Ironman. She was an experienced runner and had caught the triathlon bug two years before, building up her race experience with a series of sprint- and Olympic-distance races. Her racing had gone well, and she wanted to venture into longer distances. She was confident that with all her long-distance training, her body was becoming more efficient at burning fat during exercise.

Prior to her race taper, Maddie's training peaked at 22 hours weekly. She practiced her intake of a carbohydrate electrolyte beverage on the bike, and felt that she was becoming more efficient at using fuel during training. Maddie is very weight-conscious and takes pride in her lean physique and 14 percent body fat level, which requires keeping an eye on portions even with her heavy training schedule.

Prior to race day Maddie emphasized carbohydrates in her diet but had no formal carbohydrate-loading plan. On race morning she consumed oatmeal and a banana, and she hydrated in expectation of the day's 88°F temperature and high humidity. Having done well in the swim, Maddie started on her bike with one bottle of her favorite sports drink. She slowly consumed the 24 ounces of fluid over the 54-mile segment. At about 42 miles, her nutrition strategy—or lack of one—hit her hard, with both low blood sugar and muscle fatigue. Maddie regrouped with a sports drink and gel offered on the course. She slowed below pace for the remainder of the bike leg and managed to pull it together for the run thanks to her extensive running background.

Maddie took two weeks to fully recover from the race and vowed to develop a more structured race nutrition plan for next season. Among the areas that Maddie planned to work on was devising a structured carbohydrate-loading plan with a sports dietitian. Maddie also wanted to increase her intake of carbohydrates before the race through a carbohydrate-loading meal plan but wanted suggestions for how to do this without having digestion problems. Finally, she vowed to learn about her personal sweat and electrolyte losses during training and focus on carbohydrate replacement on the bike so that she would be better prepared for the run leg of her next race.

NUTRITION FOR CYCLING
(ROAD CYCLING, MOUNTAIN BIKING, TRACK CYCLING, AND CYCLOCROSS)

Cycling is undoubtedly one of the most physically challenging sports that an athlete can pursue. It requires muscular strength, power, and endurance. Cyclists complete long aerobic training rides to prepare for competition, but they also incorporate a significant amount of anaerobic exercise into a program that includes intervals, sprints, and weight training. It is important that cyclists develop both the aerobic and anaerobic systems in order to compete at their best. Tactical savvy is also essential to success in cycling.

USA Cycling (USAC), the official cycling organization recognized by the U.S. Olympic Committee, has a membership of over 66,000 and sanctions more than 2,600 events across the country annually in a variety of formats from early spring to late fall. These competitions include road races varying in length from 15 to 80 miles, criterium racing, and time trialing. The sport of mountain biking is also popular, and in some areas of the country, track cycling is available. Cyclocross is a traditional off-season option, and many cyclists choose to participate in strength training during this

Focus on muscle building and increasing strength during the off-season.

Periodize nutrition based on your training cycle and body composition goals.

Start weight-loss efforts early in the season and employ a gradual calorie restriction.

Recalculate sweat rate as the season progresses and the weather changes.

Pre-ride eating increases muscle and liver glycogen stores, providing fuel for the ride.

Base pre-race meal timing on the intensity and duration of the race as well as the start time.

time of year. Thousands of other cyclists participate in recreational long-distance rides, some at a serious and focused level.

Road racing requires muscular endurance, the power to undertake surges in speed, and the ability to sprint at the end of a race. Depending on the level at which you compete, road races may last from 45 minutes to several hours. The ultimate in road racing is professional stage racing, particularly the 21-day Tour de France. Mountain bike racing requires mainly muscular endurance, but it also requires power for climbing steep hills and for sprinting at the finish. Cyclocross events are shorter but very intense and require superb bike-handling skills, the ability to ride well on varying terrain, and excellent technique in such skills as dismounting and mounting the bike. Although track racing demands mostly power from the cyclist, a good training program for this event incorporates long endurance rides. Of course, many recreational riders also complete long bike rides, especially in the warmer months, thus altering their nutritional requirements.

Cyclists typically train once daily but incorporate longer rides lasting several hours weekly, particularly on the weekends. Training can also include high-intensity rides as well as anaerobic threshold training, interval training, and sprint workouts, with the training becoming more specialized as the cyclist builds to his or her event during race season. It is not unusual for cyclists to train for 10 to 20 hours weekly during heavy training cycles. The training programs are unique to each discipline within cycling, but no matter which discipline a cyclist chooses to specialize in, meeting specific fuel demands for the type of training program and the period of training allows the cyclist to have optimal energy for both training and daily recovery.

TRAINING NUTRITION

TRANSITION PHASE (OFF-SEASON)

In the transition phase of a periodization training schedule, cyclists may train on the road, indoors on a wind trainer or rollers, or in an indoor cycling class or clinic. This off-season period is also a time to concentrate on strength training. Cyclists who live in warmer climates may put in some steady miles, but overall the volume and intensity of their training on the bike decrease at this time. Some choose to take a short break from cycling during this time and participate in other sports in order to cross-train.

If you strength train, proper nutrition can make the most of your program. Strength training helps you maintain lean body mass that is normally lost with the aging process.

It also improves your aerobic performance and helps prevent injury. Depending on your level of aerobic exercise, however, your overall calorie and carbohydrate requirements may be lower than at the height of the season. Training in the off-season simply does not require as much energy as training more than 15 hours weekly and completing rides lasting several hours.

You do need to consume enough calories to build muscle (see specific guidelines in Chapter 6). It takes 350 to 400 additional calories daily to build 1 pound of muscle, along with specific timing of protein intake around the resistance training sessions. If you are trying to shed pounds during the off-season, strict dieting can hamper your muscle-building efforts. Your protein intake should not increase significantly while weight training and may even be a bit lower than during the build cycle of the regular training season, though novice weight trainers may have slightly higher protein requirements. Protein requirements of 0.5 to 0.8 gram per pound of body weight are easily met with a well-balanced diet and nutritious food choices.

Muscle glycogen is an important energy source during weight training, so arrive for training sessions in a well-fueled state. To support your muscle-building efforts, aim for 10 to 20 grams of high-quality protein combined with 35 grams of carbohydrates within the hour before weight training. You can consider consuming a sports drink during training to maintain blood glucose levels, supply your muscles with fuel, and maintain adequate hydration. You should also practice recovery nutrition after a hard weight training session, combining both protein and carbohydrates to support muscle repair and rebuilding and to stimulate the replenishment of glycogen in your depleted muscles.

If you train outside during the colder months, you still need to replace fluid losses from sweating, though these losses may not be as significant as in hot and humid weather. If you are dressed warmly, you can lose up to 2 quarts (about 2 L) of fluid per hour through sweating. During cold-weather exercise, try to drink at least one full 20-ounce (500 ml) water bottle per hour. If the thought of a cold sports drink makes your teeth chatter, prepare your drink with warm or hot water. Hot decaffeinated tea mixed with plenty of honey can provide a carbohydrate boost. You can even dilute sweet drinks such as hot chocolate or hot apple cider for a warming treat while training. These warm liquids provide several advantages. They are easier to drink when it is cold outside, they provide a feeling of warmth, and they increase blood flow to the extremities by dilating blood vessels. Too, your body does not need to expend extra energy to warm them as it does with cold liquids. For the same reasons, keep any food you bring with you as warm as possible. Cold weather does create a greater demand for calories. Be sure to consume some carbohydrates while training, as shivering uses up fuel. So do your muscles during these winter sessions. In fact, long, low-intensity "fat-burning" rides slowly drain carbohydrate stores at a steady rate. It may be a good idea to eat close to your exercise session as this can have a warming effect. Make this meal or snack predominantly carbohydrates.

PREPARATORY PHASE (EARLY SEASON)

As spring draws near, most cyclists begin looking ahead to the racing calendar. The great outdoors begins to beckon to you for more miles, greater intensity, and perhaps even an early-season race or two. It is now time to carefully match the calories you burn on the bike with those you consume both on and off the bike. You may come into early-season training a bit heavier than your ideal racing weight and may be tempted to diet to shed a few pounds. Resist the temptation to reduce calories too severely, however, or to refrain from eating altogether during longer rides. Although these techniques may produce quick weight-loss results, they can also produce negative results, such as poor recovery, hypoglycemia during training, and intense hunger and subsequent overeating. Ultimately, restricting calories too much can hold you back in training. You don't want to end up feeling tired and overtrained just at the time when you were hoping to whip yourself into shape. After long rides, pay attention to the immediate post-exercise recovery nutrition guidelines outlined in Chapter 4. Refer to Table 4.4 for guidelines in matching your nutritional intake to your training volume and intensity.

BUILD PHASE

When training and racing season is in full gear, the number of calories your body burns—and its carbohydrate expenditure—become significant. Review Chapter 4 on daily recovery nutrition to ensure that you match your training with your carbohydrate intake and round out meals with adequate protein and fat. It can be difficult for cyclists to meet their energy and carbohydrate needs by consuming only three meals daily. Plan on snacks and possibly even incorporating high-calorie sports nutrition supplements into your diet. Some cyclists need more than 4,000 to 6,000 calories on heavy training days, an impossible food-consumption task without careful planning. Most successful cyclists are constantly grazing during the day. Large meals may make you feel heavy and sleepy, whereas several steady meals and snacks keep the recovery process going throughout the day.

Recovery Nutrition

Recovery nutrition is essential after long or intense training rides. You need 0.5 gram of carbohydrates per pound of body weight and smaller amounts of protein within 30 minutes after exercise to recover. When you train in hot and humid weather, make sure that you also consume sodium afterward to replace electrolyte losses and optimize fluid replacement. Have these recovery snacks readily available after rides. Fluids are an important part of your daily training diet. Carry or have fluid with you everywhere you go, on public transportation, in the car, and at your desk. Keep drinking, and make sure that you produce several full bladders of light-colored urine daily. Follow the daily hydration guidelines presented in Chapter 1. Check your weight before and after hard training to determine your sweat rate, and consume 24 ounces (720 ml) of fluid for every pound lost. If you are losing greater than 1 to 2 pounds (about 0.5 to 1 kg) of fluid weight during training, you are not keeping up with your fluid requirements as well as you should in training sessions. You may have a high sweat rate, or you may need to refine your drinking skills on the bike. You should also recheck your sweat rate at different points throughout the season, as it may increase as your fitness level improves, as the weather heats up, and as you become acclimated to the warmer weather. Refer to Appendix F, "Sweat Loss Calculator," to estimate sweat losses throughout the year.

Iron Intake

Cyclists should pay close attention to their iron intake. They can lose large amounts of iron through sweating and may have elevated iron requirements from their heavy training. Female cyclists should be especially careful to include good iron sources in their diet because of higher iron losses, though male cyclists are susceptible to being deficient as well. Have a physician monitor your iron stores, and supplement safely if necessary.

Bone Health

Cycling is not considered a weight-bearing sport, thus cyclists need to pay close attention to maintaining good bone health and preventing osteoporosis. This includes both men and women. While the causes of osteoporosis are multiple, consistent weight-bearing exercise and adequate calcium intake are two of the cornerstone recommendations for preventing this debilitating condition. Cyclists should incorporate weight-bearing exercise into their training year-round and consume at least 1,000 milligrams of calcium daily. If your diet does not provide this amount of calcium, a calcium supplement can make up the difference.

Body Fat Levels

Body fat levels are a big concern for cyclists. Many successful elite and professional competitors are extremely lean, but they also put in long hours of training, which is the most effective way to safely reach low levels of body fat. Severe dieting or attempts to become too lean too fast can result in fatigue, loss of muscle mass and power, and possibly overtraining. Some cyclists may have unrealistic body fat goals, and though losing excess body fat may improve climbing, it likely will have little impact on time trialing and sprinting. Striving for too low a level of body fat can compromise energy levels and even your health. Follow the guidelines for sensible weight loss presented in Chapter 6, and remember that a good cycling program requires quite a bit of energy to be successfully maintained. Be patient, and let the weight take care of itself with good training and proper eating.

HYDRATING AND FUELING ON THE BIKE

Cycling is a unique endurance sport in that refueling while you train is a relatively simple task in contrast to swimming or running, which present challenges in this regard. No other endurance sport keeps your gastrointestinal system so stable or so conveniently allows you to carry your food and fluids. This is fortunate, as the fluid and carbohydrate demands during training are high. Cyclists experience significant fluid losses, though they may be unaware of this as their sweat can evaporate quickly in the wind. This wind effect can also keep you from overheating and hide your need for fluid. Start training with a moderate volume of fluid to distend your stomach and enhance emptying, and start drinking as soon as you settle into the rhythm of your training ride. Aim for 4 to 8 ounces (120 to 240 ml) every 15 to 20 minutes, or the amount appropriate for matching or minimizing your sweat losses. Set your watch or heart rate monitor to remind yourself to drink on schedule. Once you become dehydrated, it will be difficult to catch up with your fluid requirements. Remember that riding in the heat, wind, or humidity also increases your fluid losses and therefore your fluid requirements.

You will dip significantly into your muscle glycogen stores during aerobic endurance rides lasting longer than 90 minutes. Muscle glycogen is also rapidly used for fuel when you complete interval and sprint training sessions, and it can reach low levels within even 1 hour of this type of training.

To obtain both fluid and carbohydrates, it makes sense to consume a sports drink during almost any type of training ride. Cyclists seem to be highly susceptible to "bonking," or reaching low blood glucose levels. Consuming a sports drink will maintain blood glucose and provide your muscles with a fuel source when they run low on glycogen. If you anticipate a longer training ride, consume a sports drink from the start. You can also bring along gels, bars, or bananas, which can be consumed with water if you need an occasional change from liquid carbohydrates. Just as it is difficult to catch up with your fluid needs when you are already dehydrated, it can be challenging to consume carbohydrates when your blood sugar is already low, so hypoglycemia is best prevented.

Because food and fluid can be carried on your bike, you can pack large fluid bottles filled with a sports drink. For longer rides, pack powdered drinks and reconstitute them in your emptied bottles along the way. You can plan out a route where water fountains are available or where water or sports drinks can be purchased. Bladder systems work well during more technical, off-road rides because they allow you to drink without taking your hands off the handlebars. You can also pack gels and bars in your jersey pockets or tuck them conveniently in the leg of your cycling shorts. If you find the taste of sports drinks too sweet in hot weather, look for milder or unflavored drinks. You can also alternate a good full swig of a sweet sports drink with a gulp of water on occasion.

Some cyclists believe that consuming plain water during long rides early in the season encourages more fat burning during the ride. This practice likely can only be tolerated for a limited time at very low intensities, however. Moreover, it takes more time to recover from a carbohydrate-free ride than it does to recover from a ride that includes refueling, so if you try to lose body fat this way, plan accordingly. You may need more time between training sessions, or you may decide that this strategy is not worth the stress that it places on your body. Don't plan on having good energy levels during the end of such a ride. You should never skip carbohydrate consumption on a ride when your primary goal is a good solid training experience designed to prepare you for a race.

Another technique for preparing yourself nutritionally is to eat and drink adequate amounts of fluid before a long training ride. Start with a good breakfast 2 hours beforehand, and consume plenty of carbohydrates according to the guidelines presented in Chapter 5. If you train in the evening, make sure you have a substantial afternoon snack providing 50 to 100 grams of carbohydrates 1 to 2 hours beforehand. Before very early morning rides, you may not have time for a good breakfast. But at least take a few minutes to down something simple, such as juice and toast. A small dose of pre-training carbohydrates is better than none at all, but make sure you consume carbohydrates during the ride to offset low morning liver glycogen stores.

DISCIPLINE-SPECIFIC GUIDELINES

What you eat in the days and hours before a race can have a positive performance impact. Smart pre-race eating provides several performance benefits. In particular, cyclists lower their chances of developing hypoglycemia, or low blood sugar (bonking), along with the accompanying feelings of fatigue, poor concentration, and light-headedness. Eating right for the race tops off your muscle glycogen stores and provides your exercising muscles with fuel during the race. Eating before racing helps to settle your stomach and prevent hunger pains during long races. Following the proper pre-hydration strategies before competition decreases your risk of developing dehydration during the race. You will also benefit psychologically from knowing that your body has been properly fed and you are as race-ready as you can be.

Cyclists should arrive at any race lasting longer than 60 minutes with adequate body stores of carbohydrates. Depending on your racing schedule, rest or taper for 24 to 48 hours and consume a diet adequate in carbohydrates. You can load up on carbohydrates before longer criteriums, time trials, road races, and a full race schedule of track cycling. It is especially important to rest and replenish your stores before a series of races that will take several days to complete. (See Chapter 5 for tips on carb loading.)

The foods you choose, the amounts you consume, and how you time your pre-race meal will largely be determined by your race start time, the type of race in which you are competing, and personal tolerances. For races lasting longer than 60 minutes, consume 30 to 60 grams of carbohydrates per hour during the race to prevent hypoglycemia and provide muscles with fuel later in the race. However, fluid consumption during a race is not as simple as fluid consumption during training. Depending on the type of race, bike racing often requires that you respond to sudden changes in speed, race tactics, and varying terrain.

ROAD CYCLING

Training Nutrition

Because of the nature of road cycling and the distance of the races, high training volumes are not uncommon in the sport, even for cyclists new to the racing scene. Early in the season, cyclists constrained by cold weather may participate in indoor wind-trainer sessions, indoor cycle classes, and weight training sessions.

Serious cyclists need to consume adequate carbohydrates for daily recovery, as well as protein to prevent muscle tissue breakdown during the long race season. Calorie requirements may be best met with three meals and several snacks daily. Adequate nutritional in-take is also essential to maintaining a strong immune system during the season. Cyclists often attempt to achieve low body fat levels to improve their power-to-weight ratio for climbing. Weight loss is best accomplished early in the season, and peak levels of leanness can be achieved through quality training. Both male and female road cyclists should take care to have adequate intakes of iron and monitor iron status during the season.

Competition Nutrition

During a full season of racing, a cyclist may compete almost weekly and even participate in a stage race. Cyclists should start all road events with good fuel and fluid stores. Road race start times can be as early as 8:00 a.m. and as late as 4:00 p.m. on a full day of racing that includes the various racing categories. You may have to travel to the race and eat your pre-race meal in the early-morning hours on the road. For road races that last longer than an hour, you should rest from training and consume adequate carbohydrates for 24 to 48 hours before the race. Most cyclists prefer to consume their pre-race meal 2.5 to 3 hours beforehand. As mentioned in Chapter 5, consume about 1 gram of carbohydrates per pound (2.5 g/kg) of body weight at this meal, more if tolerated. Small amounts of low-fat protein and tiny amounts of fat can also be included if your tolerances allow. Be sure to provide enough time for digestion to compensate for pre-race nerves.

Plan ahead for your race start time. If you have an early start time, it may still be worth eating 2 hours prior to exercise and then having a good warm-up. You can make this meal high in easy-to-digest carbohydrates such as liquid carbohydrates and sports nutrition supplements. If you need a smaller meal, consume ample amounts of a sports drink in the hour leading up to the race for both extra carbohydrates and hydration. Later morning starts may allow time for a large pre-race breakfast 3 or even 4 hours be-forehand. Top off this meal an hour before exercise with an easily digested item provid-ing 50 to 75 grams of carbohydrates, such as an energy bar and a banana, and consume plenty of fluids. Late-afternoon start times may allow you to sleep later and have a large pre-race breakfast followed by a snack. Or consider having an early breakfast and then a small meal 2 hours prior to the start time. Experiment with various start times and meals in training. Try to mimic the start time scenario of the most important races of the season during training so that you feel comfortable with your decisions on race day.

Plan for your warm-up. Make sure to drink adequately during your warm-up. Aim to drink a sports drink in the hours leading up to the race. Start the race with some fluid in your stomach to prime the stomach for gastric emptying during the race.

Begin fueling and hydrating early. During road races, make an effort to maintain good hydration levels as soon as you settle into the race. If the race lasts more than 60 to 75 minutes, a sports drink can maintain blood glucose levels and prevent glycogen depletion, ensuring adequate stores for your muscles later in the race. Make sure to drink gulps when the pace is relatively steady, as surges in the race may preclude drinking on the bike at key moments. Large volumes of fluid leave your stomach more rapidly than sips, and the pressures of racing are not conducive to steady sipping. Practice your drinking technique in training as much as possible—trying to mimic race conditions—and follow the pre-hydration guidelines from Chapter 5, starting 36 to 48 hours before the race.

During longer road races you may wish to try more concentrated sources of carbohydrates such as gels and pieces of energy bars. Just be sure to consume them with at least 6 to 8 ounces (180 to 240 ml) of fluid. If you are racing in very hot weather, sports drinks are your best choice, but you may need some plain water as well. Some very disciplined elite racers have trained their stomachs to consume one full bottle every half hour. Practice will also improve your ability to drink at very high intensities. Aim for at least 30 to 60 grams of carbohydrates per hour from the various products you consume and tolerate while racing. Commit to a specific number of bottles for the entire race, and try to drink on schedule. Practice your technique for receiving additional food and fluid in the feed zone.

If you are competing over a weekend in several back-to-back daily races, make sure to pay close attention to recovery nutrition. Stage races place plenty of stress on your fuel and fluid reserves. Pack supplemental products to ensure that you meet your carbohydrate needs and replenish glycogen stores prior to the next start time. It is essential that your recovery nutrition begin immediately after the race with ample carbohydrate intake combined with some protein. You should eat every 2 hours after completing a stage and even continue to fuel with a light snack before bedtime. When eating at restaurants, emphasize concentrated carbohydrate sources such as pasta, rice, potatoes, breads, and cereals. Pack some of your favorite high-carbohydrate snacks and supplements for the race, and stay away from unusual foods to avoid any gastric surprises during the event.

CRITERIUM RACING

Criteriums, or circuit races, are exciting to watch—they are often shorter in length than road races and higher in intensity, and are held on spectator-friendly courses. They require good bike-handling skills for cornering and surges in effort to keep up with breaks and maintain a good position during the race.

When preparing for a criterium, the pre-race meal and snack timing are especially precarious. You definitely want to allow enough time for digesting the pre-race meal, probably at least 3 hours to compensate for the very high-intensity pace of a criterium. Start the race optimally hydrated, as drinking during criterium racing can be difficult. To keep blood glucose levels steady, you can even down a carbohydrate gel in the 30 to 60 minutes before the race starts.

Consider keeping a sports drink in your water bottle, even for shorter races. The flavor can stimulate your desire to drink, and the carbohydrates keep blood glucose levels nice and steady, maintaining your brain's fuel supply as you navigate the criterium course. Drink whenever the opportunity presents itself, and become accustomed to drinking at higher intensities. Practice recovery nutrition after criterium racing, and make sure that you consume sodium and fluid after racing in hot weather.

TIME TRIALS

The individual time trial is often called the "race of truth," as it pits lone cyclists against the clock. Here the fastest cyclist over a given distance, whether a point-to-point race or multiple laps on a circuit, is the winner. Results are often determined by a fraction of a second, and riders do not have the benefit of drafting off another rider. Riders start one by one at specific intervals and complete the course as quickly as possible.

In the team time trial, teams race one at a time and work together to complete the course in the fastest time possible. Drafting plays a role as riders take turns "taking a pull" at the front, allowing the riders behind to do 30 percent less work at the same speed.

Time trials require rest and adequate consumption of carbohydrates. Your competition efforts will take mental concentration and steady-state exercise in the crouched position. A full stomach could interfere with being comfortable in this position. Allow at least 2 to 3 hours of digestion time following your pre-race meal. Rest and consume adequate carbohydrates for at least 24 hours prior to the time trial. Pre-hydrate, and consume a sports drink leading up to your start time for both the 40K individual time trial and the 50K or 100K team time trial.

You may consider consuming only water for a 20K time trial, as maintaining blood glucose may not be as much of a challenge for this distance when a proper pre-race meal is safely digested in your system. Choose a drink that stimulates your drive to drink. A sports drink is not necessary for shorter time trials, but it will not be detrimental, either. Sports drinks should definitely be used for efforts lasting longer than 1 hour. Make sure that your stomach does not get too bloated, and consume your fluid in sips. Practice consuming fluids in the crouched position so that you can drink as efficiently as possible during your time trial. You may want to try a bladder hydration system that will allow you to hold a more steady position on the bike while drinking. After the time trial, rehydrate and practice recovery nutrition.

TRACK RACING

Track racing takes place indoors or outdoors on a velodrome. Cyclists compete on fixed-gear bikes without brakes, and they are forced to pedal even when slowing down. Track cyclists use large gears, which take enormous amounts of power, and athletes competing at the elite level hit high speeds, with the top levels coming close to 50 miles per hour. Competitive track cycling includes very short individual and team sprints that last for less than a minute as well as longer sprints, such as the 500- and 1,000-meter time trials and the Kieren (2,000 meters), which lasts for about 2 minutes. Middle-distance events, which last for several minutes, include individual races (3,000 meters for women and 4,000 meters for men) and the 4,000-meter team pursuit. "Track endurance" events range in time from over 15 minutes to over 45 minutes and include races such as the Scratch Race (10K for women, 15K for men), the Points Race (25K for women, 40K for men), and the Madison (50K for men).

Training Nutrition

Training programs are specific to the types of events being raced. Sprint track cyclists usually have high levels of muscle mass and low body fat levels, and they strength train to build lean body mass. Their training rides generally consist of short, high-intensity repetitions with adequate periods of recovery. Training sessions are longer, with some endurance rides, when preparing for longer sprint events. Endurance road cyclists often compete in the longer track races, developing their sprint training for these events.

For training, sprint track cyclists need to maintain a caloric balance and a carbohydrate, protein, and fat mix that will optimize the power-to-weight ratio by keeping muscle mass and keeping body fat levels down. Too much calorie restriction can result in inadequate carbohydrate intake for the volume and intensity of training and can cause loss of lean body mass. Instead of undereating, these cyclists may need to engage in cross-training sessions to decrease body fat levels. Endurance track cyclists tend to have a lighter and leaner build than road cyclists.

Competition Nutrition

Because of the highly intense nature of track racing and the number of races an athlete may complete in a day, meal and snack timing for race day is a complicated matter, and good planning is essential. Although inadequate body fuel stores are not a performance-limiting factor for a single sprint event, the fuel demands of competing in successive multiple events can be high. Prior to the event, carbohydrate loading is not necessary, but you should eat adequately in the days leading up to competition and maintain adequate muscle glycogen stores for the start of a competitive day. Your pre-race meal should consist of comfortable and familiar carbohydrate foods. Endurance track cyclists should keep the carbohydrate amounts high to top off glycogen stores for their event. If you race in the evening, what you eat earlier in the day is essential for maintaining fuel stores for the later start. Make sure that your last meal is at least 3 hours before the start of your warm-up. You can consume easy-to-digest carbohydrate supplements such as gels and bars 1 or 2 hours before the start to keep blood glucose levels steady, especially if you compete in longer track events.

Track bikes do not have bottle cages, and it is not practical to hydrate during these short, high-speed races anyway. But it is important to pre-hydrate leading up to the warm-up with water or a sports drink. Look at the timing of your race schedule. Hydrate between races with a sports drink to offset fluid losses and keep blood glucose levels elevated for each race. If your schedule allows for some digestion time, plan to consume some easy-to-digest carbohydrate foods between events. Gels can provide a quick carbohydrate hit between sessions when more solid items would not be tolerated. Energy bars can also be useful for fueling and refueling, providing protein as well as carbohydrates for longer time intervals between events. Liquid meal replacements can be consumed sometime in a full day of track racing. Hydration throughout the day should be steady, particularly in hot environments.

OFF-ROAD RACING

Mountain bike racing is performed on varying terrain and includes climbs, descents, and challenging single-track sections. What started as a fun recreational sport is now included in the Olympic Games. Competitive races include a number of disciplines. Cross-country events can be point-to-point races, with distances ranging from 15 to 62 miles (25K–100K), or they can take place on a circuit course with a loop of at least 3 miles. In the circuit events, riders complete a predetermined number of loops based on their racing category, with races lasting from 1 to more than 2 hours. Short-course circuit events are also available. Mountain bike races can be timed, and they can be quite long. Some go as long as 12 to 24 hours. These longer races can be completed solo or in teams.

Besides a solid endurance base, cross-country mountain bikers develop a high level of skill, and their training combines road and off-road riding, with the mix changing throughout the season. Downhill mountain bikers complete the majority of their training on the trails, and they may include aerobic work and a strength component in their training to develop power.

Many recreational mountain bikers ride off-road regularly. Others may have to travel some distance to spend a day training or competing off-road. Elite cross-country riders tend to be lean and strong, as an excellent power-to-weight ratio is optimal for hill climbing.

Training Nutrition

The volume and intensity of training required for cross-country mountain bike racing call for a diet matched to energy expended in calories, carbohydrates, and protein. These athletes should plan an optimal daily training diet when preparing for races and events. Recovery nutrition is essential after hard workouts and between twice-daily training sessions. High-intensity sessions deplete muscle glycogen stores quickly and should be followed by proper recovery nutrition and daily fueling. Nutritional guidelines should also be followed before and after weight training sessions (see Chapter 6). Recreational riders can match their intake to training levels as well. Although they would be expected to have somewhat lower levels of energy expenditure than focused racers most of the time, they may have periods of high-volume exercise on the bike on some excursions.

Achieving an optimal level of body fat can improve performance when climbing, but body-composition goals are best achieved through a combination of quality fueling and training. Calorie restriction that would compromise recovery is not recommended and could ultimately hurt your performance if you attempt to lower body fat too much. Dieting could also result in the loss of power if there is loss in muscle mass and inadequate body fuel stores for rides and races.

During rides lasting over 1 hour, plan to hydrate and fuel with a sports drink. Off-road fluid supplies can be carried in a back-mounted hydration system, and two water bottles can be mounted on the bike. Other portable sources of carbohydrate are gels, energy bars, and blocks.

Competition Nutrition

Race start times in the various off-road categories are generally staggered throughout the day, so it is very important that you time your pre-race meals and snacks carefully for your start. Your stomach can experience some jostling during a mountain bike race or when you ride over tricky terrain, and race day nerves can also affect your digestion. Focus on consuming optimal amounts of carbohydrates, sodium, and fluids the day before, the night before, and the morning of the race.

You can carbohydrate-load for long race events by consuming 3 to 5 grams of carbohydrates per pound (7–10 g/kg) of body weight. Keep protein portions moderate and fat intake low in the 24 hours prior to the event. Hydrate enough that your urine is pale yellow in color, and salt your food if you are a salty sweater and anticipate racing in hot and humid conditions. Consume your pre-race meal about 3 hours before the start time (see Chapter 5 for more on the pre-race meal size), and include tolerable amounts of low-fat protein. Although early-morning starts may necessitate that you simply get up early and consume the pre-race meal in the appropriate time frame, later start times can be trickier. For example, for a noontime start you may need to consume a hearty breakfast 4 to 5 hours prior to the start, and then a small to moderate carbohydrate snack 2 hours before the start. Plan ahead for your race start and experiment with food choices, portions, and timing. You should also consume a sports drink to steadily hydrate in the hours leading up to the start. Many mountain bike racers like to down a gel in the 30 to 60 minutes before the start for one last carbohydrate boost.

It is more difficult to drink fluids during mountain bike races than during road races, so it is important to start the race well hydrated. Consume 8 to 20 ounces (240–600 ml) of fluid 2 hours before the start, and an additional 8 ounces (240 ml) in the hour before the start, to prime your stomach and improve stomach emptying during the race. In many sections of the race it may be impossible to let go of the handlebars. Make a conscious effort to drink during gradual climbs, dirt roads, paved sections of the course, and relatively comfortable descents. During tricky descents or when climbing over rough terrain, you will be less inclined to drink. If you have an opportunity to preview the course before the race, try to determine which sections are more conducive to refueling and rehydrating.

Many mountain bike racers use a bladder hydration system so that they will have access to at least one source of fluids without having to let go of the handlebars. These systems provide adequate fluid for the first one or two laps; after that, you can consume a sports drink from a water bottle or have a friend pass you a bottle in the feed zone. Set a goal to consume a certain amount of fluid per lap as dictated by your sweat rate—a bottle per lap may work well. Sports drinks work best because of the carbohydrates they contain. Aim to consume 30 to 60 grams of carbohydrates per hour from your sports drink. For longer races you may want to consume a carbohydrate gel, but during hot races keeping up with your fluid needs is essential. Choose a sports drink or gel relatively high in sodium if you are a salty sweater.

24-HOUR RACES

Twenty-four-hour races require riders to complete as many laps of a cross-country circuit as possible within a 24-hour time frame. Riders may compete solo or in groups, with the groups ranging in size from two to ten. Each individual lap can be completed in anywhere from 45 to 90 minutes depending on the level of the rider and the distance of the lap. Obviously, solo riders have a daunting nutritional challenge ahead of them. Team members have time between laps to rehydrate, refuel, digest, and even nap. The larger the team, the more time individual riders have for recovery. Because they get a break to rest, riders in 24-hour races can monitor their weight for sweat loss to prevent becoming dehydrated and even to prevent overhydrating.

Solo Riders

Solo riders need to contend with the challenge of riding the entire race with only short stops or slowdowns through the transition zone to refuel and rehydrate. Keeping up with fluid, carbohydrate, and sodium requirements while working within gastrointestinal tolerances during an ultraendurance race can be challenging. Carbohydrate loading in the 2 to 3 days before the race is recommended to arrive at the start with full body fuel stores. Sports drinks provide a good balance of fluid, carbohydrates, and sodium, and the relatively high-sodium options are recommended for a race of this duration. Depending on the course profile, riders can drink regularly every 15 minutes or on specific sections of the course that are conducive to drinking, such as fire roads and the start/finish of the loop. Riders should be familiar with their rate of sweat loss at the planned race pace and in various weather conditions. Other sources of carbohydrates that work well are gels, energy bars, bananas, and high-sodium items such as salted crackers. Bring a variety of foods to the race, as your tastes and cravings change throughout the long race. A variety of sports drink flavors that you have tested during training can also prevent flavor fatigue. Choose more solid items carefully, as you are racing the entire time and your stomach can become more sensitive as the race progresses. Consume solid bites or more concentrated drinks as needed for a carbohydrate boost. Cola can provide a caffeine boost during the race to help with mental focus and concentration.

Pairs

Teams of two generally trade places every one to two laps, allowing one rider to rest and refuel while the other is on the course. Depending on the length of the lap and the speed of the rider, the resting rider may have 60 to 120 minutes or more to refuel in preparation for his or her next turn on the bike. A sports drink high in sodium should be consumed on the course. Riders can bring gels, bars, jam sandwiches, a variety of fruits, and dry cereals to eat between laps as tolerated. Experiment with various carbohydrate food items while simulating race conditions to see what works best for you.

Small Teams

Riders on teams consisting of three or four members have longer recovery times between laps than pairs, often at least 2.5 hours, and sometimes even 3 to 4 hours. Although these team members should still focus on maintaining their fluid, carbohydrate, and sodium intake on the bike, there is less pressure to keep up with rehydration and refueling on the bike in this kind of race. To allow plenty of time for stomach emptying, digestion, and absorption of nutrients, however, riders should consume both food and fluids immediately after coming off the bike. Try solid items such as sandwiches, pasta, energy bars, and fruit. Keep taking fluids up to your next lap, but don't overhydrate, and be careful not to overeat. Consume protein foods wisely, keeping portions small, and avoid fat because it takes longer to digest. Include items that are high in sodium, such as broth and other soups, as well as a variety of flavors and choices over the 24-hour period.

Large Teams

Teams of six or more riders have time to digest between laps. They can keep their hunger under control and their blood glucose levels steady by eating a large carbohydrate snack 3 to 4 hours or more before their next lap start and a smaller snack of easily digested carbohydrates 1 to 1.5 hours before the lap start. Consumption of solid foods should decrease the closer you get to the start time for your next turn. Riders should consume some fluid during the lap and hydrate as needed at the completion of each lap.

CYCLOCROSS

Cyclocross takes place on a grassy loop, usually a few miles long, with a few short road or dirt road sections. There are numerous sections where riders must dismount to navigate man-made barriers. Muddy, wet, and snowy conditions are not uncommon for this race discipline, which is technically challenging and fast. Cyclocross training and competition are very high in intensity. Riders often train twice daily, and they need to take care to get enough calories and nutrients to support this training. But the most important nutritional considerations for cyclocross have to do with what takes place 24 hours before the race start time.

Though cyclocross race times may last only 45 to 60 minutes, it is prudent to optimize your muscle glycogen stores the day before a race. Because of the high intensity of cyclocross racing, muscle glycogen depletion can occur quickly. To boost muscle glycogen stores, allow yourself 24 hours of rest or light training, and focus on adequate carbohydrate consumption during this taper. Avoid scheduling training sessions close to race day that could result in muscle damage, as this would impair your muscle glycogen stores. If you are competing twice in one weekend, practice good recovery nutrition after the first race.

With pre-race meal timing, err on the side of caution and allow plenty of time for digestion in order to avoid "cross-gut." Pre-race nerves may further accentuate gastrointestinal upset. Most cyclocross racers prefer to allow 3 to 4 hours of digestion time and to focus on easy-to-digest carbohydrate foods. If your race begins after noon, factor in two pre-race meals. Have a large breakfast, and then a small "lunch" 3 hours prior to your race consisting mainly of carbohydrate-based breakfast foods. Drink plenty of fluids several hours before the race for optimal hydration. Many seasoned cyclocross racers prefer to stop fluids 30 minutes before a race to avoid feeling bloated on the bike. Gels and sports bars can also be consumed in the 2 hours before race time if well tolerated.

At the starting line, your nutritional options are limited, as cyclocross racing is done without a water bottle cage. Many racers try a carbohydrate gel at the starting line or halfway through the race for a carbohydrate boost, as the risk of bonking during cyclocross seems to be high. Even with a bottle hand-up once per lap, you may be able to manage only a few gulps of fluid because of the course and race dynamics.

DOWNHILL RACING

Downhill races typically last from 2 to 5 minutes over a 1.5K to 3.5K course. Racers need to navigate a mix of rapid descents and technical sections over single tracks, rocky tracks, and forest roads. The "4 Cross" is a downhill event in which four riders compete against each other and pass through a series of gates, with riders typically taking 30 to 40 seconds to cover the course. In the "Dual Slalom," two riders race head-to-head down two parallel slalom courses, with runs lasting 20 to 45 seconds. And in the "Observed Trials," competitors navigate a series of obstacles, and points are deducted for mistakes.

When you are preparing for a downhill event, it is important to make sure you are well fueled, well hydrated, and physiologically and psychologically comfortable at the starting gate. Although each individual race takes only a matter of seconds or minutes to complete, you may do some practice runs that day, and you may have to make several runs during the full schedule of competition. Whatever your training regimen was the day before, make sure that you have matched your output with adequate carbohydrates and calories for your intake. In fact, consuming carbohydrate amounts slightly above your requirements will ensure that your glycogen stores are fully replenished for race day.

When planning your pre-race meal, allow ample time for digestion. Three hours is ideal, but if this is not practical for your start time, modify the timing and the meal accordingly. If this time interval is feasible, aim for 1 to 1.5 grams of carbohydrates per pound (2–3 g/kg) of body weight. Practice with food choices and portions before high-intensity training sessions similar to your expected competition efforts. In the hours leading up to the start time, you can maintain blood glucose and fluid levels by sipping a sports drink. Try consuming gels to maintain adequate blood glucose levels, which are imperative for focus, quick decision making, and skillful bike handling.

You may need to consume a steady supply of easily digested carbohydrates throughout the day to maintain your energy levels through multiple runs. High-carbohydrate energy drinks, sports drinks, gels, and energy bars make good choices, so plan ahead and organize your nutrition supplies. Fluid losses may be exacerbated in downhill racers who wear heavy protection equipment and clothing that covers arms, legs, and hands, so steadily hydrate throughout the day of competition.

RECREATIONAL DISTANCE CYCLING

Recreational cyclists often ride a significant number of weekly miles, though they may exercise at lower intensities than cyclists preparing for competition. However, if your goal is to complete a century or another long ride in a specified period of time, there is a sufficient amount of high-intensity training in your weekly program to make it worth your while to pay special attention to nutrition. Overall, your diet should emphasize the carbohydrate amounts that match your training for both shorter weekday rides and longer rides. Especially with the longer rides, you need to focus on replenishing your muscle glycogen stores. After very long rides, recovery nutrition is helpful not only for replenishing these stores but also for minimizing your fatigue over the next several days.

If you ride after work or commute back and forth to work on your bike, make sure that you always carry adequate fluids and focus on hydration both on and off the bike. Pale urine indicates that you are well hydrated.

When preparing for longer weekend excursions, including centuries, resting for 24 to 48 hours before your ride and consuming a diet rich in carbohydrates will fill up your muscle glycogen stores. Eat a meal high in carbohydrates several hours before the ride to replenish your liver glycogen. When you ride longer than 90 minutes, even at lower intensities, make an effort to consume 30 to 60 grams of carbohydrates per hour from sports drinks to maintain your hydration and blood glucose levels. Because you will likely be riding at a relatively low intensity in comparison with competitive cyclists, consuming solid foods and gels along with water during the ride may be simply a matter of taking an enjoyable and relaxing break.

One of the benefits of being part of an organized ride is the accessibility of the fuel stations that supply water, fresh fruit, sports drinks, treats, and a variety of easily digested carbohydrates. You can also pack some of your favorite on-bike foods and store them in your jersey pockets and in various bike bag options. Experimentation will teach you what foods work best for your stomach. It is best to start refueling early to prevent hypoglycemia. If you do start to manifest some of the symptoms of hypoglycemia, slow down and take in some carbohydrates.

Aim for a steady supply of fluid and fuel. Know your sweat rate for the conditions and intensity at which you plan to ride. One quart (960 ml) of a sports drink provides around 56 grams of carbohydrates. Add semisolid and solid items carefully, and take in these products with at least 8 ounces of water. If you consume several hundred calories at a rest station, make sure that you give yourself a bit of digestion time at rest. Seasoned cyclists can learn to increase their tolerance for more solid items on the bike, but keep in mind that hydration with a sports drink is always your first priority.

ATHLETE PROFILE

Finding a Balance Between Fueling and Staying Lean: Jake

Jake is a young cyclist competing in college with aspirations of going pro. Knowing that many top cyclists strive to be lean to improve both their strength-to-weight ratio and their climbing ability, Jake had his body fat checked by the exercise physiology department at his college: it measured 7 percent with calipers at 183 pounds. Jake wanted help lowering his percentage to the 5 percent many cyclists aim for, and he was interested in sample menus and advice on increasing the variety of foods in his diet. He decided that he would benefit from seeing a sports dietitian.

Jake kept a journal of his current diet, which the sports dietitian reviewed. It showed he incorporated many high-quality foods in his diet but that the quantities were inadequate for recovery and for the volume and intensity of his training. Based on his current training cycle, the sports dietitian developed meal plans and menus for each type of training ride that Jake currently completes. This includes early-morning sessions, interval workouts, and longer training rides. Each meal plan provides a specific amount of calories from carbohydrates, proteins, and fats. The sample menus outline how Jake should time meals and snacks and what portions he should consume around training. Jake had

been limiting his carbohydrate intake in hopes of burning more body fat and losing weight. Because of this practice, the sports dietitian specified the amounts of fluid, carbohydrate, and electrolytes he should consume during interval training and longer rides.

Jake was surprised at the increase in his food intake. He had thought that being lean and teaching his body to burn more fat were the two most important nutritional strategies that he could follow to improve his performance. The sports dietitian carefully laid out the principles of training nutrition for Jake and explained that an increased intake, particularly from carbohydrate, would provide more fuel for training, replenish muscle fuel stores, and allow him to train harder and longer, particularly on rides taking several hours.

Jake embraced the new nutrition program, began planning ahead for meals and snacks, and now brings sports drinks on his rides. He also now consumes more food and fluids before his morning training rides and consumes more carbohydrates on the bike, and he has expanded his portions at meals following longer rides. In two weeks' time, Jake reported that his energy level had improved significantly and that he was recovering better from tougher training rides. He reported a

continues

Finding a Balance (continued): Jake

2-pound (about 1 kg) weight gain, which the sports dietitian attributed to better fuel stores rather than any unwanted gains in body fat. Jake found that with the improved diet he had better strength for climbing as well. He also learned new recipes and foods to prepare and has been able to expand the variety in his diet.

Despite Jake's minor weight gain, his body fat showed a slight decrease when retested. His daily recovery was good, and testing indicated that his power had improved. Jake plans to continue his present nutrition program in preparation for a summer race series.

NUTRITION FOR
DISTANCE RUNNING

10

AT A GLANCE
KEY POINTS

Fluid and electrolyte replacement is imperative when running in hot, humid climates.

Carb replacement is key to maintaining a desired pace and completing longer runs.

Train with the sports drink offered on the course, and refine drinking skills.

Practice your pre-race eating and fueling plan during weekly long runs.

Prioritize recovery nutrition after hard training runs, after long runs, and if training twice daily.

Runners should determine they have adequate iron stores and increase as needed.

Follow a carbo-loading plan 2 to 3 days before a long-distance race.

Participation in the sport of running currently stands at an all-time high. The number of marathon finishers in the United States exceeded 500,000 in 2010. In 2010 the majority of large marathons reported being sold-out or enjoyed record fields. In fact, the average running time for the marathon is getting longer, reflecting the extent to which participation in this race has expanded. The half-marathon distance has the highest level of participation of any distance race, with more than 1.4 million finishers in 2010. Much of this increase has been fueled by charity and non-charity training programs, as well as destination events, runners moving up or down from the marathon, and women's participation. Running is no longer just for the lean and elite—people of all ages and fitness levels are joining in and becoming healthier in the process.

Other popular race distances are 8K (4.8 miles), 5 miles, 10 miles, 15K (9.3 miles), and 20, 25, or 30K (12, 15, or 18 miles). There are also ultradistance events, such as 50K (31 miles), 100K (62 miles), and 100-mile events. Although these do not attract as large a number of participants, they are as popular as ever, with more than several hundred certified ultrarunning events in 2010.

Distance runners tend to improve their performance with age, and many run and train for more than a decade before they reach their best running times. Recreational runners are often satisfied to simply run for optimal fitness and health and enjoy the social aspects of running. Whatever a runner's level of training and competition, paying heed to nutritional considerations can enhance his or her participation in the sport. For recreational runners, that might mean simply feeling better and enjoying greater health benefits. For elite runners, proper nutrition can provide just the boost in performance that is needed to reach top goals.

TRAINING NUTRITION

Because there is such wide variation in running—with some runners just starting out at the 5K level and others running marathons or ultradistance events—training programs vary widely. Some runners may have just signed up for their first charity run, while others are planning to race in a dozen or more events during the year, perhaps at a variety of distances. Even an experienced marathoner may choose to compete in an early-season 10K race and a half-marathon while building up to the marathon of his or her choice for the season. Because of the broad range of competitive goals, training programs are somewhat specific to the athlete. Running sessions may include longer runs designed to develop aerobic endurance, on the one hand, and intense runs and interval work designed to improve the anaerobic system and speed, on the other. Training nutrition has to take all this into account and be flexible enough to be adapted to any level.

COMPETITIVE SEASON

Most large road races are scheduled from spring to late autumn, though some winter-season marathons are held in warmer parts of the country. The schedule of big-city marathons—such as in Boston, Los Angeles, Chicago, and New York—extends from April to November. Cross-country high-school and collegiate racing has a fall season, with many participants competing in winter and spring-season track. Elite runners may compete in a number of races of varying distances over the season, with some key events for preparation and peaking.

Events in hot weather usually have early-morning starts to avoid the heat. Late-season marathoners may train in hot conditions but find that race temperatures can be a wild card, with unseasonable cool or hot temperatures. Weather considerations affect the nutrition plan for race day.

Distance racing is mainly an aerobic activity, with elite runners completing a 10K race in less than 30 minutes and a marathon in just over 2 hours. Recreational runners can take more than twice as long to complete these events. Despite their aerobic natures, there are times when these races require more anaerobic effort, such as in a surge, hill, or sprint finish. Successful runners have a high maximal aerobic capacity and an economical running style, low muscularity in their upper body, and a low level of body fat.

Many factors affect the outcome of a race, including fluid and electrolyte balance and the availability of carbohydrate fuel. Typically runners go more slowly in races in heat and humidity to compensate for their absorption of environmental heat. Smaller runners are more protected from overheating.

With daily and perhaps twice-daily training sessions, attention should be placed on recovery nutrition, pre-run fueling, and fueling during the run, particularly when two hard sessions take place back-to-back. Careful preparation for the long run is crucial to successfully complete their training and be prepared on race day.

FUELING FOR TRAINING

Eating too much too close to training or competition for your own personal tolerances is probably the biggest nutritional mistake that you can make as a runner. Because running jostles your gastrointestinal system, GI disturbance is a more common problem in running than in other endurance sports. Timing your pre-exercise meals is important for feeling "light" during your run and avoiding unpleasant symptoms such as a sloshing stomach, bloating, cramping, and diarrhea.

Prior to a short, relatively easy run, what you eat before training may simply be a matter of comfort and fending off hunger or hypoglycemia. It is not uncommon for runners to train in the early-morning hours. Some experiment and find that having something light, such as juice and a plain piece of toast, works best at this time. Regardless of your tolerances, make sure that you drink water or even a sports drink to hydrate. On long morning runs, consider taking a fluid bottle or fluid belt with you. Consuming a sports drink maintains blood glucose levels in the latter part of a longer run, but even on shorter runs it is good practice. It prepares you for longer races, and it helps in any run that occurs after you have not eaten for several hours, whatever the time of day.

Consuming regular meals and snacks replenishes your fluctuating liver glycogen stores and consequently helps maintain steady blood glucose levels throughout the day and during training. For afternoon or evening runs, try to time your meals carefully and eat 3 or more hours before running. Leave enough space between meal or snack times and training times, especially for high-intensity runs and speed work. Emphasize carbohydrate sources that are easily digested. You may want to consider a liquid sports supplement, a meal-replacement product, or an easily digested gel before longer training sessions. Real food products also work well if you have experimented and determined your own tolerances.

FUELING FOR THE LONG RUN

Experiment with pre-race eating before your long weekend run. This practice sets the stage for race day—it is particularly important to know your tolerances and preferences when racing a distance of 10 miles (16K) or longer. Although it may be tempting to sleep as late as possible before a long early-morning run, the pre-exercise meal is necessary for filling both liver and muscle glycogen stores. Liquid meals may work best, but you can also experiment with carbohydrate foods that are low in fiber. Knowing what works for you in training will help lighten pre-race nerves and help you feel more comfortable about your nutritional choices on the big day.

Ideally, take in as much carbohydrate as you can tolerate up to 1 gram per pound (about 2 g/kg) of body weight 2 hours before the long training run. Although you may leave a longer time interval after eating before a race start, this is still essential practice for having a quality and well-fueled long run. If you decide to eat even closer to the long training run, lower your carbohydrate intake to half a gram per pound (about 1 g/kg) of body weight. Food choices should be kept simple. Two hours prior to a long run, a 160-pound (73 kg) runner could consume more than 100 grams of carbohydrates from 2 slices of toast topped with 2 tablespoons (40 ml) of jam, plus 12 ounces (360 ml) of orange juice. After this meal and leading up to the run, 24 ounces (960 ml) of a sports drink would provide an additional 40 grams of carbohydrate or more.

Some simple morning noshes that sit easy in your stomach and pick up your run include:

- ½ bagel with 1 tsp. (8 ml) peanut butter and 1 tbsp. (20 ml) jam with 8 oz. (240 ml) juice
- ½ cup instant oatmeal with 4 oz. soy milk and 1 tbsp. (20 ml) raisins
- 1 medium-sized high-carbohydrate energy bar and 1 banana
- Pretzels and hummus with a glass of juice

- Liquid meal replacement
- Crackers with a nut spread and banana
- Smoothie with milk, yogurt, and fruit
- Tortilla with peanut butter and raisins
- Chocolate milk and grapes
- Toasted waffle with syrup and fruit
- Bowl of rice and juice

Of course, coffee or tea, or a glass of water, can be included with all of these suggestions. Even with a good morning carbohydrate boost, longer or higher-intensity morning runs may call for use of sports drinks. Experiment with pre-run foods and fluids, as well as with water or sports drinks during your run, to determine what provides the best energy boost within your tolerances.

HYDRATION AND FLUIDS

Runners should focus on consuming fluids throughout the day and maintaining adequate hydration. Light-colored urine indicates that you are well hydrated. Try to consume about 8 to 12 ounces (240 to 360 ml) every hour when not training, and practice the pre-hydration guidelines outlined in Chapter 5. Find the best timing to prevent sloshing in your stomach during training. It is helpful to hydrate well during the day, but step up your fluid intake within an hour of your run. Some of your early-morning carbohydrate food choices can also be hydrating fluid choices, such as a high-carbohydrate sports beverage, a sports drink, juice, soy milk, or dairy milk. Hydrating before a morning run, especially a run of more than 45 minutes, is important, so consume what you can beforehand as your stomach and time allow.

RECOVERY NUTRITION

Hard training runs, and particularly twice-daily sessions, require that you pay attention to recovery nutrition. Running can cause some damage to muscle fibers, which can delay glycogen recovery. Carbohydrate intake immediately after training will start the process of muscle glycogen resynthesis and prevent the gradual process of muscle glycogen depletion that can occur over several days' time or longer. Consume 0.5 gram of carbohydrates per pound (1 g/kg) of body weight immediately after exercise and plenty of fluids for recovery. You can also add 10 to 20 grams of protein, as this may aid in muscle repair. Monitor your weight before and after running to determine sweat losses, and consume 24 ounces of fluid for every pound lost. Consuming sodium after training, particularly in hot weather, can aid in the rehydration process. Make sure that you continue to rehydrate the rest of the day, and use your weight as a gauge of hydration.

After a morning run, you could consume a breakfast of cereal, milk, and fruit with a glass of juice. After an evening run, a recovery drink can hit the spot. Don't forget to consume the same amounts of carbohydrates and protein again in 2 hours to continue the recovery process. This could mean a mid-morning snack of yogurt and fruit, or a dinner containing carbohydrates from rice, pasta, potatoes, or some type of whole grain. Remember that thirst is not the most sensitive indicator of fluid needs. Continue to rehydrate in the hours after the run.

Runners training in hot weather may find that their appetite is limited immediately after training. Smoothies are a refreshing and hydrating choice that packs in plenty of carbohydrates and protein. Frozen fruit is also appealing, as are frozen yogurt and similar cold treats, including sorbet and sherbet.

Runners who incorporate high mileage for distance running need to pay close attention to recovery nutrition. If you plan two training sessions in one day, be sure to refuel immediately after the first training session. Then, consume a meal or snack every 2 hours until the next workout, taking care to choose easily digested foods as the time for the next run approaches. If the second workout is a weight training session, consume the recommended amounts of protein and carbohydrate beforehand, as outlined in Chapter 6.

BODY COMPOSITION

Elite distance runners are typically lean and thin, most likely due to a combination of genetics and a high volume of training. Runners at any level, aware that carrying "dead weight" does not enhance performance, may develop weight-loss goals. An important first step when losing weight is to have your body composition assessed. If you are already lean, decreasing body fat levels further may offer no performance improvement. If your body type just is not that of an elite runner, dieting offers no further benefit. It is better to focus on proper nutrition strategies to fuel and hydrate your body for optimal performance. Serious runners should aim for a target weight that is not unrealistically low and that can be maintained without excessive training or stringent dieting. An overtrained or underfed runner does not produce his or her best performance. It is best to focus on sensible weight-loss strategies such as those outlined in Chapter 6.

Choose a body-composition assessment method that you can use at regular intervals throughout the season. Look at the big picture when setting your weight-loss and body-composition goals. Gradual weight loss is less likely to compromise your performance, energy levels, and recovery than rapid weight loss requiring a higher level of calorie restriction. If you have a modest amount of body fat to lose, lose it earlier in the season, well ahead of your important race dates. If you have only a small amount of body fat to lose, stick to quality eating, and let quality training take care of the body fat.

THE IMPORTANCE OF IRON

Distance runners, especially females, seem to be at higher risk of developing compromised iron status. Left untreated, iron deficiency can lead to anemia, which clearly impairs exercise performance. But even before it reaches the stage of anemia, iron deficiency appears to affect training and performance in some athletes. Clearly, iron deficiency needs to be corrected before it progresses.

Iron deficiency should be treated with a diet high in heme iron. Good sources are listed in Table 3.6 and include lean red meat, chicken, and fish. Nonheme iron can also be emphasized and consumed with a food rich in vitamin C to enhance absorption. For example, you can consume iron-fortified cereal with orange juice, mix beans and tomatoes in dishes such as chili, and include a baked potato and broccoli at the same meal. Iron-fortified breads and cereals are a major source of iron in the diet. If you purchase natural foods that are not iron-fortified, you may be inadvertently reducing your iron intake. To maximize your iron absorption from foods, do not consume them with foods that inhibit iron absorption, such as coffee, tea, or an excessive amount of bran. Bran products contain phytates, which inhibit iron absorption. Phytates are also found in nuts, seeds, wheat cereals, peanut butter, and soy products. If you don't eat adequate amounts of heme iron, consider taking a low-dose iron supplement as part of a multivitamin providing 15 milligrams of iron daily.

It makes sense for runners, especially females, to screen for iron deficiency once yearly. Low levels of serum ferritin may warrant safe and monitored supplementation to bring levels back up into the middle range. Occasionally, increases in serum ferritin result in a slight increase in hemoglobin, indicating that a mild anemia may have been present. Some athletes may benefit from a slightly higher level of hemoglobin. An iron treatment dose is often more than 50 milligrams daily, and up to 300 milligrams daily for more severe anemia. But don't start taking therapeutic iron doses without first seeing a physician. Some individuals are susceptible to hemochromatosis, or iron overload, in which excess iron is deposited in the liver and other internal organs, causing serious damage. Too much iron when it is not really warranted can also decrease absorption of other important minerals like copper and zinc. Also, never self-diagnose an iron deficiency just because you are feeling run-down and tired. Fatigue can be related to a number of health, nutritional, and training factors.

When you have true anemia, a physician can prescribe a therapeutic dose of iron. Liquid ferrous sulfate is well absorbed. You can increase your dose slowly to minimize any gastrointestinal side effects of taking the supplement. Ferrous gluconate is often better tolerated than other forms of iron. Take your supplement on an empty stomach with a dose of vitamin C or a glass of orange juice. Iron supplements should be taken separately from calcium supplements to prevent a decrease in iron absorption. Your physician can monitor your serum ferritin and hemoglobin levels for several months afterward and continue, adjust, or discontinue supplementation as appropriate.

COMPETITION NUTRITION

Competition day has its own special nutrition considerations. Hydration is critical for all entrants in any running event, and fueling during the race is also essential for any race lasting longer than 90 minutes. The pre-race meal is also a key consideration, as races often have early-morning starts, race nerves can affect food tolerances, and early-morning liver glycogen stores are typically low. The perfect pre-race meal will prevent hunger before and during the race, be easily digested, and top off blood glucose levels before the start.

5K, 8K, 10K, AND 10-MILE RACES

Because of the typical times in which races ranging in distance from 5K to 10 miles will be completed, these races will not significantly challenge your muscle glycogen stores if you have eaten properly in the 24 to 48 hours before the race. You do need to arrive at the starting line not only with properly fueled muscles but also with replenished liver glycogen stores and a content and settled stomach. A pre-race meal can help keep blood glucose levels steady throughout your warm-up and race and prevent feelings of hunger. Of course, you will want to be cautious when choosing your pre-race foods and timing your meal. Experiment in training with timing and portions, and consume easily digested carbohydrate foods and/or liquids that you know you can tolerate. Determine your best pre-race food and fluid tolerances through practice and experimentation prior to early-morning runs.

Once you address your fueling needs, your major nutritional risk during a race of this length will be dehydration. Faster runners competing in cool weather in the shorter distances are unlikely to waste time to stop and drink. But as race finish times increase and the temperature rises, optimal pre-race hydration becomes even more crucial. You need fluid when you wake up in the morning, and you can lose fluid in the hours prior to the race through sweating and urination. Gauge your fluid status by monitoring the color of your urine. Drink adequately to fill and empty your bladder before the race. Consider your warm-up time, travel time to the race, and waiting-around time, and use these moments to drink plenty of fluids, without overhydrating.

You may want to experiment with a sports drink for both fluid and a carbohydrate boost before racing, sipping it in the time before the race. Carbohydrate-sensitive athletes can experiment with this pre-race strategy in training. Fluid intake during the race should benefit racers running for more than an hour. Stick with about 16 to 32 ounces (480–960 ml) per hour. You may want to consume only water during a 5K or 10K, but a sports drink is fine if it appeals to you. Slower finishers in the 10-mile race should consider hydrating with the sports drink provided at aid stations.

HALF-MARATHON (21.1K) AND 20K, 25K, AND 30K RACES

Races ranging in distance from 20K to 30K (or 12–18 miles) present their own set of nutritional challenges and definitely require an on-course fueling and hydration plan. For some top competitors, the half-marathon—a 13.1-mile race—does not present a significant fuel challenge, as the race is completed in less than 90 minutes. However, the vast majority of runners will complete the half-marathon in more than 90 minutes, and perhaps even in 2 to 3 hours. What matters for any of these race distances is that you are aware of your projected race time and plan your nutrition program leading up to the race accordingly.

For most competitors, all of these race distances require carbohydrate loading the day before the race, careful pre-race meal planning, and refueling with a sports drink to compensate for sweat losses. Taper your training up to 2 days before the race, and boost your carbohydrate intake to 3 to 4 grams per pound (6.5–9 g/kg) of body weight. Stick with low-fiber carbohydrate sources, keep protein portions low to moderate, and keep fat intake very low. Follow the same plan the day before the race, but have your large meal fairly early so that you wake up hungry and anticipate your pre-race meal.

In your pre-race meal, emphasize easily digested carbohydrate foods. Liquid sources low in fiber should be well tolerated. Aim to consume 30 to 60 grams of carbohydrates during any race lasting longer than 90 minutes. Sports drinks are generally the best-tolerated source of carbohydrates, but many runners have also experimented successfully with gels during longer races. Choose gels that contain sodium, and make sure that you take them with at least 8 ounces of water.

MARATHON (42.2K)

The marathon—a 26.2-mile race—requires careful nutritional planning on the part of even the most elite competitors. Lasting more than 2 hours for the world's top runners, the marathon is most challenging at about the 20-mile mark, when "hitting the wall," or running low on muscle glycogen, becomes a real possibility for any race participant. Having a nutrition strategy that puts your fuel gauge on full at the starting line is essential. This means knowing how to carry out a successful carbohydrate-loading plan during the pre-race taper.

Carbohydrate loading is synonymous with the marathon. The principles of carbohydrate loading, and the most current research-based guidelines, are provided in Chapter 5. After your last long run prior to the marathon, pay close attention to matching or even slightly exceeding your carbohydrate requirements for the remainder of your training during taper week. For maximum glycogen stores, an intake of 4 to 5 grams of carbohydrates per pound (9–11 g/kg) of body weight has been recommended, or about 500 to 700 grams daily. However, carbohydrate loading does not necessarily require enormous amounts of food and calories. On rest days, your calorie needs may not be especially high, and you simply need to eat enough carbohydrates to fill up your glycogen stores. This may only necessitate that a greater percentage of your calories be derived from carbohydrates, preferably those low in fiber.

During this critical time, make sure that noncarbohydrate foods do not crowd out the foods high in carbohydrates. Exceeding your protein and fat requirements serves little purpose during the 48 hours preceding a marathon. Just keep reasonable amounts of

FLUID AND SODIUM BALANCE FOR LONG-DISTANCE RUNNING

Hyponatremia, or low blood sodium levels, seems to be more prevalent in the marathon than in other long-distance events, likely due to the high level of participation and the high percentage of first-time participants in the longer event. Ultra-marathoners are also at risk of developing hyponatremia given their distance. Some hyponatremia-related fatalities have occurred in marathons over the past several years, though recently the numbers have decreased, but problems related to overhydration and dehydration during competition persist. For this reason, it is important to have a tested hydration, fueling, and electrolyte-replacement plan. The increased number of participants who are racing recreationally and taking longer than 4 to 5 hours to complete the race may translate into more sweating and sodium loss for these competitors. The fitter a runner becomes, the more he or she sweats. So as runners new to distance racing increase their fitness and training levels, their sweat levels increase as well, causing greater sodium losses. Hyponatremia seems to occur more often in women than in men, and women are signing up for marathons in increasing numbers.

But hyponatremia may also be caused by excessive consumption of fluid, which dilutes the concentration of sodium in the blood. Women generally have lower sweat rates than men and consequently lower fluid needs during a distance race, and women who do not realize this can drink too much, reducing their sodium levels. Women also have lower blood volume than men, and when they overdrink, they overfill more rapidly. Drinking a sodium-free fluid does not adequately replace the sodium lost in sweat as the marathon progresses.

Part of the problem seems to be that marathoners often receive the message that they need to drink a lot of fluid. Rather than taking the time to determine their own personal sweat rate by weighing themselves before and after training (see the sidebar "Estimating Your Sweat Losses" in Chapter 5 for the proper procedure), they may drink too much, often consuming a sodium-free fluid such as water. It is easier to drink when running at a recreational pace than when running at the elite level, and recreational runners often slow down to fill up at the water stops. It is ironic that most of the winners of any given marathon are probably the most dehydrated finishers on the course. At their fast pace, they not only have limited time for drinking but also likely produce a higher amount of sweat. Even marathoners finishing in the 3- to 4-hour range are likely to sweat more than they replace. Finishers taking 4 to 6 or even more hours to complete a race are much more likely to

continues

FLUID AND SODIUM BALANCE FOR LONG-DISTANCE RUNNING *continued*

overhydrate. To prevent overhydration and hyponatremia during a marathon, practice the following precautions:

- Determine your sweat rate during long training runs. Check your weight before and after training, and measure your fluid intake during the run with a graded water bottle. If you are gaining weight during long runs, you need to decrease your fluid intake.
- Use a sports drink during all your long runs, and practice training with the sports drink offered on the course.
- Choose a relatively high-sodium sports drink if you are a salty sweater, as evidenced by salt marks on your clothing. Check the sodium content of the drink to be offered on the race course.
- Develop and practice a drinking plan for your long runs, based on the information you learn from monitoring your weight before and after training.
- Consume a sodium-containing fluid after long runs based on the weight-monitoring results. Aim for 20 ounces (600 ml) for each pound (about 0.5 kg) of weight loss.
- Don't drink obsessively in the days leading up to a marathon. Hydrate so that your urine is pale yellow in color, but don't overhydrate. Remember that your sweat losses decrease considerably during your pre-race taper. Just drink to maintain a good level of hydration.
- Don't rehydrate indiscriminately after a marathon. Your risk of hyponatremia can remain high for several hours. Have a variety of recovery foods and drinks that provide sodium.

protein and fat in your diet. Have a menu prepared ahead of time to ensure that you not only choose high-carbohydrate foods but also consume enough of them. Refer to the food lists providing 30-gram carbohydrate servings in Chapter 4, and draw out some sample meals. Beware of sweet foods that may provide some carbohydrates but also plenty of fat. They may fill you up and taste good, but they won't adequately fill your muscle glycogen stores. This may also be a good time in which to consume some extra sugar and high-carbohydrate fluids such as juices and smoothies, which have the added bonus of being low in fiber. You may wish to avoid high-fiber foods for 24 to 48 hours before the event to ensure that you can "race light" and reduce gastrointestinal difficulties.

Your body stores a considerable amount of fluid when you carbohydrate-load. Don't be alarmed if your muscles feel a bit stiff, or if the number on your scale increases, when you are carbohydrate-loading. The additional stored water helps to delay dehydration during the race. Of course, you should also hydrate your body by drinking plenty of fluids in the 48 hours prior to the race. Keep a water bottle and hydrating fluids with you at all times. Monitor the color of your urine to ensure that it is light in color and that you are optimally hydrated but not overhydrated. During your race taper, your sweat losses go down considerably. Just make sure you rehydrate sufficiently after any activity. At rest, try to stay in fluid balance. There is no need to hyperhydrate for the marathon, a practice that could actually increase your risk of developing dangerous fluid overload and hyponatremia. Several full bladders of light-colored urine should indicate that you are in fluid balance.

Plan to consume a high-carbohydrate breakfast the morning of the race. You can minimize your overnight liver glycogen losses by consuming a late-evening snack; however, eating the right pre-race meal, and timing it appropriately, can be much more effective in refilling your liver glycogen stores and helping you maintain blood glucose levels when racing. Eating properly is far superior to not eating the morning of the race. Eating breakfast also settles your stomach and prevents hunger during your warm-up and at the starting line. Some runners may prefer to have a liquid meal replacement or breakfast shake in order to avoid eating solid foods before starting several hours of hard running. Experiment during long training runs to determine your favorite and best-tolerated pre-race meal. If you are traveling to the race, you may want to pack some of your favorite race foods to supplement your restaurant diet. Avoid trying new foods in the days leading up to the race. If you will be running in hot weather, or for several hours, increase your salt intake prior to the race to prevent a decrease in blood sodium levels while racing.

What you consume during the marathon is just as important as what you had beforehand. Meeting your fluid needs while running in competition is also crucial. The faster you run, the more heat you produce and the greater your risk of dehydration. Even if your marathon starts in the early morning to avoid excess heat, be prepared for temperatures to rise in hot climates. Running longer than 90 minutes will also challenge your body's carbohydrate stores, no matter how careful your pre-race eating. Focus early in the race on consuming carbohydrates in order to delay depletion of your glycogen stores. Sports drinks are your best-tolerated option and provide both needed fluid and carbohydrates.

Aid stations are generally provided every mile in a marathon. Find out ahead of time what sports drink will be provided at the race and drink it during training to develop a taste and tolerance for the product. You need to average about 4 to 8 ounces (120 to 240 ml) every 15 to 20 minutes, or consume the amounts that most closely match your sweat rate or minimize your sweat losses. Depending on your sweat rate, which you should know beforehand from monitoring during training, you may only need to drink at every other aid station. Practice drinking and running in shorter early-season races. Even seasoned racers do not consume the full amount of liquid provided in the cup, but you can practice your technique. Pinch the cup to form a funnel, and take two gulps. If you have to slow up in order to drink, you will still improve your race time by consuming adequate fluids and carbohydrates.

Many runners also consume carbohydrate gels during a marathon. Make sure that you consume a gel packet with 8 ounces (240 ml) of water. If you think that you will require several energy gels during the race, consider carrying them in a waistband or waist pack. Your goal is to consume at least 30 to 60 grams of carbohydrates every hour. Practice with gels during training. By race day, you should have mastered the best fluid- and fuel-replacement techniques to support your individual preferences and tolerances. You should also be flexible enough to consume the products offered on race day and adjust your plan as needed during the race.

ULTRARUNNING

Ultradistance races typically start at 31 miles but can also be 50, 62, or 100 miles. Other races are organized around a time frame, whereby you run as far as possible for 12, 24, or 48 hours. For races of these lengths, nutritional factors can determine whether you complete the race. Runners training for ultras extend the long weekly run that is the core of marathon training and put in high mileages on a regular basis. Besides building stamina and mental fortitude, these training runs give you the opportunity to develop your skills in fueling and hydrating for the long haul.

For competition, the taper presents the opportunity to carbohydrate-load, as discussed earlier in this chapter and in Chapter 5. Eat a large snack the night before the race, and have your tried-and-true pre-race breakfast already planned out. Use liquid supplements as needed to be optimally fueled and hydrated before the race. Increase your salt intake to compensate for salt losses during the race, as the long running times and constant fluid intake can increase the risk of hyponatremia. Many ultrarunners do finish races with some weight gain, lower sodium levels, and even hyponatremia.

Dehydration can prevent an ultrarunner from completing a race. Drink at least 20 ounces (600 ml) of fluid per hour, or more or less depending on your sweat rate. Know your sweat rate for your race pace and various environmental conditions (for method,

RUNNING AND GASTROINTESTINAL DISTRESS

Runners seem to be more susceptible than other endurance athletes to gastrointestinal (GI) distress and diarrhea during training and racing. The causes of these problems are unknown, but they may be related to the constant jarring and repetitive motion of running. GI upset may also be related to the intensity of your running, decreased blood flow to the GI tract, and dehydration. Some runners may be able to identify specific foods that aggravate GI problems.

Drink plenty of fluids before and during exercise to prevent dehydration and maintain adequate blood flow to your intestinal system. Start drinking early to prevent dehydration. Some runners have benefited from lowering their fiber intake close to exercise. You may even want to reduce your fiber intake at dinner the night before an early-morning run. Caffeine, particularly from coffee, is known to have a laxative effect. Limit or avoid caffeine, as well as artificial sweeteners such as sorbitol and aspartame, which may aggravate symptoms, if they seem to cause problems for you. Make sure that you are not taking any medications or over-the-counter supplements that aggravate GI symptoms, and if you are experiencing chronic GI difficulties, see a physician to eliminate the possibility of intestinal parasites and other medical problems such as irritable bowel syndrome, celiac disease/ gluten intolerance, and other gastrointestinal disorders. Some runners may need to experiment with removing specific foods from their diet to determine which items may be aggravating their symptoms. Some items that you may want to consider limiting are:

- Fiber, especially the day before and day of long or high-intensity runs
- Lactose from milk, milk-based products, and ice cream
- Fructose such as in dried fruit, fruit juices, and certain fruits such as apples, pears, and grapes
- Sorbitol
- Excess caffeine, especially in timing around the more intense or longer runs

You can also experiment with pre-run meal timing and food choices in that meal. Remember that although fueling before a run is important, plenty of time should be left for stomach emptying. Some runners may tolerate liquid choices, easily digested energy bars, and gels more easily than other foods before a run.

see the sidebar "Estimating Your Sweat Losses" in Chapter 5). Set your watch if you need to remind yourself to drink, and have a predetermined fluid schedule outlined. Carry a sports drink for both carbohydrates and fluids, and make sure a specific number of bottles will be available to you at each aid station. Because of the length of the race and the degree of hunger that can set in, ultrarunners often take in gooey carbohydrate gels or the more solid and chewy carbohydrate blocks and other semisolid items, such as energy bars, to fuel and settle their stomach. Experiment with these supplements. You may also want to consume liquid meals for a caloric boost during sections of the race where you power-walk, as well as electrolyte tablets and drinks to prevent hyponatremia.

The foods and fluids provided on the race course can vary greatly. You may find fruit, pretzels, cookies, potato chips, M & Ms, peanut-butter-and-jelly sandwiches, salty broth, and/or baked potatoes at aid stations. Find out what will be available on the course and practice with these foods during training. Be sure to take along some tolerated salty food items and salt tablets to replace sodium losses during the race.

Start replacing fluid, carbohydrates, and sodium early so that you can finish the race. Know your sweat rate at the planned race intensity and in various race conditions. Once you become depleted, it can be difficult to dig yourself out of a nutritional hole. If your stomach feels bloated and is not emptying properly, you may be dehydrated. If your stomach does become overfull and you vomit, start consuming a sports drink slowly to rehydrate. It will empty from your stomach as quickly as water and provide needed carbohydrates and sodium.

Sodium losses vary greatly among individuals and in various weather conditions. Experiment in training with use of salt tablets to determine what works for you. Salty foods such as soup or broth may be available at aid stations for some electrolyte replenishment. Keep any salt tablets that you carry with you away from moisture so that they do not break down before you ingest them. Wrapping them in plastic should work. Make sure that you ingest them with plenty of water. If you determine that you are losing weight during the race at check-ins, rehydrate with sodium-containing fluids that increase fluid retention. If you determine that you are gaining weight during the race, then lower your fluid intake and up your intake of sodium-containing products.

Drinking your calories is often your best option. Experiment with various drinks and flavors to prevent taste fatigue, and try to consume more than 250 calories per hour. Besides sports drinks, you may benefit from more concentrated sources such as high-carbohydrate supplements and meal replacements. These products are not as hydrating as sports drinks, but they provide needed carbohydrates. If you use these products, they will empty more comfortably from your stomach if you are well hydrated. Having access to a variety of foods during the race is a good idea because it gives you different options to choose from, which may make it easier for you to keep up with your calorie and fluid needs. It is fine if you decide not to use some of them—they will at least be there if you need them. They not only provide variety but may satisfy a craving or two along the way. Caffeine-containing soft drinks can provide an energy and mental boost later in the race. During long races, mental fatigue can occur, and a nice glucose boost from carbohydrates may be just what you need.

ATHLETE PROFILE

Fueling for the Long Run: *Lauren*

In contacting a sports dietitian, Lauren had two goals. One was to learn how to fuel before, during, and after her long runs in preparation for her first marathon, and the other was to lose 10 pounds in the 20 weeks leading up to the race. She had completed one half-marathon and was eager to take on the longer distance. Lauren was aware that dropping some weight would improve her running speed and tolerance of the heat. Her race was planned for September, and race day temperature was a wild card, with a history of both very cool and very warm temperatures.

Lauren weighed 140 pounds (64 kg) and had a body fat level of 25 percent. Her sports dietician determined that losing 10 pounds (4.5 kg) would place Lauren at a body fat level of 20 percent. Lauren and the sports dietitian decided on a weight-loss goal of 1 pound (0.45 kg) weekly for the first 6 weeks. Her training was just beginning to build during this time and this rate of weight loss was not expected to compromise her recovery.

Because Lauren's training schedule included both long and short runs, cross-training, and speed work, she was given meal plans for various workout days. Each plan was based on that day's training and total energy requirements, with a 500-calorie deficit for weight loss. Meal and snack timing for the day was also outlined to provide steady fuel during the day, and before, during, and after training.

Lauren was given instructions on how to calculate her sweat rate. She was advised to do this during an hourlong run and to keep close track of the amount of fluid she consumed during the race, as well as any changes in body weight before and after the run. Learning that she consumed fluid at 50 percent of her sweat rate, she was instructed to refine her drinking practices during the long run. She was able to do this easily as her long run was completed with a training group who supplied a sports drink along the run. As the temperature increased, so did her sweat rate, and she was able to increase her intake steadily during the training season.

As Lauren's long runs progressed in length, the sports dietitian developed a high-carbohydrate menu to be consumed the day before so that Lauren could begin the run on optimal muscle glycogen stores. She was also advised of pre-run meals that she could consume several hours before a long run.

Lauren reached her weight goal in 13 weeks. During this time she built her endurance and reported good recovery from her long runs. She also learned about carbohydrate loading for the long runs and the race, and refined her strategy for replacing carbohydrate, electrolytes, and fluid during training.

NUTRITION FOR SWIMMING

Individuals of all ages and abilities are involved in the sport of swimming at the recreational and competitive levels. Swimmers train with local clubs, on high-school teams, and in college under the National Collegiate Athletic Association (NCAA). The NCAA has a strong swimming program, with over 9,000 men and over 11,000 women participating in the sport (including diving) during the 2009–2010 season. U.S. Masters Swimming offers training and competition opportunities for athletes ranging from nineteen to eighty-plus years old and includes more than 50,000 members across the nation. Many masters teams train at local YMCA pools or at high-school and university pools, but competitive swimming also includes open-water and long-distance swimming.

Competitive swimming at the high school, collegiate, and Olympic levels requires a serious commitment to training. These swimmers may complete anywhere from six to twelve sessions every week, each covering a training distance of 1,000 to 2,000 meters (for a sprinter in the taper phase) to 10 kilometers (for a distance swimmer in the base phase of training). Elite swimmers also incorporate land-based aerobic training, such as running and cycling, into their programs, as well as weight training. Swim training programs can vary greatly, however, depending on the swimmer's age, fitness level, competitive goals, and race events and distances. Elite swimmers

Swim training times and workouts are often demanding in contrast to the brevity of competition times.

Swimmers sweat, though sweat rates are often lower than those seen during land training.

Sports drinks, gels, and blocks provide fuel during hard training sessions and maintain blood glucose levels.

High school and collegiate swimmers should develop nutrition plans for early-morning and after-noon training sessions for constant refueling.

Pack snacks and fluids for meets, and time portions around projected swim times.

tend to have pronounced upper-body muscle development. Successful swimmers can achieve high power outputs along with a highly refined technique. This requires good muscular development in the upper body, and also in the lower body to achieve a good kick.

Collegiate swim training is often very demanding and, in sharp contrast to the brevity of the competitive events for which these swimmers train, can require long periods of time in the pool. Races are typically divided into sprint (50–100 m), middle-distance (200–400 m), and distance events (800–1,500 m). Times range from just over 20 seconds for sprint to 7 to 8 minutes for middle-distance and 14 to 16 minutes for the longer events. Competitive swimming requires high rates of energy production, and sprint events are largely anaerobic.

Collegiate swimmers can train up to 20 hours per week during the height of the season. They may schedule two sessions daily—one in the early morning or afternoon and another in the evening—to accommodate school and work schedules, although they may decrease their training load to 8 hours weekly out of season.

Masters and club swimmers are a diverse group, but even those who do not compete at meets are often serious about training. Masters swimmers may train at high intensities and anywhere from 1 to 2 hours daily. They may also participate in open-water events and in triathlons and various forms of land training. The amount of time that masters swimmers put into their weekly training varies greatly but often reaches levels that warrant an endurance training diet. Like athletes at the high-school, college, and elite levels, masters swimmers will find that paying proper attention to nutrition will enhance their health, their fitness, and their performance in swimming.

TRAINING NUTRITION

Swim training intensities can include both aerobic and endurance-based training as well as anaerobic training sessions of interval work at different percentages of maximal heart rate. Clearly, swim workouts can rely heavily on muscle glycogen stores for fuel. Swimmers who regularly fail to replenish these stores after hard training sessions may find that they eventually become unable to complete sessions. Inadequate recovery can be compounded over the long haul. Even swimmers who frequently cross-train, thus drawing on different muscle groups, may find that the benefits afforded by proper endurance nutrition are worth the effort it takes to pay attention to dietary matters.

Swimming competition itself often lasts only seconds or minutes, making competition highly anaerobic, though aerobic metabolism becomes more significant as the distance of the event increases. Olympic-level races last from 20 seconds to 15 minutes. Because of these relatively short race times at high intensities, swimming competition requires a unique set of nutritional strategies. Buildup of lactic acid, rather than depletion of fuel stores, is likely to be the limiting performance factor. Of course, an exception would be long-distance swimming, which draws more on the aerobic system and presents a real challenge to muscle fuel stores. Regardless of the competitive event, serious training requires adequate recovery nutrition.

RECOVERY NUTRITION

Energy

Calorie requirements for swimming increase as the volume and intensity of individual training sessions and of the program as a whole increase. Because of the wide range of training programs found among swimmers of all ages and competitive levels, calorie intake will vary from one athlete to the next. Refer to Chapter 4 for calorie recommendations. Moreover, an athlete's calorie requirements will vary from day to day depending on the intensity and distance of his or her swimming and cross-training efforts. Match your calorie intake to your training for the day for optimal recovery, and pay close attention to eating well when you have several heavy training days in a row. An athlete who does not do so too often finds that fatigue and subpar performance can even halt training after just a few days of high-intensity effort.

Both male and female swimmers have special needs during their teenage years. Adolescent male swimmers, on the one hand, sometimes experience a period of heavy growth and muscular development that can result in significant short-term increases in energy needs. When combined with swim training, these growth spurts can use enough calories to outpace average intake, and during these times, it is best for optimal swimming performance if the athlete knows how to plan and carry out a healthy eating plan rather than just filling up on pizza and other fast foods. The danger for adolescent female swimmers, on the other hand, is falling prey to society's ideals of thinness, which can lead to inadequate calorie intake. Hormonal changes during these years can mean an increase in body fat for young women, and female swimmers may struggle to maintain low levels of body fat despite a high training load. But the energy needs of serious swimmers can exceed several thousand calories daily, as swimming may burn anywhere from

500 to 700 calories per hour. If excess body fat is truly a concern in regard to health and performance, following sensible weight-loss strategies may be warranted (see Chapter 6). Generally speaking, distance swimmers often have higher levels of body fat than sprinters. Swimmers should consider whether and how leanness could benefit them individually. Some body fat in the right distribution may, in fact, enhance buoyancy in the water.

Carbohydrates

Adequate calorie intake is of course synonymous with consuming enough total carbohydrates for optimal recovery. Swim training typically lasts from 60 to 120 minutes per session. But it is not just long, steady-state sessions that can use up this important and limited fuel supply; shorter sessions of high-intensity interval or speed work can also deplete muscle glycogen stores. Match up your daily carbohydrate intake with your training as outlined in Chapter 4. After strenuous training sessions, consume adequate carbohydrates for recovery, aiming for 0.5 gram of carbohydrates per pound (about 1 g/kg) of body weight, or about 50 to 75 grams of carbohydrates, immediately after exercise to begin the synthesis of muscle glycogen before your next training session. You can combine these carbohydrates with small amounts of protein, if desired, but make sure carbohydrate intake is your first priority. Convenient items that can be brought to the pool for consumption include energy bars, high-carbohydrate supplements, bagels, crackers, juices, and fruit.

Fluid Requirements

Swimmers training in the steamy environment of a heated indoor pool or outdoors in the hot sun can have moderate sweat losses that may not be obvious to them because they are wet anyway. Just how much a swimmer sweats in the water varies depending on individual sweat rates and fitness levels. Nevertheless, sweat rates are also affected by water temperature, air temperature, and humidity, particularly in an outdoor pool.

Limited data currently indicate that sweat losses in the pool are moderate compared with those in other types of endurance training, even for athletes who spend a significant amount of time traveling up and down the pool. Though these sweat losses are not as heavy as those measured in cyclists or triathletes, they should still be replaced through fluid intake during training. As in any sport, one of the best techniques for monitoring your fluid loss is to weigh yourself before and after training (see the sidebar "Estimating Your Sweat Losses" in Chapter 5). For every pound of weight lost, drink 24 ounces of fluid during and after training. Sweat rates vary among individual athletes: Though average fluid losses among swimmers may be moderate compared with those of land athletes who train in the heat, some individuals may have higher sweat rates than others.

Fortunately, swim training presents a convenient opportunity to replace fluids whether the sweat loss is modest or significant. Leave your fluid bottle at the end of your lane for relatively long or intense swim sessions. Concentrate on taking gulps every 15 minutes or whenever the nature of the training session allows you to take a quick break without disrupting your interval work. Gauge whether your drinking habits are keeping up with your losses by weighing yourself before and after training. Sweat losses are expected to be higher during anaerobic threshold sets than during steady swimming, but knowing your individual sweat rate in different types of sessions is the key.

When you monitor your before and after weights, check that you don't overhydrate. Because sweat losses are somewhat diminished when swimming, very motivated drinkers may exceed their fluid losses. For training sessions lasting more than 1 hour, and for shorter sessions that are high in intensity, consume a sports drink. These drinks provide carbohydrates to maintain adequate blood glucose levels and supply your muscles with fuel when body stores run low. Sports drinks can easily meet both your carbohydrate and fluid requirements if consumed in adequate amounts. They also increase the drive to drink and enhance fluid absorption. Hydrate leading up to practice, and consume 20 ounces of fluid for every pound (600 ml for every 2 kg) of weight loss during training.

NUTRITION ISSUES FOR SPECIFIC GROUPS

High-School Swimmers

Many dedicated swimmers are in adolescence and experience dramatic physical changes in their bodies during this time. In order for them to reach their full growth potential, the energy demands of both growing and training must be met. This is especially true of adolescent boys, as mentioned earlier, who often require frequent meals and snacks in order to maintain both weight and growth. They should also include high-quality protein in their diet and may require up to 0.75 to 0.9 gram of protein per pound (1.6–2 g/kg) of body weight per day. These elevated protein requirements are easily provided in a well-balanced diet, particularly if energy needs are met. Protein supplements are not necessary for a high-school swimmer's diet.

Swimmers who struggle to meet caloric requirements may simply find that their busy training and school schedules limit the amount of time they have to eat. Planning is essential for these high calorie-burning athletes. Close attention should be paid to recovery nutrition after early-morning training. Packing foods and fluids high in carbohydrates when getting ready for school is essential. If the schedule and classroom setting allow, a mid-morning snack will aid the recovery process. Lunch should not be some fatty choice from the school cafeteria; rather, it should be planned out and should consist of high-quality protein, adequate carbohydrates, and reasonable amounts of good fats. A pre-exercise snack is also useful for maintaining energy levels and steady blood glucose levels for afternoon training. Of course, a variety of foods is essential for a balanced diet, and young athletes should be sure to make good food choices to support muscle growth, recovery, and top performance.

Adolescent swimmers should consume water during breaks in training, or sports drinks for training lasting longer than 60 minutes. Sports drinks maintain hydration levels and provide fuel for athletes who have not eaten for a few hours. High-intensity training sessions can also warrant the ingestion of sports drinks to provide glucose for fuel.

Consuming a high level of calories can ensure a diet adequate in vitamins and minerals, if planned wisely, but adolescents have higher calcium and iron requirements and need to plan accordingly. It is easy to fall short of these nutrients. Good intakes of calcium along with optimal training can help a young athlete achieve peak bone mass, reduce risk of stress fractures, and minimize the effects of bone loss later in life. Good sources of calcium should be emphasized in the diet (see Table 3.5). Iron intake is a particular concern for adolescent girls, who have increased iron losses with menstruation. Food sources high in iron should be emphasized in the diet (see Table 3.6). A multivitamin providing the RDA for iron may be beneficial, but higher doses should not be taken without a physician's supervision.

Overall, high-school athletes should minimize their reliance on fast foods as much as possible to limit their intake of fatty foods and hydrogenated and saturated fats. Packing fruits to supplement school lunches is one good option. Low-fat milk and yogurt may also be available at most school cafeterias. Athletes can pack healthy low-fat lunches consisting of sandwiches, fruit, and other carbohydrate items such as pretzels and granola bars. Their parents should become involved in meal planning and assist them, especially when it comes to meals served at home. Their dinners should include quality protein sources and whole grains. An evening snack can provide additional nutritious calories.

Swimmers struggling with body weight management issues despite their high energy output during training should not try to conform to an ideal promoted by the media and other elements of society. Young women especially need to realize that their body fat levels are likely within a healthy range. They should appreciate that success in competition is related to a number of factors and not solely based on low body fat levels. Following sensible strategies for controlling weight at a healthy level is best. It is especially important to avoid extreme diets, such as ones that eliminate almost all fat or restrict calories to an unreasonable level for keeping up with growth and training needs. In some cases, rigid dieting can lead to disordered eating or even full-blown eating disorders. Parents, coaches, and caregivers should be aware of the signs and symptoms of these disorders and provide and seek help if needed. (For more specific weight-loss guidelines for endurance athletes and more information about eating disorders, see Chapter 6.)

Collegiate Swimmers

Swimmers in college are limited by the NCAA to 20 hours of training per week during the regular season. Training often consists of two practice sessions daily. These athletes frequently weight-train, and running is often part of their training program.

Collegiate swimmers must meet high energy and carbohydrate requirements and carefully practice the principles of recovery nutrition, particularly when training twice daily. Inadequate carbohydrates between an early-morning and late-afternoon training session can compromise performance. Carbohydrates should be consumed immediately after training and should be followed by a high-carbohydrate meal or snack. They can also be consumed several hours prior to exercise to replenish liver glycogen stores and provide fuel for the second training session. Collegiate swimmers, like all athletes, should monitor their fluid losses during training by checking body weight before and after exercise, and they should drink water and sports drinks during high-intensity workouts or sessions that are relatively long in duration, as well as during strength training sessions, to replace their fluid and carbohydrate losses. The real challenge for collegiate athletes, however, is meeting their nutritional requirements when eating at the college dormitory or preparing meals in their own apartments.

COMPETITION NUTRITION

One of the ironies of competitive swimming is that hours and hours of preparation week after week and month after month culminate in races lasting just seconds or minutes. However, although each race may be brief, swim meets may be held over several days' time—and international events can last even longer. Swimmers often compete in multiple heats and events over the course of the entire event. It is not unusual for a swimmer to

DINING AT THE DORM

Eating dormitory food can present a new challenge to the college athlete accustomed to family-style home-cooked meals. Although an athlete may be able to keep foods in his or her dorm room and may have the opportunity to purchase foods near campus, the majority of his or her nutritional needs will have to be met at the dorm dining hall during breakfast, lunch, and dinner. Dining hall hours may be limited, however, and it can be difficult to co-ordinate class, training, and meal times. Dining hall hours may not always be sufficient to accommodate a heavy schedule. The serious swimmer may not be able to meet his or her calorie requirements in just three meals daily—but falling short can lead to weight loss or suboptimal recovery from daily training. Athletes may also be overwhelmed by the variety of foods offered in a dorm cafeteria. If they are not familiar with sensible sports nutrition principles, they may not feel confident that their food choices match their training requirements. They may have no idea of how to estimate their carbohydrate needs, and even if they do, it may be difficult to know what ingredients are contained in various entrees offered. The food-preparation techniques used in the kitchen and the fat content of certain items may be a mystery, as the popular terminology for dorm protein offerings—"mystery meat"—implies.

It is also possible to overeat at a dining hall, where portions and choices are unlimited. Moreover, many athletes may snack while studying and feel that they have fewer food restraints imposed upon them than they did at home. They can begin to feel somewhat out of control in regard to their food choices. Food may also be a large part of the social life at school, and it can be all too easy to consume excess calories when a typical evening includes going to a party, visiting the snack bar at the student union, or dropping in at the local pizza parlor or pastry-laden coffeehouse.

Nevertheless, with knowledge and planning, eating in the dorm cafeteria can support a healthy sports diet. Athletes should educate themselves about the carbohydrate content of various foods and balance these items with quality protein sources and healthy fats (see tables in Chapter 4). For example, a grilled chicken breast with rice, a steamed vegetable, and a salad topped with olive oil would make a good meal choice for a college athlete. Athletes should understand that they can include some fat in their diet. It is a matter of balancing their fat intake with the day's other food choices and the training plan for the day and the rest of the week.

When eating in a dorm, survey all the choices before deciding what to consume. Don't just pile up on everything; rather, try to balance the meal by incorporating items from several food groups. Remember that the menu in the cafeteria is provided on a cycle. Your favorite foods and other interesting items will come around again. Treats can be part of the diet as long as they are well-chosen items and in reasonable portions. It can be tempting to stay in the cafeteria and socialize with friends. However, this can lead to eating when you are not hungry. Let your food choices be well informed and based on rational decisions, and avoid the overeating that can happen when emotions or social situations govern eating habits.

For those athletes who cannot meet their nutritional requirements with the three daily meals offered, several options exist. Many cafeterias permit snacks such as sandwiches, fruit, or yogurt to be taken from the dining hall for consumption later. You can also keep a small fridge in your dorm room and stock fruit, yogurt, milk, cereal, and granola bars. You may decide to purchase snacks on campus between classes as your schedule permits. Fruit smoothies make excellent recovery snacks and may be available at a juice bar. Purchase your favorite sports drink, if possible, to minimize fuel depletion, enhance your workouts, and ultimately improve your recovery. (See also the section "Eating Well on Campus" in Chapter 14.)

compete in a heat in the morning and a final later that day or have several races scattered throughout one day. It may be necessary to travel to races either by car, bus, or plane, and traveling not only can cause fatigue but also can take a toll on one's eating habits.

CARBOHYDRATE LOADING

Before swimmers arrive for a competition, they likely have tapered their training for several days, increasing their muscle glycogen stores. If so, they have a better chance of being race-ready and well fueled. Although an athlete's calorie needs may decrease somewhat, or even greatly, depending on the extent of the taper, it is still necessary to eat enough carbohydrates to ensure plenty of available glycogen. A high percentage of the pre-race diet should therefore come from carbohydrates. Carbohydrate stores can be filled with 24 hours of proper eating on a high-carbohydrate diet combined with rest.

Swimmers who follow a longer race taper should decrease their total calorie intake over that time period to prevent unwanted gains in body fat.

The pre-competition meal should replenish low liver glycogen stores in the morning and increase blood glucose levels. Swimmers may have to carefully time their food and fluid intake throughout the competitive day in order to replenish stores between heats, semifinals, and finals. Some well-tolerated choices are sports drinks, fruit juices, and gels when there is only a short period of time between races. For longer time intervals, swimmers can consume bagels, English muffins, energy bars, fruit, or sandwiches. Swimmers normally complete light warm-ups prior to competition and a swim-down after the event to improve recovery, so take all of this into consideration when planning your snacks and fluids for a competition day. Well-tolerated protein choices can augment this carbohydrate intake. Good choices include lean turkey, yogurt, dairy products and soy milk, and energy bars with a high protein content. If traveling to competition, bring some of your favorite and well-tolerated competition foods with you. In addition, drink fluids steadily—without overdrinking—but be aware that if the competition is being held in a warm and humid environment, you will need to increase your fluid intake accordingly. Your urine should be pale in color if hydration levels are adequate.

LONG-DISTANCE SWIMMING

The fuel demands of long-distance swimming are high, and swimmers specializing in this niche should consume adequate snacks and meals before and after all training sessions. They should also hydrate with a sports drink during their long training swims in order to provide fuel when muscle glycogen stores run low and develop a tolerance for these products, which will become even more essential when racing. Their carbohydrate intake should match their swim training volume, as outlined in Chapter 4.

Long-distance swimmers need to take extra care that they start any race, whether a 10K, which is now an Olympic distance, or a 25K—or even a 75K or an 88K, which are possible on the World Cup circuit—optimally fueled and hydrated. Typically these races take about 1 hour for every 5 kilometers, with women at a slightly slower pace than the men, which puts 10K finishes at over 2 hours and 25K finishes somewhere around 6 hours. Other race distances can take 7 to 10 hours to complete.

Because of the high fuel demands of distance swimming, competitors should carefully consume a high-carbohydrate diet during the race taper. High-carbohydrate supplements can make the carb-loading phase simpler, and swimmers should make sure they maximize this opportunity, as outlined in Chapter 5. Sports drinks, energy bars, and concentrated carbohydrate foods are all beneficial in preparing for these long events. Drink lots of fluids in the days leading up to the race, and carefully plan your pre-race meal. Carbohydrate-containing liquids and easily digested foods will fill your liver glycogen stores before the race and raise your levels of blood glucose.

Swimmers should be accustomed to taking and consuming "feeds" during a race. Events at the 5K and 10K levels have feeding stations, and athletes swimming these distances can be optimally fueled with a sports drink. Feeding cups typically provide 8 to 10 ounces (250–300 ml) of fluid, such as a sports drink, and can be consumed at each feeding station as needed, ideally every 15 minutes. An athlete's fluid requirements can be higher in hot weather than in cooler temperatures or cooler water conditions.

In events covering more than 10 kilometers, there should be a feed support boat. Swimmers should have a predetermined feed schedule, but they should be prepared to modify this schedule during the race as needed. Aim for 60 to 75 grams of carbohydrates per hour, or 0.5 to 0.6 gram of carbohydrate per pound of weight (1 to 1.4 g/kg), and practice rolling on your back and drinking. Gels can be carried in your swimsuit or provided from the support boats. Have solid foods available to eat when you tire of drinking. Try cut-up energy bars or even a few bites of a banana. Aim to obtain feeds every 20 minutes.

Be aware of how air and water temperatures can affect your food and fluid needs during the race. Colder water temperatures make you burn fuel more quickly as your body attempts to keep itself warm. This may increase your need for carbohydrate sources such as gels and for a variety of solid items. Without proper fueling, strong hunger pains can set in. Hot-water feeds can also be warming during the swim. In warmer water, your fluid needs increase during competition. Try to keep your hydrating fluids cool in warm weather and be aware of your sweat rate in these conditions.

ATHLETE PROFILE

Nutrition to Beat Illness: Erica

Erica is a collegiate swimmer who had suffered frequent upper respiratory infections early in the current training season. She often missed workouts when she was sick or had lackluster training due to fatigue. Wondering if her frequent illnesses might be related to some nutrient missing in her diet, she decided to visit a sports dietitian for a nutritional evaluation.

Erica told the sports dietitian that she was living in an apartment with several other swimmers and prepared her own meals, and that she trained twice daily, in the early morning and late afternoon, before settling down for a long evening of homework. The dietitian took a food recall from Erica to determine the general outline of her daily diet, including food choices and meal and snack timing around training.

The sports dietitian found several areas requiring significant improvement in Erica's diet. Erica did not consume any foods or fluids before swimming, and she trained for 90 minutes on only 16 ounces of water. She was advised to consume a high-carbohydrate-protein sports shake before training, providing 50 grams of carbohydrate and 15 grams of protein in 16 ounces of fluid, in the 30 minutes before training. Erica found that she could tolerate this supplement, and also started consuming 24 ounces of sports drink in the early training session. These strategies helped to maintain blood glucose levels during early-morning training.

Erica was also not eating enough food, mainly carbohydrates between her morning and afternoon training sessions. So she increased her post-swim breakfast intake with an ample portion of a high-calorie cereal, milk, fresh fruit, and fruit juice. She chooses lunch fare that includes whole-grain bread, pasta salad, vegetables, and fresh fruit. Before her afternoon training she now downs an easily digested energy bar. She began to focus on daily hydration throughout the day, making sure that she brings a water bottle to classes. Erica also fuels with a sports drink during her 2-hour afternoon practice.

The sports dietitian increased Erica's dinner portions because her caloric intake was 1,000 calories below her daily training energy requirements. She emphasized lean proteins at dinner, as well as nutrient-dense grain sources, vegetables, and healthy fats. Fruit and yogurt were suggested as an evening snack when studying.

After two weeks of better fueling, Erica reported better energy levels during training, improved recovery, and an overall better sense of well-being. She reported no further respiratory infections for the next 8 weeks. Erica felt confident that her upgraded sports nutrition plan would support her training and health in the coming months.

PART IV
SPECIAL NUTRITIONAL CONSIDERATIONS

Meeting and Managing the Challenges

Part IV addresses some of the special nutritional considerations that endurance athletes may encounter during the course of their training program and competitive season. These challenges require nutrition strategies that go beyond those of optimal fueling for good health, training, and competition. Nutritional considerations for specific population groups such as the young athlete, masters athlete, and pregnant athlete are also provided.

Chapter 12 addresses clinical or health concerns, including conditions that require very specific nutritional modifications, such as celiac disease, food allergies, irritable bowel syndrome, and diabetes. Integrating nutritional strategies for these conditions into the sports nutrition guidelines outlined in Parts I to III allows the athlete to train and compete as desired, and to manage these conditions along with any appropriate medical treatment.

In Chapter 13, we look at some unwanted conditions endurance athletes may experience related to their training, such as muscle cramping or a fragile immune system. Here we review nutrition strategies that can be practiced around training that can help prevent and treat specific conditions. Too, we explore how to recognize and capitalize on the physiological differences that exist between male and female endurance athletes.

Finally, Chapter 14 describes some of the challenging environmental conditions that an endurance athlete might encounter, such as temperature extremes—including training in very cold and very hot temperatures—and training and racing at altitude. Nutritional adjustments specific to these environmental conditions can support the athlete in training and recovery, as well as help him or her withstand the elements when competing or participating in an event.

AT A GLANCE
KEY POINTS

Young athletes need
adequate energy for growth,
as well as for training and
recovery.

Masters athletes may need
to adjust caloric intake as
they age.

Pregnant athletes need
adequate energy and
protein on top of training
requirements for each
trimester.

Certain gastrointestinal-
related conditions can be
treated by removing specific
foods from the diet.

Poor performance and
increased risk of injury are
examples of the damaging
effects of eating disorders.

Female athletes are at
risk for compromised
bone health related to
inadequate caloric intake
and compromised hormonal
status.

THE ATHLETE WITH UNIQUE NUTRITION CONSIDERATIONS

All endurance athletes should aim for a balanced and nutrient-filled training diet, but some athletes may have health considerations that require diet modifications or treatments as well. For example, many endurance athletes follow a vegetarian diet, or an athlete may have celiac disease or diabetes. Younger and older endurance athletes, too, have special nutrient considerations specific to their stage of life that need to be incorporated into the training diet outlined in this book. Many endurance athletes have gastrointestinal complaints, and the diagnosis of irritable bowel syndrome appears to be increasing, as does the incidence of food intolerances. In addition, certain athlete populations are at increased risk of low bone mass, an important health risk that can lead to serious health concerns later in life.

SPECIAL POPULATIONS

THE VEGETARIAN ATHLETE

Vegetarians are individuals who have consciously made the choice to completely exclude animal foods from their diet, or to include only specific animal foods, such as dairy products, eggs, or fish, and obtain a significant portion or all of their protein from plant foods. Whether these dietary modifications are for health, environmental, ideological, or taste-related reasons, vegetarians need to pay close attention to their nutrition program to ensure adequate protein consumption and sufficient intake of specific vitamins and minerals. Vegetarian athletes must deliberately design a well-balanced diet suited to their training program.

As touched upon in the sidebar on p. 39, "vegetarianism" is an umbrella term that incorporates a range of dietary exclusions. A plant-based vegetarian diet may refer to one of the following descriptions:

Semi- or Near-Vegetarian: Includes fish, poultry, eggs, and dairy products but no red meat

Pesco-Vegetarian: Includes fish, dairy products, and eggs

Lacto-Vegetarian: Includes dairy products

Ovo-Vegetarian: Includes eggs

Ovo-Lacto Vegetarian: Includes dairy products and eggs

Vegan: Includes no animal foods whatsoever

The idea that being a vegetarian and being a competitive athlete are mutually exclusive is a myth. Indeed, there are many benefits to becoming a vegetarian when the diet is varied and well balanced, and there are plenty of world-class athletes who don't eat meat. Vegetarians have many whole foods to choose from and a high number of vegetarian options at supermarkets. Many studies have shown that vegetarians have a lower incidence of cancer, heart disease, diabetes mellitus, and hypertension. Vegetarians often consume more fiber, less saturated fat and cholesterol, and higher amounts of unsaturated fats in their diet. Because of high fruit and vegetable intake, vegetarian diets are generally higher in antioxidants and phytonutrients. The higher fiber intake of a vegetarian diet can help to control calorie intake, which may benefit some individuals. Endurance athletes, however, typically have high energy requirements, particularly during specific parts of their training cycle. Plenty of endurance athletes are vegetarians, and they can learn to increase calories and protein without too much added fiber around training sessions and during heavy training cycles.

As a vegetarian, you need to carefully choose foods that provide specific nutrients in your diet. These nutrients include protein, of course, but also iron and zinc, and—particularly if you exclude dairy products—vitamin B12, calcium, and vitamin D.

Throughout this book, the unique considerations of vegetarian athletes are addressed in regard to specific nutrients. Of course, any athlete can choose to include more plant sources of specific nutrients—including high-quality plant proteins—in his or her diet. Plant foods are filled with health-promoting minerals and other nutrients. A plant-based diet also supplies plenty of carbohydrates for replenishing body fuel stores after training. Filling up on whole grains, fruits, and vegetables benefits any endurance sport athlete. Milk and yogurt, though sources of high-quality protein, add good amounts of carbohydrate to your diet as well.

Like a diet containing meat and other animal protein, a vegetarian diet can support training efforts, or it can be overly restrictive, poorly planned, and counterproductive.

THE YOUNG ATHLETE

What keeps a young endurance athlete strong, fast, and injury-free? A solid training program, focus, and the proper diet. High-school athletes perform better and feel better when they know when, what, and how much to eat for training and race day. The proper diet balance for athletes at any age provides energy, promotes recovery from training, and ensures optimal fuel for race day. However, young athletes are growing while training, and they need more food, more fluid, and more vitamins and minerals than other kids their age. They also need to pay close attention to the timing of their food and fluid intake, particularly around training sessions.

Nutrition Basics

In both childhood and adolescence, physical activity and growth play major roles in total energy requirements. Children especially experience rapid growth and form muscle and bone. Generally, females have their most rapid increase in height between 10 and 13 years of age, and males between 12 and 15 years of age. The main nutritional goal is to promote normal growth and development, and energy intake should be adjusted to also meet the requirements of exercise programs. During adolescence, females gain lean body mass and body fat, and males gain mostly lean body mass. Many young endurance athletes pattern their diet after that of their parents, and this is a key opportunity to model optimal eating habits. Adolescents should eat to satisfy their requirements for growth and training, but given the current rate of overweight in this population, still be cognizant of appropriate portions.

Key nutrients for the young endurance athlete are carbohydrates, proteins, fats, fluid, and vitamins and minerals. They function as a team, with different foods supplying different combinations of these nutrients.

Carbohydrates

While it is not clear from research that young endurance athletes benefit from carbohydrates in the same manner as do adult endurance athletes, carbohydrates are necessary for optimal performance and energy and also provide important fuel for the brain. However, at least 50 to 60 percent of the calories that a young athlete consumes should come from carbohydrates. All carbohydrates are converted to glucose. When glucose is not used for immediate energy needs, it is converted to glycogen, which is stored in the muscles and liver. These stored carbohydrates, or glycogen, are the most valuable fuel source for a young endurance athlete. No matter what the intensity or duration of a workout, carbohydrates are burned for fuel. Wholesome carbohydrates such as whole grains, fruits, and vegetables come packaged with vitamins and minerals. Sugars and processed carbohydrates should be kept to smaller amounts in the diet as they are not as high in nutrients. Because children derive a significant amount of energy from snacks, whole grains and fruits should be emphasized as choices.

Protein plays an important role in muscle building and repair after exercise and should supply about 20 percent of a high-school endurance athlete's calories. Lean protein should be emphasized over fatty choices to limit unhealthy saturated fat in the diet. Growing athletes should derive 20 to 30 percent of their calories from fat to meet the remainder of their energy needs for development. Healthy fats provide essential fatty acids and fat-soluble vitamins.

Vitamins and minerals are small but powerful nutrients that help us process calories from food, build strong bones, prevent disease, and keep our immune system healthy. Consuming a variety of foods provides a variety of vitamins and minerals. Calcium and iron are key nutrients for the child and adolescent.

Calcium is crucial to adequate development of bone density. Young athletes cannot always relate to the adverse health effects of low calcium intake in adulthood, but they can be at increased risk of stress fractures during the training and competition season. Both dairy (milk, yogurt, cheese) and nondairy (green leafy vegetables) sources of calcium can be emphasized in their diet. Refer to Table 3.5 for good sources of calcium. Protein and vitamin D also play important roles in bone mineral health, and young athletes may need to take a supplement to augment their vitamin D intake from food to reach the recommended 600 IU.

Inadequate iron intake can lead to iron deficiency and anemia as well, which can affect muscle metabolism and brain function in the young athlete, and lead to fatigue. Iron intake is especially important in girls after the start of menstruation, and anemia can develop in boys during growth spurts. Young female athletes may also reduce their iron consumption when they restrict energy intake because of concerns with body image and the end of their growth spurt. Refer to Table 3.6 for good sources of iron.

Fluid and Hydration

Fluid is the most important nutrient for young athletes, as they are more susceptible to heat illness than adults when active in hot weather. Learning how much to drink, when to drink, and what to drink influences a young athlete's performance more than any other nutrition strategy. Not following proper hydration guidelines can greatly impair performance and even place the young athlete in life-threatening situations.

Sweating keeps the body cool during exercise, and fluid lost needs to be continually replaced. Although environmental factors affect everyone, children produce more metabolic heat per pound of body weight during exercise and have a reduced sweating capacity, which decreases their ability to lose heat through sweat evaporation. Like adults, young athletes usually do not have a strong drive to drink fluids during exercise.

Dehydration can result from inadequate fluid intake. Dehydration can progress from mild to severe, so young athletes should learn to start pre-hydrating for exercise, and learn to replace fluid losses during training. Early symptoms of dehydration include thirst, headache, and fatigue, as well as nausea, dry mouth, and clammy skin. As dehydration progresses, body temperature increases, and other symptoms can be dizziness and weakness. When dehydration is severe, heatstroke occurs and sweating stops, and the athlete is greatly disoriented.

The body needs about 64 ounces (1,920 ml) of fluid daily to maintain normal hydration. Fluid lost through sweating also needs to be replaced. Water should be the primary fluid consumed in the daily diet, though skim milk is also an important fluid source that provides calcium and vitamins A and D. Soda and other sweetened drinks should be absent or very limited in the diet as they provide calories and very little nutrient value and are often consumed in super-sized portions. Juice should also be limited because it is often a large source of calories and not appropriately portion-controlled. One hundred percent fruit juices should be limited to 4 to 8 ounces (120 to 240 ml) daily. Foods can provide up to 20 percent of daily fluid needs.

The Current Daily Reference Intakes for water are 56 ounces (1.7 L) at four to eight years of age; 70 and 80 ounces (2.1 L and 2.4 L) for girls and boys, respectively, at nine to thirteen years of age; and 77 and 110 ounces (2.3 L and 3.3 L) for girls and boys, respectively, at fourteen to eighteen years of age. Of course, these needs can change with heat, humidity, altitude, and activity.

To prevent significant dehydration from exercise, young athletes should be taught to drink on a schedule before, during, and after exercise to prevent dehydration. They can be provided with individual drinking containers that have markings to demonstrate how much they are drinking. Young athletes should drink according to the plan shown in Table 12.1, which is based on body weight.

Young athletes should drink before exercise so they start fully hydrated. Education on drinking at regular intervals during and after the activity is also important. Like adults, children should not wait until they are thirsty to consume fluids. Research indicates that when young athletes consume a sports drink, they stay better hydrated, because it contains flavor and sodium to encourage drinking and consequently they ingest a more optimal volume of fluid. The electrolytes in the sports drink also maintain a more optimal fluid balance in the body than does flavored or plain water. Sports drinks should be consumed during training sessions lasting over 60 minutes, and children can be educated on their appropriate use before, during, and after exercise.

Eating Breakfast and Snacks

Breakfast is an important meal for the young athlete. Depending on their sport and training schedule, young athletes may train early in the morning. Often, workouts begin after consuming only a small pre-exercise snack due to timing constraints, rendering breakfast an important recovery meal. Many common breakfast foods provide carbohydrate and some protein. Young athletes may be able to consume a healthy breakfast

TABLE 12.1 HYDRATION STRATEGIES FOR ACTIVE KIDS

FLUID TIMING	HOW MUCH FLUID	
	LESS THAN 90 LB. (41 KG)	GREATER THAN 90 LB. (41 KG)
1 hour before activity	3–6 oz. of fluid (90–180 ml)	6–12 oz. fluid (180–360 ml)
During activity (every 20 minutes)	3–5 oz. fluid (90–150 ml)	6–9 oz. fluid (180–270 ml)
After activity	8 oz. (240 ml) per 0.5 lb. (0.25 kg) fluid loss	12 oz. (360 ml) for 0.5 lb. (0.25 kg) fluid loss

offered at school, but many may need to pack a breakfast to be consumed right after practice. A combination of a whole-grain cereal, skim milk or yogurt, and fruit makes an optimal recovery breakfast.

Snacks provide a good portion of a young athlete's energy and nutrient intake and may be required to continue the nutrition recovery process after an early-morning training session. Consuming a morning snack between classes or in class as allowed can continue to replenish liver and muscle glycogen. Young athletes who train in the afternoon should also consume an afternoon snack beforehand to provide fuel for the session. Again, healthy snacks can be emphasized, as well as foods tolerated close to exercise. Ideally, the athlete will pack a snack, as school vending machines are likely to offer less healthy choices. A sports drink for afternoon practice can also be packed in liquid or powder form. Meals, snacks, and fluids should be determined ahead of time for the busy young athlete and kept at a safe temperature with a cold pack and insulated lunch sack.

Preventing Overweight and Obesity

About one in three American children and teens is overweight or obese, about triple the rate since 1963. This is leading to a broad range of health problems that previously were not seen until adulthood, such as high blood pressure, type 2 diabetes, and elevated cholesterol. Overweight and obese children are more prone to low self-esteem, negative body image, and depression.

In children and adolescents, body mass index (BMI) is used as an assessment tool, and it correlates well with the level of body fat. Being "at risk of overweight" is defined at the 85th to 95th percentile for BMI for age, and "overweight" is defined as being at the 95th percentile or above. Assessment of body composition can help determine if a child or teenager is truly overweight; this is especially important in athletes who may be muscular and incorrectly defined as overweight.

Because the causes of overweight in children and adolescents are multifactorial, such as the great availability of energy-dense foods and increasing portion sizes, even those who are active can be at risk. Overweight or at-risk children are not advised to "go on a diet," but rather to emphasize nutrient-dense foods over energy-dense foods to promote growth, weight maintenance, or appropriate increases in weight along the growth curve.

Body Image

As children grow and develop, body image concerns also develop. This is especially a concern among female adolescents, as over one-half of them report a history of dieting.

Athletes may also strive for a low weight and decreased body fat level in an attempt to improve performance. While the causes are multifactorial, an eating disorder often starts with dieting or can be triggered by comments from coaches, peers, and teammates related to weight. Dieting in girls can lead to a number of health problems, including low bone mass. Please refer to the sections on eating disorders and the female athlete triad later in this chapter for more information on these related topics.

Young Athletes and Alcohol

Underage alcohol intake can be a problem in many ways. High-school athletes participating in endurance sports should be aware of alcohol's harmful effects. Parents of teenagers should emphasize that alcohol consumption not only is illegal but can result in long-term health risks. Too, young athletes need to understand that alcohol and hangovers affect performance. Alcohol can disrupt fluid balance and temperature regulation, impair fine motor skills, and cause subpar practices and competitive performance.

Race or Competition Day

High-school athletes should develop a race nutrition plan during the training season. Refer to Chapters 8 through 11 for sport-specific nutrition guidelines for competition.

Nutrition Education

High-school athletes can benefit greatly from nutrition education under a registered dietitian who specializes in sports dietetics. Nutrition lectures presented by the dietitian can review sports nutrition fundamentals, help plan appropriate team meals, and demonstrate the importance of eating well. Sports dietitians can also develop personalized nutrition plans for young athletes who desire more detail and guidance in their training nutrition program.

THE MASTERS ATHLETE

Endurance sports are heavily populated by "masters athletes," with age-group wins in triathlon, age-category racing in cycling, and long-distance running heavily dominated by athletes in their thirties and forties. Because of the high level of participation of these seasoned athletes, some of the physiological and nutrition adjustments that come with healthy aging are important to understand.

Lean Body Mass

One of the most significant physiological changes that occurs with aging is a slight decrease in muscle mass after age thirty. Weight training can offset these muscle losses and provide the masters athlete with the benefits of maintaining strength and power. Muscle is metabolically active tissue. Weight training can strengthen weak body areas and improve one's strength-to-weight ratio. Masters athletes who are dedicated to resistance training should refer to the corresponding nutrition guidelines provided in Chapter 6.

Energy Requirements

Because of the large range of training commitments and schedules found among masters athletes in any endurance sport, calorie and carbohydrate requirements vary. It is the intensity and volume of training that dictate the best nutritional plan. Masters athletes should be aware that their nutritional requirements can change throughout the year as they make seasonal adjustments in training volume and focus. As athletes age, a decrease in calories may be necessary to maintain a healthy weight. However, the quality of the diet should not be compromised. Nutrient-dense foods become an even more important component of the diet when calorie requirements decrease.

Although aging is typically regarded as a function of chronological age, the number of years a person has been alive may be a very poor predictor of functional age. Functional age refers to the quality of life that an aging person can enjoy as related to his or her fitness level, strength, and management of health risk factors. Masters athletes in their fifties and sixties often outperform sedentary persons in their twenties. But even well-conditioned and -trained athletes will experience a decline in aerobic power after age thirty to thirty-five. VO_2max declines after age twenty-five, but at a slower rate in active individuals than in sedentary ones. Muscle strength plateaus at age thirty-five to forty and then declines, though muscle strength can be maintained and improved with a good resistance training program. Masters athletes who adopt a healthy lifestyle can derive very tangible health benefits from these good habits and their training. These benefits may include more favorable blood lipid profiles and lower risk of developing hypertension, diabetes, and osteoporosis.

Specific Nutrients

It is thought that for the most part, older athletes should follow the same recommendations for carbohydrate, protein, and fat intake as younger athletes with comparable training programs. Aging may increase the need for calcium in women in particular to prevent osteoporosis (though men can also develop this debilitating condition). Vitamin D requirements increase after age seventy, and vitamin B6 requirements increase after age 50. Continuing to choose nutrient-dense foods throughout a lifetime is useful for meeting the increases in vitamin and mineral needs that occur with aging, without adding unwanted calories to the diet. Masters athletes concerned about adequate vitamin and mineral intake can take a balanced low-dose multivitamin-and-mineral supplement. This supplement should also provide the daily value of vitamin B12 for individuals over age sixty, since gastric acid levels decrease with aging, reducing absorption of B12 by the body. Calcium supplementation may also be beneficial to meet higher calcium needs. Postmenopausal women and older men may not need as much iron, and should have iron levels checked to determine if their multivitamin should or should not contain iron, as excess iron has been linked with cardiovascular disease.

Calcium needs increase with age among both men and women. One study conducted at Tufts University that included both men and women over age sixty-five found that an average intake of 1,350 milligrams of calcium (500 of which came from a supplement), combined with a diet high in protein, produced higher bone mineral densities in the test subjects after three years. Lower calcium intakes—of 850 milligrams daily—did not work synergistically with the protein to improve bone density. Researchers are still trying to determine the underlying mechanisms and why the high protein intake was not accompanied by increased calcium excretion in the urine. The bottom line from this study is not that older individuals should eat excess protein but rather they should meet their calcium requirements and maintain good protein intake within the recommended ranges for health and training. For calcium supplementation, the form recommended for older individuals is calcium citrate, which does not require stomach acid for absorption (we produce less stomach acid as we age).

Older athletes should also pay attention to fluid intake. Thirst sensation declines in older individuals, affecting their fluid regulation. At the same time, their fluid requirements actually increase, because more water is needed to remove waste products from their system as kidney function declines with aging. Generally, older athletes can tolerate exercise in the heat but should drink as much fluid as possible before and after the exercise session. They should aim for the high end of recommended fluid intake amounts during exercise, consuming 8 ounces (240 ml) every 15 minutes. Older athletes should also pay close attention to warning signs of dehydration and be aware of how any medications they are taking may affect heat regulation.

Fiber is also an important nutrient for older athletes. Not only does fiber help lower blood lipid and keep blood glucose levels stable, but it can also decrease risk of diverticulitis. Refer to Chapter 2 for good sources of fiber; both soluble and insoluble sources are important.

THE PREGNANT ATHLETE

Many pregnant athletes desire to maintain a high degree of fitness during pregnancy and often return to training and competition as quickly as possible. It is no longer unusual for Olympic or professional athletes to have a child and resume training at a high level soon after the baby's birth. Although these athletes may be most concerned about consuming an adequate number of calories for a healthy and appropriate weight gain, the nutrients consumed while planning a pregnancy are also very important.

Much confusion surrounds exercise recommendations during pregnancy. The American College of Obstetricians and Gynecologists (ACOG) first published guidelines in 1985, then in 1994, and again in 2002, and many of the earlier recommendations have become dogma that does not reflect more accurate updates. Research has not legitimized the fear that high-intensity exercise is harmful to the mother and fetus. However, the American College of Sports Medicine recommends that women who plan to continue their regular pregnancy exercise program should not exceed pre-pregnancy intensity levels. An endurance athlete who enters pregnancy in a high training state may be able to continue her exercise program for some time. The ACOG also recommends that women should avoid "exercise to exhaustion"; the Rate of Perceived Exertion (RPE) can be used as a guide to exercise intensity. Pregnant athletes should be aware that it will take lower levels of effort to attain the same RPE as pregnancy advances. Pregnant endurance athletes should discuss exercise guidelines with their obstetrician.

It is a good idea to see your physician before trying to conceive to discuss how to get the best nutrition during this time. He or she may recommend taking a prenatal multivitamin-and-mineral supplement in order to obtain folic acid and other important nutrients. Folate (found in food sources) and folic acid (from supplement sources) deserve serious attention by women athletes even contemplating pregnancy. An adequate intake of folate, about 400 micrograms daily, prior to conception and during the first several weeks of pregnancy, can help prevent birth defects such as spina bifida. Folate is used for the synthesis of DNA, the building block of all cells. During the first twenty-eight days of pregnancy, cells divide rapidly and form the neural tubes that become the baby's brain and spine. Many American women fall short of the recommended 400 micrograms of folate.

Good food sources of folate include asparagus, lentils, spinach and other leafy green vegetables, dried beans such as kidney beans, and orange juice. Grain products such as bread, pasta, rice, and enriched flour have been fortified with folic acid for several years, and a decrease in these types of birth defects has been the result. Many health experts also recommend that any woman who may become pregnant take a multivitamin providing 400 micrograms of folate.

During the first three months of pregnancy, it is normal to have no weight gain or perhaps a small gain of up to 5 pounds. After the first trimester, a weight gain of up to 1 pound weekly is normal. Generally a total weight gain of 25 to 35 pounds is recommended. Underweight or lean women may be advised to gain more weight, for a total of about 28 to 40 pounds. Adequate weight gain comes down to finding the right balance of calories to build your own tissue during pregnancy, to support the growth of the baby, and to meet your energy needs from exercise in order to prevent having a low-birth-weight baby or a premature delivery. Starting in the second trimester, pregnancy requires only an additional 300 calories daily above your usual energy needs and another 10 to 12 grams of protein. These additional amounts are easily met with an increased food intake—for example, 8 ounces of milk and a small turkey sandwich.

The expectant mother's weight gain comes from growth in her own body tissues, the baby's body weight, and tissues that support the baby's growth. It includes an increased blood volume, body fluid, and breast tissue as well as the placenta, umbilical cord, and amniotic fluid. Body fat stores increase in anticipation of lactation, which requires at least an additional 500 calories daily above normal nonpregnancy requirements in the third trimester.

Your physician will monitor not only your total weight gain but also your pattern of weight gain to make sure that it is appropriate. Weight recommendations in pregnancy are based on body mass index and range from 25 to 40 pounds (11–18 kg). The lower the BMI, the higher the recommendations for weight gain. For example, a female endurance athlete may have a BMI of 19 and be advised to gain 28 to 40 pounds, whereas a BMI of 20 to 26 requires a weight gain of 25 to 35 pounds. While pregnancy is often characterized as "eating for two," the increase in energy requirements is not that significant. Energy needs do not increase significantly in the first trimester, increase about 300 calories daily above baseline in the second trimester, and increase by 500 calories above baseline in the third trimester. Since the endurance athlete may continue to train during this time, energy needs can remain high. However, with a possible decrease in exercise volume and intensity, there may need to be an adjustment in caloric intake despite the additional energy needed for maintaining a pregnancy.

Fluid requirements also increase during pregnancy, and it is critical to maintain proper hydration during exercise and training. Pregnant athletes need about 2.5 to 3 quarts (about 2.5 to 3 L) of fluids daily plus whatever is needed to account for sweat losses during exercise. It is essential that you begin your training sessions well hydrated if you are pregnant. Overheating could have serious negative effects on the unborn baby. Increases in fetal temperature when a mother is ill and has high fever in the first trimester have been associated with birth defects. Plenty of fluids should be consumed several hours before exercise, and at least 4 to 8 additional ounces (120 to 240 ml) should be consumed every 15 to 20 minutes during exercise. Pregnant women have a lower sweating threshold and begin to sweat sooner during exercise to dissipate heat.

Carbohydrates can be consumed several hours before exercise to prevent hypoglycemia. Sports drinks, carbohydrate gels, and energy bars can be consumed during exercise to maintain blood glucose levels, but make sure they do not contain extra vitamins, minerals, or herbal additives. Your training diet and your prenatal vitamin-and-mineral supplement should be more than adequate to meet your nutrient requirements; do not take more vitamins and minerals than your doctor recommends. Herbal products and teas have not been tested in pregnancy and should be avoided.

Do discuss your intake of iron and calcium with your doctor or sports dietitian to make sure you are getting enough of these important minerals during your pregnancy. Iron requirements double during pregnancy owing to a pregnant woman's expanded blood volume. Most pregnant women receive adequate iron in their prenatal vitamin-and-mineral supplement, but some require an additional iron supplement in order to prevent anemia. Anemia can result in fatigue, shortness of breath, and increased delivery risks. The baby also runs the risk of developing anemia if iron stores are too low, and athletes may already have low iron stores. Your doctor should check your iron levels early in your pregnancy and again at regular intervals until the birth. Be sure to include plenty of high-iron foods in your diet (see Table 3.6).

Calcium plays an important role in every woman's health and deserves extra attention during pregnancy. Calcium requirements increase to 1,200 milligrams daily during pregnancy. As the baby builds bone, the mother's bones serve as a calcium source. If her diet is inadequate to supply the baby's needs and maintain this calcium reservoir, the risk of developing osteoporosis later in life increases. High-calcium food sources are listed in Table 3.5. You can also consider taking a separate calcium supplement during pregnancy to meet your elevated requirements. But do consult with your doctor or dietitian first. Certain nutrients and foods should be limited during pregnancy. Excess vitamin A intake from oversupplementation can increase the risk of birth defects. Intake from a supplement should not exceed 5,000 IU of vitamin A daily. There is also no room for alcohol in the diet, as it can produce severe negative effects for the baby, such as fetal alcohol syndrome. Caffeine should be restricted to no more than 300 milligrams daily or avoided altogether. Avoid saccharin, and limit other artificial sweeteners as much as possible. Limit soft cheeses such as brie, camembert, blue cheese, and feta cheese because they can increase the risk of bacterial contamination. In general, pregnant women should be careful about food safety, never eat raw fish, and make sure that all meats are well cooked. Avoid any unpasteurized milk products and raw eggs.

Fish can also be contaminated with mercury, which can have adverse effects on the developing baby, though there are many benefits to the unborn baby receiving the DHA fatty acid found in fish. Fatty fish such as swordfish, mackerel, shark, bluefish, tilefish, and striped bass should be avoided completely. Other high-mercury fish to avoid are marlin, red snapper, trout, fresh tuna, and white canned albacore tuna. Lobster can also be high in mercury and should be avoided. Limit your consumption of canned light tuna to less than 6 ounces weekly, and your total fish intake to 9 to 12 ounces weekly. Sole, tilapia, scallops, shrimp, canned salmon (wild Alaskan), and catfish are relatively low in mercury. Eat low-fat fish, and trim excess fat as much as possible. Several prenatal vitamins include 300 mg of DHA as well to easily supply this important nutrient during pregnancy.

After the birth, lactation and breast-feeding will increase your daily energy requirements 500 calories or more above your nonpregnancy requirements. Fat stores accumulated during pregnancy serve as an important energy source for lactation, but your diet should be rich in nutrients during the breast-feeding period. Your fluid needs will also be high during this time. Weight loss can occur gradually with lactation, but it is best to try not to lose more than 1 pound weekly, as an overly restrictive diet will decrease the quantity of milk that you produce. Maintain the high calcium and iron intakes that you established during your pregnancy, and ask your doctor about whether you should continue taking your prenatal multivitamin-and-mineral supplement. Limit alcohol and caffeine intake, as they can enter breast milk. It may be best to nurse before exercise due to transient changes that occur in breast milk with exercise. When women train at very high intensities or complete interval training, higher levels of lactic acid in the breast milk may result, resulting in altered taste of the milk.

CLINICAL CONDITIONS

IRRITABLE BOWEL SYNDROME

Irritable bowel syndrome, or IBS, is a collection of symptoms that occur in the digestive tract when an individual's nerves and muscles don't work correctly. It is a fairly common condition affecting up to 20 percent of the world's population. It is more common in women and generally occurs before age 35.

Common symptoms of IBS include cramping, abdominal pain, diarrhea, gas, bloating, constipation, mucus in the stool, and frequent changes in bowel habits. IBS is often considered a diagnosis of exclusion and is often diagnosed when other gastrointestinal conditions have been ruled out. It is a functional disorder, as there are no abnormal medical tests or visual abnormalities. In IBS there is disorder of intestinal motility, making intestinal time too fast or too slow, resulting in frequent bowel movements or constipation, or both. IBS sufferers are more sensitive to pain from gas-producing foods.

Although this disease comes in many shapes and forms, the universal complaint is bloating, affecting over 90 percent of sufferers. A GI infection can lead to IBS, as can hormonal changes during a woman's menstrual cycle. IBS also seems to run in families.

IBS is a chronic condition with no cure, but several treatments can help IBS sufferers feel better. These include diet modifications, medications recommended by a physician, and some dietary supplements. Stress can aggravate IBS symptoms.

For the endurance athlete with IBS, sorting out dietary modifications that are effective must be done in conjunction with adopting an optimal training diet and sports nutrition supplements needed for fueling and recovery. Not managing IBS symptoms could interfere with both training and competition goals, so it is important to seek the assistance of a sports dietitian who is also familiar with IBS.

If dietary, medical, and other health care measures don't bring any symptom relief, there may be other underlying conditions, such as celiac disease (discussed below). Another is small intestinal bacterial overgrowth (SIBO), whereby bacteria that belong in the large intestine take residence in the small intestine. Finally, there may be food allergies or unusual food sensitivities (also discussed below).

The Diet Connection

Uncovering the diet connections for each individual with IBS can be tricky. Possibilities include specific foods or groups of foods, portions of certain foods, and the conditions under which these foods are consumed. These are some common food triggers, and there can be many reasons why some foods trigger IBS symptoms.

Malabsorption

Malabsorption occurs when something interferes with absorption of nutrients from the foods we eat in the small intestine. Food that is not absorbed properly makes its way from the small intestine to the large intestine. In the large intestine, bacteria that reside there get busy fermenting the food, producing gas and bloating. There are a number of carbohydrates that can be particularly troublesome in IBS; they are referred to as FODMAPs carbohydrates. Decreasing intake or load of these carbohydrates in the diet can help the athlete manage his or her IBS symptoms.

FODMAPs Carbohydrates

Your first question regarding these carbohydrates is likely to be "What is a FODMAPs?" Good question, and hang on tight, as it is a bit of a tongue twister. FODMAP is an acronym for Fermentable Oligosaccharides, Disaccharides, Monosaccharides, and Polyols. These are a collective group of carbohydrates often malabsorbed in the intestine. Two of the most troublesome FODMAPs are lactose and fructose; next come fructans, polyols, and galactans.

Lactose

Lactose is the sugar found in milk and related dairy products, and it can be a real nuisance in IBS. Symptoms of gas, bloating, and diarrhea can occur within 30 minutes to 2 hours after consuming these foods. Lacking the enzyme lactase is the cause; lactase breaks down lactose into glucose and galactose so they can be easily absorbed into the small intestine.

Even if you are lactose-intolerant, you may have a threshold of lactose absorption, meaning that you can tolerate small amounts of lactose. Milk, evaporated milk, and dry milk products provide the largest amounts of lactose. Soft cheeses contain moderate amounts of lactose, while hard cheeses contain little to no lactose. Lactose can be hidden in waffles, pancakes, cereal, salad dressing, and some breakfast cereals and may not be easily discerned from label reading. If you omit or limit dairy products, make sure that you meet your calcium and vitamin D requirements (see Chapter 3). Cheese substitutes and nondairy milk substitutes (such as soy, rice, and nut milks) are available and often are fortified with calcium; lactose-reduced milk is also available and may be tolerated. These products are also a source of carbohydrate for your training diet.

Fructose

Fructose, the sugar found primarily in fruits and honey, can cause symptoms in IBS sufferers. Here the problem is not lack of an enzyme but rather a lower threshold of fructose absorption. While diets rich in fruits offer many health advantages, you may need to limit specific fruits. Added fructose and high-fructose corn syrup (HFCS) may also contribute to problematic symptoms, and they may even be responsible for the increasing incidence of IBS. Agave syrup, which has gained popularity as a sweetener, contains a high amount of fructose. Some experts estimate that up to 50 percent of IBS sufferers experience fructose malabsorption.

Look at food labels for HFCS, fructose, and crystalline fructose. Fruits that are especially high in fructose include apples, coconut milk, dried fruit and fruit juices, guava, mangoes, honey, pears, and watermelon. Fruits that contain more glucose than fructose are ripe bananas, blackberries, strawberries, raspberries, blueberries, grapefruit, grapes, kiwifruit, oranges, and lemons. Often it is a matter of dosing, just as with lactose, to find your tolerance threshold.

Endurance athletes with a high fructose sensitivity may need to consume fructose-free sports drinks and gels during training and competition to prevent unwanted GI symptoms.

Fructans

Fructans are composed of fructose chains, and we lack the necessary enzyme to break the fructose chains. Fructan-rich foods include asparagus, beer, garlic, leeks, onion, and wheat. Inulin and fructooligosaccharides (FOS) are often added to various foods to increase fiber content and are rich in fructans. Wheat is the biggest source of fructans in the American diet, and minimizing wheat-containing foods may be an effective strategy against IBS. Besides controlling portions, you can also substitute wheat foods with wheat-free alternatives.

Polyols

Polyols are known as sugar alcohols and can have a laxative effect. Fruits that naturally contain polyols include apples, apricots, cherries, nectarines, peaches, pears, plums, and prunes. Polyols are also used in sugar-free products—check labels for mannitol, sorbitol, xylitol, isomalt, lactitol, and maltitol.

Galactans

Galactans contain chains of the simple sugar galactose. As with fructans, we lack the enzyme to break them down. Galactan sources include Brussels sprouts, cabbage, chickpeas, kidney beans, lentils, soy foods, and wax beans.

The more FODMAPs carbohydrates you consume, the more likely they will have an effect on your intestine. A food diary can help in assessing which of these foods aggravate IBS symptoms. You can also work with a dietitian familiar with IBS to follow a trial low-load FODMAPs diet and do a food challenge series to assess tolerances.

IBS and Fiber

Fiber is an indigestible complex carbohydrate, and it's a bit tricky when it comes to IBS. If constipation is the major IBS symptom, adding more fiber can be helpful. For the individual with diarrhea, adding fiber would only aggravate existing symptoms. It may also be helpful to focus on the type of fiber consumed.

Fiber comes in two forms, soluble and insoluble. Most fiber-containing foods have a combination of both types. Soluble fiber forms a gel in the gut and slows down the digestive process. Recent studies have found that persons with IBS better tolerate this fiber, which is found in oats, barley, beans, and fruits. Insoluble fiber speeds up gut transit time and can aggravate symptoms. It is best to increase water-soluble fiber slowly over a few weeks' time so that your gut can adjust and benefit from the increase. For some IBS sufferers, specific fiber supplements can be helpful. Psyllium husk is a source in many water-soluble fiber supplements.

IBS and Fat

Besides eating healthy fats for your heart and adequate essential fatty acids as outlined in Chapter 3, you may need to determine your own fat threshold. Dietary fats in particular can trigger the reflexes that cause an overreaction to eating. Every time we eat we stimulate something called the gastrocolic reflex, which controls the movements and contractions of our intestines. Dietary fats, more than proteins and carbohydrates, get this gastrocolic reflex going. Fat-rich foods also require more stomach acid to be broken down for digestion. Managing your fat intake can help you manage your IBS symptoms.

Probiotics

You may find it interesting and even a bit gross to know that you have over 2 pounds of bacteria living in your small intestine. There are over 400 different types—both good and bad bacteria. Maintaining proper balance between the good and the bad is key. Many diet and lifestyle factors can diminish some of these good bacteria, and adding more of the good can be helpful in many GI conditions, including IBS.

Many studies have evaluated probiotic use in IBS, and the most effective seems to be bifidobacterium infantis 35264, which has been shown to reduce pain and gas. Other strains have been helpful in regulating constipation. It may be beneficial to include a variety of probiotics in your diet, as there appears to be a synergistic effect. The two most common sources are lactobacillus and bifidobacteria; both can be consumed in food and supplement form. Lactobacillus acidophilus is found in yogurt. Look for yogurt made with "live and active cultures." Culturelle® and Align® are supplements in pill form that are commercially available probiotics backed by a number of scientific studies indicating various health benefits. Some probiotic supplements are also available in powder form.

Prebiotics

Prebiotics are undigested food that provides fuel for probiotics residing in our intestine. Inulin and fructooligosaccharides are oligosaccharides (the O in FODMAPs). Neither one is absorbed, and they could be problematic for individuals with IBS, so prebiotic use should be individualized for the person with IBS. Watch out for supplements that contain both probiotics and prebiotics, as you may want to take the probiotic-only supplement.

The bottom line is that planning and making time for healthy meals and snacks are as important for IBS management as they are for an optimal training diet. This allows for consumption of high-quality foods, limited intake of processed foods, and more relaxed mealtimes combined with appropriate supplementation and medical management as needed.

FOOD ALLERGIES AND SENSITIVITIES

Chances are you know someone who has a food allergy, particularly a peanut allergy. Food allergies often produce dramatic results in the sensitive individual, and reactions can be severe. There is definitely an increased interest today in food allergies, but there is no clear agreement on the true prevalence of food allergies, with estimates ranging from 1–2 percent to less than 10 percent of the population. Although it appears the incidence of food allergy is increasing, it may be the increased awareness of the condition and the availability of more diagnostic tests.

Food allergies may also often be confused with *food intolerances* and *food sensitivities*, but they are really a different type of response in the body. Food sensitivity, or adverse food reaction, is a generic term that refers to any bothersome reaction that occurs after the ingestion of a food. It can be a food allergy or a food intolerance. Food intolerance occurs when your body has a negative reaction to food that does not involve the immune system but can involve the digestive system. The reaction is caused by a component of the food that has not been digested completely (such as lactose intolerance) or that cannot be processed properly by the body.

In contrast, food allergy occurs when your immune system reacts symptomatically to a food, usually one containing protein, that your body recognizes as foreign. Your body responds by making antibodies to stop the invasion of these perceived allergens. Symptoms can be diverse and include skin-related reactions such as eczema or hives; digestive issues such as abdominal pain, nausea, or vomiting; lung-related reactions such as asthma, stuffy or runny nose, or earache; or all body systems simultaneously, often referred to as *anaphylaxis*. This latter reaction can be severe and life-threatening; it commonly occurs after consumption of peanuts or shellfish.

Eight foods account for 90 percent of all food allergies: eggs, fish, milk, peanuts, shellfish, soy, tree nuts, and wheat. The FDA requires that foods containing any of the top eight allergens include them in bold print on the ingredients list. The majority of IBS sufferers feel that food contributes to their symptoms, and food allergies could trigger IBS symptoms. Individuals with a wheat allergy may also need to sort out if they have a true wheat allergy or an intolerance to gluten (found in wheat), or have celiac disease, which is a distinct type of immune system reaction. For more on celiac disease, read below.

Physicians can order various skin and blood tests for food allergies and sensitivities. Another process that helps in determining food allergies and sensitivities is an elimination diet.

The Elimination Diet

The comprehensive elimination diet is designed to clear the body of foods and chemicals that you may be allergic or sensitive to, and at the same time improve your body's ability to handle and dispose of these substances. The theory behind the diet is that these food modifications will allow your body's detoxification processes to rest and recover and then begin to function efficiently and effectively again. Because the body is not continually exposed to various toxins, they can be more easily eliminated.

Generally the comprehensive elimination diet is well tolerated and can be extremely beneficial to an individual with multiple food allergies, sensitivities, and intolerances. You can begin an elimination diet to determine what specific foods may be causing unwanted reactions and symptoms. While the comprehensive elimination diet is a "clean" whole foods diet, it is probably best followed in the off-season and early in base season when there is less focus on a detailed training diet.

Individual responses to the diet are highly variable; there is no "typical" or "normal" response. More often than not, individuals report increased energy, improved well-being, and decreased muscle or joint pain. However, some people report initial reactions to the diet, particularly in the first week, with symptoms such as changes in gastrointestinal function, headaches, joint and muscle stiffness, and light-headedness. Symptoms rarely last more than a few days. An elimination diet can be followed for 21 to 28 days.

This diet will eliminate the suspect main eight allergens as well as gluten, additives, preservatives, colorings, and artificial sweeteners. Caffeine is also eliminated, as are hydrogenated oils and high-fructose corn syrup. A dietitian can guide you in meal planning for an elimination diet and provide simple recipes and food-shopping tips. It can be beneficial to keep a food journal at this time to record not only the foods consumed but also your symptoms.

The comprehensive elimination diet can be followed for 2 to 4 weeks before beginning reintroduction guidelines. When reintroducing foods, it is best to test them in their purest form. A reaction test has you consume each food component three different times on a test day at about 4-hour intervals, while monitoring for symptoms. The challenge can be stopped if any symptoms are clearly developing from the foods. Two days of one specific food challenge are usually adequate, but if the results are unclear, the same food challenge can be repeated for up to 4 days. A food journal should be kept and each food graded on a pass/fail system. If there is no response to a food, you can then proceed to the next food challenge. The duration of the food challenge phases depends upon the response to specific foods and how quickly foods can be identified as reactive.

Once you are aware of what foods need to be avoided or greatly reduced in your diet, you can then develop a sports nutrition training plan for the upcoming season, if necessary, with the help and guidance of a sports dietitian.

Celiac Disease/Gluten Intolerance

Celiac disease, also known as gluten-sensitive enteropathy, is a chronic autoimmune intestinal disorder that can manifest in genetically susceptible individuals. The development of celiac disease requires a combination of genetic, environmental, and immunological factors and may be triggered by a gastrointestinal or viral infection, severe stress, or surgery. World prevalence of celiac disease is estimated at 1 out of 266 persons; in the United States it is estimated that 1 of every 100 persons has celiac disease, which is similar to data from European countries. Several decades ago, celiac disease was thought to be a rare disorder, usually diagnosed in early childhood. Celiac disease can occur at any age, including in the elderly.

Persons with celiac disease need to follow a gluten-free diet for life. *Gluten* is the collective term for specific types of proteins found in wheat, rye, and barley that damage the absorptive surface of the small intestine in persons with celiac disease. The walls of our small intestine are lined with tiny finger-like projections called villi, which are necessary for digesting and absorbing nutrients required for good health. When gluten damages these villi, they become inflamed and flattened, causing malabsorption of calcium, iron, and folate. As damage progresses, malabsorption of carbohydrates, such as lactose, and fat-soluble vitamins (A, D, E, and K), protein, and other nutrients can occur.

Understandably, chronic exposure to gluten can result in vitamin and mineral deficiencies and related diseases such as osteoporosis and anemia. There is increased risk of developing neurological disorders, other autoimmune disorders, and certain types of cancer. There is also increased risk of miscarriage, and of infertility in both men and women. Celiac disease affects many systems in the body other than the GI system, and the range and severity of symptoms can vary greatly from person to person. It is also possible to have "silent celiac disease" with no or very subtle symptoms.

The diagnosis of celiac disease is difficult because of the broad range of symptoms and their variance in severity. Celiac disease affects not only the gastrointestinal tract but other body systems as well. These symptoms can occur singly or in combination in both children and adults.

Some symptoms of celiac disease are:

- Iron, folate, and/or B12 deficiency
- Multiple vitamin and mineral deficiencies
- Abdominal pain, bloating, and gas
- Indigestion/reflux

- Nausea and vomiting
- Chronic fatigue and weakness
- Diarrhea, constipation, or intermittent periods of both
- Lactose intolerance
- Migraine headaches
- Bone/joint pain
- Easy bruising
- Swelling of the hands and feet
- Depression
- Canker sores

Diagnosis can be difficult, and many individuals suffer from symptoms for an average of 10 years before being diagnosed. Specific blood tests include IgA endomysial and IgA transglutaminase (tTG) antibody tests. These tests are not 100 percent accurate, and some persons may test negative despite having celiac disease. The only definitive test is an intestinal biopsy.

It is important not to try a gluten-free diet prior to performing a blood test or biopsy, as this can interfere with making an accurate diagnosis. Antibody levels, as well as the villi, may return to normal on a gluten-free diet and prevent a definitive diagnosis.

Once a diagnosis has been made, a strict gluten-free diet must be followed for life. When gluten is removed, damage to the small intestine heals and symptoms improve and eventually disappear. Even if the person with celiac disease is feeling well, consumption of small amounts of gluten can cause intestinal damage.

Foods to Avoid on a Gluten-Free Diet

Gluten is found in wheat, rye, and barley. Many foods made from these grains are obvious, such as breads, cereals, and pasta. However, a number of foods contain hidden amounts of gluten in the form of thickeners and stabilizers added to processed foods. If you have celiac disease, you need to become adept at reading ingredients lists and recognizing potential sources of gluten. Gluten may be lurking in many seemingly innocent products, such as deli meats, salad dressing, gravies, and soups.

Oats remain an area of controversy in the gluten-free diet. Oats present two distinct issues. First, many oats are cross-contaminated with gluten-containing grains during growing, harvesting, and processing. Recent research has found that oats can cause a specific intestinal reaction in some individuals while causing no change in others. Oats that are guaranteed to be uncontaminated are available, so advice regarding oat consumption needs to be individualized for each person with celiac disease.

Foods to Consume on a Gluten-Free Diet

Athletes with celiac disease should develop a formulary of gluten-free products that can be incorporated into their training and racing diet. Grains and starchy foods that are gluten-free include rice, corn, potato, tapioca, sago, lentils, dried beans, amaranth, buckwheat, sorghum, quinoa, and millet.

Read all ingredients lists and become familiar with company brands that manufacture gluten-free products in separate production facilities. You may need to pack gluten-free foods for travel to competition, or inquire ahead about the availability of gluten-free products. Gluten-free snack bars, sports drinks, and gels should all be on the menu. As you develop your own training nutrition meals and snacks, consuming a gluten-free diet should support your training goals, recovery, and preparation for competition, just as it would for any other athlete.

THE DIABETIC ATHLETE

More endurance athletes with type 1 or type 2 diabetes are competing successfully in endurance sports than ever before. Type 1 diabetes is an autoimmune disease that affects the insulin-releasing cells of the pancreas, so that they produce little or no insulin. Type 2 diabetes results when insulin receptors are unable to recognize insulin produced in the body, and usually occurs in overweight or obese individuals.

Team Type 1 is the first professional cycling team with riders who have type 1 diabetes; type 1 diabetics also compete in long-distance running, swimming, and triathlon. Type 1 diabetes is a condition in which the body is unable to produce insulin. Without insulin, the body is not able to use glucose as a fuel source. This section reviews the sports nutrition issues for persons with either type 1 or type 2 diabetes, though some of the strategies for specific challenges and circumstances may be more typical in type 1 diabetes. Athletes with type 2 diabetes also routinely compete in endurance events. The following advice should not replace the advice of your diabetes educator.

Endurance athletes with diabetes face fueling challenges that are unique to their disease, and they must continually monitor and manage their blood glucose levels to prevent hyperglycemia (high blood glucose) or hypoglycemia (low blood glucose). Glucose levels can fluctuate depending on exercise intensity and duration, the time of day, the athlete's emotional state, environmental conditions, and absorption rates of food and insulin. Clearly nutrition programs for endurance athletes with diabetes need to be individualized by a qualified sports dietitian and a diabetes educator, who may be the same person or two persons working as a team to support the diabetic athlete.

Because of their training demands, endurance athletes with diabetes need to fuel like an athlete, meeting specific energy and carbohydrate, protein, and fat requirements for different types of workout days, while making adjustments to insulin and medication to support their training and fueling efforts. Different fueling approaches for specific workouts can require specific adjustments in insulin.

For the daily training diet, athletes with type 1 or type 2 diabetes have the same nutritional training requirements as any other endurance athlete. Including carbohydrates with a low glycemic index may assist with blood glucose control, as they are released more gradually into the bloodstream. Blood glucose control tends to be better when a consistent meal and snack pattern is followed. Athletes with type 1 diabetes are encouraged to adjust their insulin according to their training diet, rather than modify their food intake to suit the insulin dose. In other words, they must eat like an athlete and think like a pancreas!

One of the biggest concerns for athletes with type 1 diabetes is developing hypoglycemia. This is especially true both during and following exercise if they do not make the proper adjustments in their food intake and insulin. Athletes with type 2 diabetes who do not take insulin have to worry less about hypoglycemia, depending on the type of oral medication they take, and may need to make adjustments in their oral medication with increased training. Adjustments for type 1 diabetes are much more complicated and erratic. Hypoglycemia can also develop in the 24 hours following moderate to intense training, so blood glucose must be monitored before and after exercise as well as in the hours following exercise.

One of the technologies available to the diabetic athlete is the blood glucose meter, which can provide results in five seconds. This allows the athlete to check blood glucose levels throughout the day for optimal management, but also before exercise. Ideally the athlete will start exercise at a blood glucose range between 100 and 200 milligrams per deciliter. If levels are too low, the athlete can consume an appropriate level of carbohydrates, or if levels are too high he or she may need to add more insulin. If blood glucose levels are very high and ketones are present in the urine, training may need to be postponed. These meters also provide diabetic endurance athletes with important data to understand their blood glucose responses to exercise, insulin, and food intake, so that they can learn what adjustments are optimal for them.

For workouts lasting over 60 minutes at moderate to high intensity, diabetic endurance athletes need to consume carbohydrate during training, just like any other athlete. A good start is to aim for 30 to 60 grams of carbohydrates per hour. Sports drinks conveniently provide carbohydrate, fluid, and electrolytes. Gels and sports bars can be added. Usually it is not necessary to take extra insulin if carbohydrate is consumed during exercise. Steady intake of carbohydrate is recommended, and checking blood glucose levels can help determine what adjustments in insulin are needed for specific workouts. Diabetic athletes can be educated about insulin adjustments, blood glucose monitoring, and correction factors in insulin for their training, fueling program, and optimal diabetic control.

Continuous Glucose Monitoring (CGM) devices are another important tool for athletes who want information on what is happening to their glucose levels. These devices give readings about every five minutes, provide information on blood glucose trends, and can be used as an alert, particularly during exercise, in hopes of preventing low blood glucose levels. Diabetic athletes can make adjustments in their carbohydrate intake during exercise to prevent hypoglycemia. Insulin pumps are another device for athletes with diabetes, allowing them to adjust insulin down during and after exercise to prevent hypoglycemia. These pumps allow athletes to adjust their insulin in smaller time increments for more precise dosing.

After exercise, the same recovery strategies apply to the diabetic athlete, whereby fluid, fuel, and electrolytes need to be replaced. Increased sensitivity to insulin lasts for several hours after exercise. Eating optimally after exercise can prevent hypoglycemia, and sometimes an insulin dose may need to be reduced. Monitoring blood glucose levels after exercise can be helpful.

It is inevitable that there will be some excitement and nerves in the lead-up to competition. One side effect can be release of the hormones adrenalin and cortisol, which stimulate the release of glucose from the liver and reduce the effectiveness of insulin, ultimately resulting in fluctuating blood glucose levels. Practice and try to simulate race day to set up a nutrition, medication, and monitoring plan on paper. Relaxation techniques can also help. While a type 1 athlete may decrease his or her basal insulin rate to prevent low blood glucose levels on race day, race nerves and stress hormones that increase blood glucose levels, along with pre-race carbohydrate intake, may require adjustments in the regular insulin coverage. Carbohydrate intake needed to complete the race should not be sacrificed. Basal insulin can be decreased post-race if needed to prevent low blood glucose levels. Recovery carbohydrate strategies should also be practiced post-race to prevent low levels.

Initially, athletes with type 1 diabetes may need to collect a lot of information and work closely with their sports dietitian and/or Certified Diabetes Educator. This information, combined with logical adjustments and experimentation, will allow the diabetic endurance athlete to develop an insulin/medication and fueling plan for both training and competition day.

THE ATHLETE WITH DISORDERED EATING

When you train and compete, being able to move your body quickly over a given distance for a set amount of time offers a performance advantage. Having a lower level of body fat is therefore considered to be a mechanical advantage. However, athletes can become overly focused on their weight and body fat levels. Because athletes may be driven, goal-oriented, perfectionistic, and highly competitive, some of the qualities that promote athletic success may manifest in unrealistic weight and body fat goals. Placing undue emphasis on losing a few pounds is the result. Pressure to lose weight may come from a number of outside sources, including trainers, coaches, athletic peers, and the media. Female athletes are especially at risk of becoming dissatisfied with their bodies and distorting their body image, though males are also susceptible.

Under a broad definition, *disordered eating* encompasses a full spectrum of eating behaviors, with misguided and unhealthy strategies for weight loss and occasional bingeing and purging at one end of the disordered eating continuum and full-blown eating disorders of anorexia nervosa, bulimia nervosa, and EDNOS (Eating Disorder Not Otherwise Specified) at the other end. There are many gray areas in disordered eating, and it can be difficult to differentiate where a minor difficulty ends and a true eating disorder begins. Often behavior that begins as an attempt to lose weight takes on a life of its own and develops into an unhealthy group of behaviors that qualifies as disordered eating.

Although the incidence of full-blown eating disorders is not exceptionally high in most sports, studies indicate a high incidence of disordered eating behavior and distorted concerns regarding body weight, body fat, and body shape among athletes. Common disordered eating behaviors include skipping meals, constantly weighing oneself, eating very little fat, and fearing that specific foods may promote unwanted weight gain.

Binge eating, as characterized by consuming large amounts of food while feeling out of control, can be part of disordered eating.

Another term, *anorexia athletica*, describes a syndrome characterized by disordered eating and compulsive exercising. It is associated with an intense fear of gaining weight, despite being at normal or below-normal weight, and is marked by food restriction, often to fewer than 1,200 calories per day, and excessive exercise. Bingeing, self-induced vomiting, and use of laxatives and diuretics may also occur. Some athletes are able to stop these behaviors when their participation in a sport ends. But for other athletes, the behavior continues on to develop into a full-blown clinical eating disorder.

Eating disorders are complicated and multifactorial. Psychological and emotional issues such as anxiety and depression, an inability to cope with family and personal problems, life stresses, and the pressure to be thin or lean from both the athletic subculture and society may be involved. Biochemical imbalances may also play a role. Triggers associated with eating disorders in athletes include traumatic life events such as relationship and family problems, recommendations to lose weight, prolonged periods of dieting, and a large discrepancy between actual weight and self-defined ideal weight. It is possible that individuals at high risk of eating disorders will gravitate toward certain sports, but being involved in a sport may also trigger the eating disorder in a susceptible athlete. Risk factors that are more common among athletes than among the general population include prolonged periods of dieting or weight cycling; an increase in training volume; stress related to sports and training, such as the loss of a coach; weight-loss pressures from coaches and trainers; and lack of guidance on appropriate weight and body-composition goals and healthy weight-management strategies.

Although eating disorders among men in the general population and male athletes specifically are not as prevalent as among females in both realms, they are still a concern. The figures currently available may underestimate the true prevalence of eating disorders in men. Males who develop disordered eating are more likely to previously have been overweight or even obese, and the fear of gaining weight may relate to this past experience. Male athletes may also diet in an attempt to improve performance or in response to an injury that limits training. Male athletes are in fact more susceptible than females to muscle dysmorphia, a body image disorder characterized by an intense preoccupation with body size and degree of muscularity. Individuals with this disorder attempt to increase body size and may abuse performance-enhancing drugs or dietary supplements that promise to increase muscle mass or decrease body fat. This disorder is more common in weightlifting and bodybuilding than in other sports but can affect athletes in any sport.

EATING DISORDERS

Anorexia Nervosa

- Resistance to maintaining body weight at or above a minimally normal weight
- Intense fear of gaining weight or becoming fat even though underweight
- Distortion in self-perception of one's body weight or shape
- Denial of the seriousness of the current low body weight
- Infrequent or absent menstrual periods in females who have reached puberty

Physical Characteristics of Anorexia Nervosa:

- Hair loss and growth of fine body hair
- Low pulse rate
- Sensitivity to cold
- Stress fractures, osteopenia, or osteoporosis
- Overuse injuries
- Abnormal fatigue
- Gastrointestinal problems

Bulimia Nervosa

- Recurrent episodes of binge eating characterized by a sense of lack of control and an excessive amount of food consumed within a short period of time
- Purging behavior such as self-induced vomiting and misuse of laxatives, diuretics, enemas, or other medications
- Binge-eating and purging behavior occurring on average at least twice weekly for 3 months
- Self-esteem inappropriately influenced by body shape and weight

Physical Characteristics of Bulimia Nervosa:

- Frequent weight fluctuations
- Difficulty swallowing and throat damage
- Swollen glands
- Damaged tooth enamel from gastric acid
- Electrolyte imbalances and dehydration
- Menstrual irregularities
- Diarrhea or constipation

continues

EATING DISORDERS *continued*

Eating Disorder Not Otherwise Specified (EDNOS)

This category includes disorders of eating that do not meet the criteria for a specific eating disorder.

- Episodes of binge eating without the use of compensatory behavior as seen in bulimia nervosa
- Repeatedly chewing and spitting out, but not swallowing, large amounts of food
- Anorexia nervosa–like symptoms in conjunction with regular menstrual periods
- Bulimia nervosa–like symptoms, but with the behavior occurring less frequently or for less than 3 months
- Regular purging behaviors after consuming only a small amount of food

Muscle Dysmorphia

This term describes a form of body image disturbance described primarily in male bodybuilders and weightlifters.

- Preoccupation with not being sufficiently lean and muscular
- Preoccupation with muscularity that causes significant social impairment
- Excessive exercise, preoccupation with food, abuse of steroids, and/or abuse of dietary supplements aimed at increasing body size or decreasing body fat

There are several common warning signs for eating disorders. Someone suffering from a disorder may repeatedly express concerns about body weight, refuse to maintain even a minimal weight, enforce periods of severe calorie restriction, and/or engage in excessive physical activity that is not part of a balanced training program. Other warning signs are carrying out food rituals, engaging in self-induced vomiting, and abusing laxatives and diet pills. Some of these behaviors by themselves do not prove the presence of a full-blown eating disorder, but these signs do justify further attention to the possible presence of a problem. The sidebar "Eating Disorders" describes some of the characteristics of full-blown eating disorders.

Disordered eating and true eating disorders can pose significant health risks to athletes. They can lead to poor performance related to glycogen and electrolyte depletion, dehydration, and loss of lean body mass. Nutrient deficiencies can result, as can increased

Anorexia Athletica

This term has been used to describe a condition that is not a full-blown eating disorder.

- Disordered eating in conjunction with compulsive exercise
- Intense fear of weight gain despite weighing below the expected weight for age and height
- Weight loss achieved by food restriction and extensive compulsive exercise
- Self-induced vomiting and use of laxatives and diuretics

Binge Eating Disorder

This disorder is currently a subset of EDNOS but is expected to be classified as a separate diagnostic entity.

- Recurrent episodes of binge eating during a discrete period of time and characterized by a large amount of food and a sense of lack of control
- Binge episodes that are characterized by eating more rapidly than normal; eating until uncomfortably full; eating large amounts when not physically hungry; eating alone because of embarrassment at the volume of food; feeling disgusted, depressed, or guilty after eating; experiencing marked distress regarding the binge eating
- Bingeing at least twice weekly for 6 months

risk of infection, illness, and injury. Other health-related effects are decreased metabolism, gastrointestinal complications, menstrual dysfunction in females, and decreased bone mineral density. To avoid these harmful effects, an athlete with an eating disorder requires the help of a team of skilled professionals trained in treating the condition, including a physician, a dietitian, and a psychologist or therapist.

BONE HEALTH AND THE ENDURANCE ATHLETE

Bone health has received heightened attention over the past two decades owing to the increasing rate of osteoporotic fractures and stress fractures. Exercise levels, hormone balance, genetics, and nutritional factors such as calcium intake, vitamin D status, and acid-base balance all influence the maintenance of this important body tissue. Your calcium balance depends on the amount of calcium you consume and absorb as well as the amount you lose in your urine. The athlete at risk of development of compromised bone health must take all of this into account when making decisions about his or her diet and supplementation.

Bone is a dynamic tissue that is constantly being broken down and rebuilt under the regulation of your body's hormones. When the process of bone breakdown or bone resorption (loss of bone) exceeds bone formation, overall bone loss occurs. Early in the bone loss process this can result in reduced bone mineral density, or osteopenia. If this bone loss is prolonged, osteoporosis, a condition in which low bone mass has developed and bone is fragile, can result, and there is greater risk of fracture.

AMENORRHEA AND THE FEMALE ATHLETE

The hormone estrogen plays a crucial role in maintaining bone tissue in women. When estrogen levels are low, bone serves as a source of calcium to maintain normal levels of calcium in the blood and perform important physiological functions in the body. Even if physical activity is high, low estrogen levels, as seen in amenorrhea (loss of menstrual period) and after menopause, can result in bone loss.

Female athletes seem to have a higher incidence of menstrual irregularities than women in the general population. *Athletic amenorrhea* has been used to describe menstrual imbalances in female athletes. A variety of factors have been implicated in the development of amenorrhea in athletes. It appears that the predominant factor is inadequate calorie intake. An excessive training load, or an increase in training that is not matched with proper food intake, creates a caloric deficiency that can result in amenorrhea. Of course, disordered eating or a full-blown eating disorder can also result in a chronically low intake of calories and amenorrhea. Amenorrhea may be more common in certain sports that emphasize small frames, such as running, gymnastics, and dance, but it can occur in any endurance sport under certain precipitating conditions.

Whatever the causes, it is clear that female athletes with amenorrhea have lower bone mass than athletes who menstruate regularly. About 45 percent have osteopenia, or reduced bone mineral density, whereas 12 percent have osteoporosis. It is estimated that athletes with amenorrhea can lose 2 to 3 percent of bone mass yearly. A greater incidence of stress fractures has also been reported in athletes with current or past menstrual disturbances. Athletes with these health concerns should see a sports medicine physician for assessment of bone mass, hormonal status, and appropriate medical treatment.

Researchers are looking at what can reverse bone loss in female athletes and help them build bone again. Recent data indicate that hormone replacement through the use of oral contraceptives provides minimal positive effects because it does not produce true return of menstruation, and can also provide a false sense of security for the athlete. Medications commonly prescribed for treating low bone mass in postmenopausal women also seem to have a minimal effect in this younger population group.

Since the primary cause of low estrogen levels is inadequate intake of energy or calories in relation to training, nutritional strategies have proven the most effective in improving bone mass in these athletes. First the energy deficiency must be addressed in the athlete with amenorrhea, often requiring some weight gain and restoring to a normal BMI if body weight is too low. However, some athletes may remain weight stable while increasing calories and resume normal menstruation. With adequate energy intake and appropriate training, a return to normal hormone levels may take place over a few cycles. These female athletes can benefit greatly from the guidance a sports dietitian can offer regarding appropriate calorie intake and the balance of other nutrients in the diet. If there are underlying issues with disordered eating, or a full-blown eating disorder, the treatment team should also include a psychologist.

Athletes being treated for amenorrhea should increase their calcium intake to 1,500 milligrams daily and their vitamin D intake to an amount that will optimize blood levels for maximum calcium absorption, or at least 600 IU daily. Refer to Table 3.5 for a list of foods high in calcium. If this amount cannot be achieved through diet, calcium supplements can make up the difference. Doses of 500 milligrams of calcium carbonate or calcium citrate combined with vitamin D can be taken once or twice daily. Excessive intake of protein, when combined with inadequate calcium intake, and high intakes of caffeine and sodium can also aggravate calcium absorption. Overall balance in the diet, especially adequate calorie intake, should also be restored. Weight-bearing exercise may be continued, though not at excessive levels. Data indicate that bone mass can increase 2 to 3 percent per year with energy restoration, and 25 percent over a decade through nutritional strategies that restore menstruation.

MEN AND OSTEOPOROSIS

According to the National Osteoporosis Foundation (NOF), the number of men with osteoporosis in 2011 was 2 million, and 12 million are at risk of this disease. Up to one in four men over age 50 will break a bone due to osteoporosis. Men of all races and ethnic groups are affected, though Caucasian men appear to be at the greatest risk. Men also suffer from osteoporotic fractures of the spine, wrist, and other bones, though this happens later in life than in women. Although this disease significantly affects men, however, and osteoporosis risk among women has been well publicized in recent years, it remains underdiagnosed, underreported, and inadequately treated among male patients.

BONE BUILDING AND CYCLING

It has long been known that the proper type of exercise for stimulating production of osteoblasts, the cells that build bone, is weight-bearing activity and weight training. But some endurance sports, such as swimming and cycling, do not offer these specific weight-bearing benefits.

It is not unusual during a full season of racing to hear about a pro cyclist or two breaking a clavicle or other bone in a multirider pileup. But is there something inherent to cycling that increases your risk of developing a break when you hit the pavement hard? A growing body of research indicates that being fit through cycling training alone does not guarantee optimal bone density.

Bad bones are a serious health concern. Osteoporosis is characterized by low bone mass and deterioration of bone tissue over time. This leads to fragile bones and increased risk of fracture of the hip, spine, and wrist. Osteopenia, or subnormal bone density, precedes osteoporosis.

Recent studies should convince cyclists especially to pay attention to training and nutrition strategies that maximize bone mass. A recent study at the University of Oklahoma compared the bone mass of competitive male road cyclists, most in their late twenties to early thirties, with men who exercised recreationally. DEXA bone scans indicated the cyclists had lower bone density in the spine than did controls. About one-fourth of the cyclists had bone density scores classified as osteopenia, while 9 percent had the more severe osteoporosis. Researchers could not relate these results to testosterone levels, a bone-regulating hormone in men, or calcium intake.

A recent study at the University of Colorado also produced worrisome results. Researchers measured bone density in fourteen competitive male cyclists for one year. Bone mass was found to decrease significantly from the pre-season to off-season in several locations. As a sidebar to their study, one group of cyclists was supplemented with 1,500 milligrams or 250 milligrams of calcium citrate daily. This supplementation did not af-

BONE-BUILDING TIPS

1. Add weight-bearing exercise such as resistance training or running to your training program year-round if you are a cyclist or swimmer.

2. Aim for at least 1,000 mg of calcium daily in foods and portions providing:

   300 mg daily: milk, 8 ounces; yogurt, 8 ounces; Swiss cheese, 1 ounce

   200 mg daily: cheddar cheese, 1 ounce; colby cheese, 1 ounce; mozzarella, 1 ounce; broccoli, 1 cup cooked; collard greens, 1 cup cooked; bok choy, 1 cup cooked

   100 mg daily: cottage cheese, 1 cup; dried beans, 1 cup cooked; orange, 1 large

3. If you cannot consume 1,000 mg daily from food, consider adding fortified products such as calcium-fortified orange juice. Check labels of products consumed regularly, such as recovery drinks and energy bars, for calcium content.

4. Add a calcium supplement of 500 mg daily if your food intake is not adequate or if you need higher amounts of calcium due to existing low bone mass.

5. Increase intake of food sources of vitamin D, such as fortified milk and fatty fish. Most cyclists can safely soak up 15 minutes of direct sunlight three times weekly to produce vitamin D from sunlight, but consider a supplement during the winter months or year-round. Aim for 800 IU daily.

6. A high intake of fruits and vegetables has an alkalizing effect on blood levels, as this helps to keep calcium in bone rather than increasing urine calcium losses.

7. Cigarette smoking and excess alcohol intake can negatively affect bone mass.

8. Hormone status can affect bone mass. It is established in female athletes that inadequate caloric intake can negatively affect hormone levels; more data are needed on male athletes.

fect the rate of bone loss between groups, indicating that risk factors other than nutrition played a role.

The low impact of cycling exclusively, with no other cross-training, can increase your risk of developing low bone density. One study that compared the bone density of cyclists, runners, and weightlifters found that cyclists had lower bone density than the other two groups. Triathletes have been found to modestly increase bone mass over the season.

This is where cross-training comes into consideration. Cyclists should be aware that repetitive impact activity is very important for maximizing bone mass. They should consider adding weight training and running to their program, and do these activities year-round, not just during the off-season.

Low bone density does increase your risk of getting a fracture, so if you have concerns about your bone mass, consider getting a bone density scan to establish some baseline data. If you have a slighter build or a family history of low bone density, your risk is increased. Older cyclists may have lower bone density and a higher risk of fracture even without the trauma of a crash. Female cyclists are at even greater risk of developing low bone density, and bone scans can be important in identifying this early on.

Cyclists who are heavily focused on race performance also spend many hours on the bike sweating. Sweat contains a number of minerals other than the more obvious sodium, such as calcium. Your calcium sweat losses could add up to several hundred milligrams over a long ride and increase your calcium requirements. Men are typically advised to obtain 800 milligrams daily and women about 1,200 milligrams, though cyclists with low bone mass or those at risk could increase their calcium intake from food and supplements to 1,500 milligrams daily. Vitamin D is essential to bone health, and while sunshine is an excellent source, wise use of sunscreen can block vitamin D production, and food sources are limited. Many multivitamins contain anywhere from the daily value of 400 IU to the more likely effective and appropriate dose of 800 to 1,000 IU daily. Recommendations for these two important bone-building nutrients need to be individualized for each cyclist's current bone mineral density and risk factors and blood vitamin D status.

Body mass may also play an important role. Many cyclists, despite churning out hundreds or thousands of miles each year, watch their caloric intake closely in hopes of staying light and lean for climbs. Subpar energy intake could increase bone loss in men, just as it can in women, through an impact on the particular sex hormones that affect bone mass in each gender. More research on men is needed, as well as data from other non-weight-bearing sports such as swimming.

PERFORMANCE BOOSTS AND PROBLEM-SOLVING WITH NUTRITION

PERFORMANCE-ENHANCING STRATEGIES

Endurance athlete are always looking for that extra edge obtained from some type of diet manipulation, often adding or taking away a key nutrient at specific points in a training program. Two strategies, one focused on manipulating dietary fat and the other on dietary carbohydrate, aim to increase the endurance athlete's utilization of fat during exercise.

FAT LOADING

The idea of fat loading to improve performance is provocative, as the fat stored in your muscle and adipose tissue is an abundant supply of fuel. Even the leanest athletes have adequate fat stores to fuel low- to moderate-intensity training for several days in contrast to body carbohydrate stores, and endurance training enhances an athlete's capacity to burn fat at a given intensity.

Nutritional strategies that encourage athletes to "increase fat burning," or draw upon more of your fat stores for fuel rather than carbohydrate, are often promoted, but there are several problems associated with fat loading (loading your diet with fat) to switch on this enhanced fat burning. Although following a fat-loading diet may sound like a tasty treat, it requires a level of meal-planning knowledge that is usually found only among sports dietitians. Training on a fat-loading diet can be extremely difficult. One study demonstrated that subjects responded poorly in training when following a low-carbohydrate, high-fat diet for several weeks. Diets that are very high in fat can also have detrimental health effects.

Several well-designed published studies on fat burning conducted by researchers at the Australian Institute of Sport in Canberra and other research laboratories have shed light on fat metabolism during exercise. These studies were designed to test the hypothesis that athletes may be able to adapt to a high-fat diet for 3 to 5 days prior to an event (thereby eliminating some of the risks associated with a long-term high-fat diet), followed by a carbohydrate load in the 48 hours prior to competition. The theory was that this technique would both maximize glycogen stores before competition and optimize the muscles' capacity for fat oxidation during endurance exercise. The studies concluded with a time trial performance test to better mimic real athletic conditions.

These studies indicated that several days on a fat-periodization diet could enhance an athlete's capacity for fat burning during exercise and that this effect could be maintained even after it was followed up by one day on a carbohydrate-loading diet, a high pre-exercise meal, and consumption of carbohydrates during exercise. However, the researchers did not detect measured benefits in endurance and ultraendurance performance. Fat loading also seemed to reduce the muscles' ability to break down glycogen during exercise that has high-carbohydrate fuel demands. One study measured the effects of the same fat-loading protocol on endurance exercise interspersed with periods of high-intensity exercise (as often happens in race and training situations). It revealed that there was no performance improvement and that the ability to complete sprints during the race was impaired.

Currently there is no justification for recommending fat-loading/glycogen-loading dietary protocols to improve endurance or ultraendurance performance. This nutritional strategy may even cause a performance detriment in situations where athletes need to sustain high-intensity exercise for brief periods.

"TRAIN LOW, COMPETE HIGH"

"Train Low, Compete High" is another dietary periodization strategy that has long captured the interest of athletes, and is now receiving more attention from scientists. When utilizing this technique the athlete deliberately trains with lower glycogen stores or without the support of any carbohydrate intake during training. The goal is to enhance the training adaptations that normally occur in the muscle, particularly to turn on more fat-burning properties in the muscle itself. In other words, you get a better return on your training. This sounds good on paper, but the real data are limited.

Some of the studies looking at the "train low, compete high" concept did not actually manipulate diet to lower glycogen stores, but rather training. For example, subjects in one study completed a second training session every other day, with a rest day in between, while restoring glycogen. The low glycogen comes into play when they train for the second time that day in a glycogen-depleted state. This particular study did not see significant performance improvements and was completed with untrained subjects. This is a lot different from making some manipulations with diet and training in highly trained athletes.

Two additional studies have looked at training subjects over three weeks' time. Both studies found that athletes who completed demanding interval training on low glycogen did have greater improvements in muscle markers that change with training. It should be noted that these athletes did suffer during these tough training sessions and did have lower power output during the workout. Overall, they ended up doing less work in these important training sessions. At the end of the study, the "train low" group was compared with the "train high" group. Both groups showed equal improvements on a performance test ride. So the "train low" group did not hurt their performance, but neither did they improve more than the "train high" group.

Another "train low" technique that athletes may use is to take in only water during training (rather than a sports drink) in order to limit carbohydrate. Here too the goal is to enhance training adaptations, particularly fat burning. Often, early-morning training sessions that occur before breakfast fall prey to this strategy. Cyclists or runners may opt to train low on long low-intensity rides early or for easy runs in the training season. For gentle workouts this may not be as taxing, though it would place you at greater risk of low blood glucose or "bonking" during the workout given the low level of liver carbohydrate stores from an early-morning start.

When it comes to training low and competing high, it's best to keep the big picture in mind. Key training sessions may best be done with plenty of carbohydrate so that the desired intensity and duration are achieved, thereby forcing the desired training adaptations. Other sessions may be done with less glycogen recovery and no carbohydrate intake during training, and completed successfully. Keep in mind what you want to accomplish with a particular workout. It should also be noted that harder training sessions completed with limited carbohydrate intake also place greater stress on the immune system. At this time "Train Low, Compete High" is more of an art than an actual science.

USING NUTRITION TO PROBLEM-SOLVE

Due to the nature of their training, endurance athletes often encounter problems not seen by the average gym devotee. Muscle cramps associated with training and racing in the heat can put a quick damper on training and racing, as can an injury or illness such as a cold or flu.

STRATEGIES TO DEAL WITH MUSCLE CRAMPS

Any endurance athlete who has suffered a muscle cramp probably remembers it well. These rapidly ignited and long-sustained muscle spasms can be painful and inconvenient, particularly when they occur during competition. The exact cause of muscle cramps remains a mystery, however, and research data on cramping are limited. What is known is that muscle cramping generally occurs during relatively long exercise sessions in the heat and is often associated with overexertion. Some cases of muscle cramping may be due to simple muscular exhaustion or low fuel stores; others may result from biomechanical problems or mineral and fluid deficiencies. Whatever the cause, there are some methodical nutritional steps you can take to help prevent muscle cramps that have their origin in nutrient deficiencies. You may need to experiment with these possible solutions; prevention in recurrent sufferers is often a matter of trial and error.

Although scientists have not yet figured out a way to look directly at the muscle cell to see precisely what is causing a heat cramp as it is occurring, research suggests that muscle cramps are related to salt and fluid imbalances. Muscle cramps during exercise have been linked to low levels of sodium in the blood. If there are large amounts of sodium chloride in an athlete's sweat, or an athlete replaces his or her sweat losses with low-sodium drinks or plain water, diluting the sodium in the blood, or both, the chance of getting a muscle cramp increases. Dehydration and other mineral deficiencies, such as shortages of calcium and magnesium, may also be predisposing factors.

Some age-groupers experience muscle cramps during races, especially when they do not yet have much experience in competition or do not have a well-thought-out race nutrition plan, even if they have not been prone to cramps in training. Competition in ultraendurance events also presents extreme situations that extend beyond training, and may take place in very hot and humid weather conditions. Increasing salt intake when training in hot, humid weather prior to competition can help. Maintaining hydration levels before, during, and after exercise can also help. During exercise, try to consume the amount of fluid necessary to match or minimize your sweat losses. Recheck your sweat rate for different training disciplines in varying weather conditions, and monitor the color of your urine. Sports drinks with some sodium or enhanced sodium are better than plain water for making sure you do not dilute your blood sodium levels.

It is also prudent to obtain plenty of sodium in your diet while training in hot weather. Foods that contain sodium include canned soups, pretzels, cereals, various cheeses, crackers, and yogurt. You can salt your food prior to training in the heat or on competition days. If you find yourself craving salt, your body may be telling you that it needs more. Sodium losses in 1 quart (960 ml) of sweat can range from 400 to 1,800 milligrams, or even more in some endurance athletes. Having a high sweat rate only compounds the level of sodium losses each hour during training and competition. Cramp-prone endurance athletes can use high-sodium sports drinks during training to replace sodium losses. Electrolyte tablets that contain sodium are also available for very salty sweaters. However, they should be taken with plenty of fluids and not overconsumed.

Other reasons for muscle cramping are sometimes cited, and if you are prone to cramping you may receive advice based on these theories. There has been some speculation that potassium losses can lead to muscle cramping, for example. Your diet can easily supply ample amounts of potassium. Excellent sources include all fruit juices, fruits, and vegetables, with some of the best sources being grapefruit, orange, and pineapple juice; apricots, bananas, and papayas; and greens, carrots, potatoes, and tomatoes. Milk, yogurt, and dried peas and beans are also good sources of potassium. Although sodium losses are a more likely culprit, you may want to eat generous portions of these high-potassium foods anyway, as they provide carbohydrates. A lack of calcium is also sometimes blamed for muscle cramps, though its involvement has not been conclusively proven. Although blood calcium levels do not typically fall below normal during long-distance training, low levels may play a role in cramping for some individuals competing in ultraevents. Calcium is the most abundant mineral in your body and plays many functional roles, including a role in muscle contraction. To be on the safe side, athletes suffering from muscle cramps should at least correct inadequate calcium intake. Being sure to consume enough calcium won't hurt, and it will help to preserve bone mass, if nothing else.

Good sources of calcium, including milk, yogurt, and leafy green vegetables, are listed in Chapter 3. A calcium supplement can also compensate for a low dietary intake of this important mineral. Yet another theory is that lack of magnesium, a mineral that plays an important role in muscle relaxation, may be related to muscle cramping. Good sources of magnesium include nuts, seeds, legumes, green leafy vegetables, and unrefined grains.

Make sure to test strategies for preventing heat-related muscle cramps carefully in training. Any nutritional plan for preventing muscle cramps will depend on your medical history, usual diet, and usual sweat and sodium losses. If following these nutritional strategies does not help you solve the mystery of muscle cramps, look to resources that can help you determine whether there is a biomechanical cause or problems with your stretching or training techniques.

NUTRITIONAL STRATEGIES FOR INJURY RECOVERY

You may at some point in your career as an endurance athlete suffer from strains, abrasions, bruising, or fractures. Most likely the speed at which your injury heals is of concern to you. While you may have a rehabilitation program mapped out, the calories and nutrients that you require for this program may differ from your usual eating. What is clear, however, is that protein, fat, carbohydrates, and vitamins and minerals are essential for timely and complete healing of injuries. Weight-management issues may also present themselves at the time of an injury due to a marked decrease in energy expenditure.

Often during rehabilitation an athlete fears putting on body fat. The injury often results in significant changes in energy expenditure as a result of changes in an athlete's training program. For a period of time, the volume and intensity of training will decrease, and the type of training may temporarily change. Endurance athletes become accustomed to eating enough to support a demanding training program, and when an injury occurs, it may be difficult to know how and when to cut back on this caloric intake to achieve the proper caloric balance. Muscle mass may also decrease during the recovery period, depending on the type of rehabilitation program that is prescribed. Depending on the type and extent of the injury, an athlete's caloric expenditure may decrease by several thousand calories per week. An athlete who decreases training volume by just 4 hours a week could experience a weekly 1-pound weight gain if he or she continues to follow his or her usual eating habits.

At the other extreme, an athlete who cuts back too much on calories may not be eating enough to support the healing process. When recovering from an injury, it is best not to undereat protein and calories. Protein is necessary for the growth and repair of body tissue, supports healthy immune function, and is required for the synthesis of enzymes and hormones. Undereating calories can also lead to increased incidence of infection and slower wound healing.

Regardless of the type of injury, maintaining energy balance is key. Injured athletes can keep a food record and determine their normal caloric intake. They then can trim from 200 to 500 calories or more daily to prevent weight gain if needed. Sometimes the intake of carbohydrates and protein needs to be decreased slightly to prevent a gain in body fat. Excess dietary fat that was easily burned off in training should also be reduced. But if you are recovering from an injury, avoid drastic dietary restrictions so that you don't miss out on needed nutrients. Some personalized guidance from a sports dietitian can be helpful when you are injured.

In many instances, starting a resistance and rehabilitation program provides a big advantage. Building muscle takes work and energy, allowing you to consume more calories than you would be able to consume if you simply cut back on training or stopped for a time altogether. A good rehabilitation program can thus somewhat offset the decreased caloric expenditure that typically occurs during recovery from an injury. If these weight-training sessions are intense, consuming carbohydrates during training can facilitate recovery and muscle repair.

After an initial period of healing, athletes often engage in rehabilitation programs that are just as demanding as their usual training, though the program may differ in scope and timing. Your meal plan may need to be adjusted to support energy levels at specific training times and encourage tissue repair and muscle-building efforts. Increasing your intake of certain nutrients and even supplementation may support the healing process. One of the principal functions of vitamin C is collagen synthesis, a core component of scar tissue. Collagen is also required for the formation and maintenance of connective tissue such as cartilage as well as tendons and bones. Vitamin C plays a role in red blood cell synthesis, too. Load up on some of the good vitamin C sources listed in Chapter 3. Fruits and vegetables are abundant in vitamin C and are also low-calorie foods. Increasing your intake of fruits and vegetables will also provide antioxidants and bioflavonoids that can protect your muscles against damage during exercise and further support the healing process.

Other important vitamins for a recovery nutrition plan are vitamin A, which supports collagen formation and the immune system, and the B vitamins, especially if there have been trauma and stress associated with the injury.

Several minerals, including iron and zinc, play important roles in the recovery process as well. Zinc is a component of many enzymes involved in energy metabolism and is required for protein synthesis and wound healing. Zinc from animal protein is absorbed best. Iron, of course, is needed for oxygen transport and the formation of hemoglobin and myoglobin, processes that enable the athlete to maintain a high level of rehabilitation training. Good sources are listed in Chapter 3.

Your protein and calorie requirements can change at specific phases of the rehabilitation process. However, a nutrient-dense diet is a plus at any time after an injury. A good multivitamin-and-mineral supplement high in antioxidants and bioflavonoids can also be useful at this time for the extra insurance it provides that you are getting all the nutrients you need for recovery.

STRATEGIES FOR BOOSTING YOUR IMMUNE SYSTEM

Periods of heavy training are sometimes associated with depressed immune function, and compromised immune function can be further aggravated by inadequate nutrition. Combining training with school or work can overtax your resources, stress your body, and compromise your ability to fight infection. A strong immune system should result in fewer colds and other viruses, and when you do get sick, should enable you to make a quicker recovery.

Specific foods can strengthen your immune system and help to prevent unwanted halts in your training program due to illness. Vitamin C has a widespread reputation as an immune system booster, but it is not a magic pill for preventing the common cold. It should, however, be part of your daily diet in adequate amounts. Though a daily multivitamin-and-mineral supplement may contain the Daily Value (DV) of vitamin C, don't underestimate the importance of ample food sources of this nutrient. Athletes can consume more than three servings of fresh fruit and up to 2 cups of cooked vegetables daily for ample amounts of dietary vitamin C. Megadoses of vitamin C in supplement form have not been shown to protect the immune system—250 milligrams is adequate to saturate body stores.

Fruits and vegetables contain hundreds of phytochemicals that provide many preventive health benefits and are also excellent sources of carotenoids that boost the activity of the white blood cells called lymphocytes. Beta-carotene can also be converted to vitamin A, an important nutrient for the immune system. Other nutrients important for a strong immune system are zinc, iron, and vitamins B6 and B12. A good daily multivitamin-and-mineral supplement providing 100 percent of the DVs ensures adequate nutrient intake. Megadosing with vitamins and minerals can compromise the immune system, and excessive intakes of iron, zinc, and vitamin E are not advised. A balanced diet that includes a large variety of foods provides many nutrients that work together to keep your immune system healthy, and a moderate-dose supplement ensures that you are obtaining all the nutrients that you need.

Consuming adequate calories is beneficial not only for an athlete's recovery and energy levels but also for maintaining a healthy immune system. Falling short of your calorie requirements can compromise your immune system, as can poorly planned and low-calorie diets, especially those low in protein. Diets too low in calories can result in inadequate intake of vitamins and minerals, which also decreases immunity. Training with optimal stores of glycogen obtained from a diet adequate in calories and carbohydrates not only provides fuel for your workouts but also boosts your immune system.

Levels of certain stress hormones normally rise during exercise, but athletes who train in a carbohydrate-depleted state experience a greater increase in these hormones than those who are well fueled. Your immune system appears to function best when carbohydrate is available. Consuming carbohydrates during exercise also seems to diminish some of the immunosuppressive effects of intense training. Generally, strenuous exercise suppresses immune function and gives viruses a strong "window of opportunity" after a workout to gain a foothold in your body and start an infection. Besides replacing carbohydrate during training, practice optimal recovery nutrition guidelines as well.

New research is also looking at the effect of probiotics/prebiotics and vitamin D in the immune system of athletes during periods of heavy training.

JUST FOR FEMALES

One special consideration involves in particular the female endurance athlete. Over the past two decades sports nutrition guidelines have derived from research data based on male test athletes. But there are growing data regarding the potential unique nutritional requirements of female athletes—simply by using female athlete test subjects and seeing if they respond to the same nutritional strategy in the same manner as or a different manner than male subjects.

Do the nutritional requirements of male and female endurance athletes differ? Despite the well-established physiological differences between female and male athletes, female athletes are routinely given the same sports nutrition advice as male athletes. Much of the female athlete–focused research has looked at endurance exercise, and female athletes participating in these sports can benefit from a few key findings. Recent research, including several studies from McMaster University and the University of Guelph, both in Ontario, Canada, has resulted in gender-specific guidance for women relating to carbohydrate loading, nutritional intake during training, and recovery strategies.

Training and eating properly before a race can optimize body glycogen fuel stores for female athletes just as it can for their male counterparts. In order to glycogen-load effectively, women need to consume an adequate number of grams of carbohydrates per pound of body weight. Female endurance athletes should taper and carbohydrate-load before extended competition even though they have been found to derive less benefit from the process than their male counterparts following the same glycogen-loading protocol.

Researchers at McMaster University have also studied gender differences in carbohydrate consumption during exercise, with useful results. Female athletes may not respond as robustly as men to carbohydrate loading, but they can consume sports drinks during exercise to compensate for storing less glycogen. Test subjects cycled at 60 percent VO_2max for 90 minutes while consuming an 8 percent carbohydrate beverage (1 g of carbohydrate per kilogram of body weight). When female athletes performing endurance exercise were provided with sports drinks during exercise, they oxidized, or burned, more of the sports drink than did males. Overall, however, women still burn more fat than carbohydrate during exercise than do men. Carbohydrate consumption during higher training intensities would also be expected to benefit female athletes.

Other research from McMaster University has shown that consuming carbohydrates immediately after training improves muscle glycogen resynthesis and recovery in women just as efficiently as in men. Males and females appear to store glycogen at similar rates when carbohydrates are given immediately after endurance exercise, and they benefit from this strategy equally. More research is needed to determine how this nutritional recovery strategy affects training programs specific to endurance athletes.

Another study pointed to the need for more data to fine-tune the knowledge of the unique daily nutritional requirements of female athletes and the effect of diet manipulations on performance, particularly for carbohydrate intake. Researchers had well-trained female triathletes and cyclists follow three separate protocols and consume either a low-carbohydrate diet of 1.4 grams per pound (3 g/kg) of body weight, a moderate-carbo-hydrate diet of 2.25 grams per pound (5 g/kg) of body weight, or a high-carbohydrate diet of 3.5 grams per pound (8 g/kg) of body weight for 6 days. Subjects then cycled to exhaustion. Interestingly, on the high-carb diet, subjects had difficulty consuming the prescribed amount of carbohydrates. When completing a time trial after cycling at 70 percent VO$_2$max, no significant performance differences were found among the three diets. More performance testing of various carbohydrate dietary levels in female athletes is needed. Earlier studies have demonstrated a difference in fuel metabolism between men and women, but more research is needed in this area before nutritionists can draw any real conclusions about what it all means in practical terms. In any case, nutritional recommendations may become more sex-specific in the future as awareness of metabolic differences in men and women increases.

Another recent finding is that women have a greater increase in core temperature during exercise, given similar heat exposure, than do men. The onset of sweating may occur at higher body temperatures, and sweat rates may be lower. However, there are likely more differences in sweat rates among individual women athletes than between men and women. Female athletes should still consume enough fluid during and after exercise to match their fluid losses, while staying within their gastrointestinal tolerances. Another study indicated that replacing body fluids after exercise is not affected by the phase of the menstrual cycle.

Although the protein needs of female athletes are higher than those of the general population, there appear to be no significant differences between men and women athletes in this regard. Protein intake should be based on body weight and specific training programs, and it can vary with the amount of calories and carbohydrates consumed. Of course, adequate calorie intake allows for more optimal utilization of the protein consumed.

There has been growing concern among some researchers that as a greater number of female athletes attempt to reach lower body fat levels, their health could be compromised. Women have to work harder than men to achieve the same level of leanness. When a female athlete's intake of calories is inadequate, her body may be more prone to making adjustments to defend or maintain her current weight than a male athlete's body would, given the same dietary and training factors. Current data indicate that inadequate calorie intake is the main trigger for hormonal imbalances, absence of menstruation, and compromised bone health.

Although more specific nutritional training recommendations for women need to be tested and formulated, women athletes should still practice focused strategies to ensure optimal performance. Based on the current research, female athletes can be confident that they will benefit from consistently practicing optimal recovery nutrition following hard training, glycogen loading in combination with adequate calorie intake, and consuming enough carbohydrates during training and competition to keep up their glucose levels.

NUTRITIONAL STRATEGIES FOR EXTREME ENVIRONMENTS

Endurance athletes train and race in a wide variety of environmental conditions, ranging from the dangerously hot to the uncommonly cold. Often, endurance events are not about the battle with other competitors but rather with the environment and extreme conditions. Endurance athletes can often bake and freeze all in one day. In some parts of the country, the typical weather for an event may be a yearly wild card with a wide temperature range. You may find yourself competing in humidity, at high altitude, or in the cold. It is imperative to pay attention to nutrition strategies and adjustments designed for environmental extremes, not only if you want to complete the event but if you want to finish the event safely. Following are some nutritional strategies that can help you cope with extreme conditions.

TRAINING AND RACING IN THE HEAT

Changes in body temperature out of the range of the normal state of equilibrium can be dangerous, with a high core temperature deserving special attention. Heat illness, ranging from heat exhaustion to

AT A GLANCE
KEY POINTS

Anticipate your environment, adjusting your nutrition strategy accordingly.

Heat adaptation results in greater fluid loss, which must be compensated for.

More calories are burned in cold conditions than in temperate ones.

Iron and vitamins E and C are especially beneficial when training at high altitude.

Focus on sensible, healthy lower-fat choices when eating away from home.

heatstroke, can sometimes be confused with dehydration. In the case of heat illness, your body temperature rises as you accumulate heat from both the environment and exercise. You can overheat on a very hot day, well before you become dehydrated. Preventing heat illness requires that you choose a safe exercise environment and pace yourself appropriately. Dehydration, of course, will only increase your body temperature in extreme conditions.

In addition to causing greater fluid losses and increased body temperature, training in the heat imposes other stresses on your body. When you train in hot weather, your body experiences an increased rate of muscle glycogen use, which can result in premature fatigue. So in addition to fluid replacement, you should emphasize glucose replacement to meet the accelerated fuel demands imposed by training in the heat.

Lactic acid production is also greater, and your heart rate increases to compensate for fluid losses. Consequently, training at a given intensity is harder than it would be in cooler weather.

The key to training in hot weather is to appreciate that your body must adapt to the heat. Although a few training sessions of 30 to 60 minutes each at 70 percent of VO_2max may be helpful, full adaptation to the heat takes from 7 to 14 days and is a highly individual response. After 10 days of training in the heat, the sweat response adapts in several ways: you start to sweat sooner, you sweat more, you sweat over more of your body, and your sweat contains fewer electrolytes, decreasing your sodium losses. Other adaptations are an increased blood volume and decreased sodium excretion in the urine. After 10 days of training in the heat, your sweating capacity during exercise can double.

Though these adaptations are essential to cooling your body, they do result in greater fluid losses. Clearly, if these fluid losses are not replaced, you run the risk of becoming dehydrated and the benefits of heat acclimatization are lost. Because your sweat capacity is greatly enhanced after adapting to the heat, dehydration can occur quickly. Weigh yourself before and after training to determine the amount of fluid lost in a typical training session (see the sidebar "Estimating Your Sweat Losses" in Chapter 5). Try to consume 24 ounces (720 ml) of fluid for every pound (about 0.5 kg) of weight lost to replace both sweat and urine losses.

Keeping up with fluid loss is often a matter of logistics. Make it a priority to bring fluids with you, and set your watch to remind you to drink at specific intervals. Sports drinks are a great choice. Besides providing carbohydrates, they provide the important electrolyte sodium. Sodium and chloride, which form salt, are the major electrolytes lost in sweat. When you go out for a very long training session or compete in races lasting several hours, you may be at risk of developing hyponatremia, or low blood sodium levels. Hyponatremia results from losing large amounts of salt through sweating or from replacing fluid losses with plain water, diluting the sodium concentration of your blood.

To prepare for these sodium losses, you can increase your intake of salty foods for a day or two before a long training session or race, unless this is medically contraindicated. Avoid drinking plain water when a sports drink or sodium-containing gel plus water can be consumed to maintain blood sodium levels. If plain water tastes better in the heat, consider one of the sports drinks with little or no flavor. These products are often very appealing in hot weather. Drinking cold or icy fluids feels good in the heat and may help prevent overheating. Though more studies are needed, cold beverages may keep down core temperatures.

Sweeter products or something a bit salty may stimulate your desire to drink. Cool drinks are usually more palatable. Sodium stimulates your drive to drink and enhances the rehydration process. Sweating results in large fluid losses and relatively small sodium losses for most endurance athletes, but some athletes are salty sweaters. As mentioned, consuming large amounts of plain water after exercise can dilute your blood before your full blood volume has been restored. This dilution effect shuts down the thirst mechanism, and you urinate to bring your blood concentration back to normal. The end result is that you will produce a large amount of diluted urine before you are fully rehydrated.

Here are some nutritional strategies for beating the heat:

- Know your sweat rate after you have acclimated and the conditions in which you will train and compete.
- Drink on a schedule and use a higher-sodium sports drink.
- Add electrolyte tablets and mixes to your sports drink to compensate for very high sodium losses.
- Practice and refine your rehydration techniques and skills.
- Start out with a full tank of body fuel and fluid.
- Be prepared to carry what you need or to plant or purchase ongoing supplies during the workout.
- Replenish with fluid, sodium, and carbohydrates promptly after completing the workout or event.

HYDRATION AND FUELING IN THE COLD

Many endurance athletes train outdoors almost year-round, which in many parts of North America means training in the cold. Perhaps you run or bike outdoors, or you may cross-train in a winter sport such as Nordic skiing or snowshoeing. Weather conditions are often less than ideal, and in the cold you must still maintain a safe core temperature.

There are several methods by which your body can prevent excess cooling. First, you may find yourself shivering, which raises the body's resting rate of heat production. Your nervous system can also increase the metabolic rate to produce more heat. Finally, the blood vessels in your extremities vasoconstrict to prevent further heat loss. Body fat and proper clothing also help to insulate your core from the cold. The goal is to produce heat faster than heat is dissipated.

It is important to start training sessions in the cold well hydrated. Dehydration impairs your ability to train and perform, just as it does in the heat. There are several physiological mechanisms through which your hydration can become compromised in cold weather. One such mechanism is cold-induced diuresis. When you exercise in the cold, the vasoconstriction that occurs causes your blood pressure to increase, and there is an increase in the blood pressure in your kidneys, which causes you to urinate and lose fluid and sodium.

Water loss in the cold also occurs when you inhale cold air. Your lung passages warm the air and saturate it with water. When you exhale this air saturated with water, there is fluid loss. Fluid losses from your lungs can add up to over 1 quart (about 1 L) daily when you are outdoors for a day of training in the cold. These losses increase with intense exercise.

Even in the cold air, an increase in your body temperature during exercise can result in sweat losses. Dressing for cold-weather training and keeping your body warm with insulating clothing also enhance sweating. Sweat losses in cold weather can reach up to 2 quarts (approximately 2 L) per hour during moderate to intense exercise when you are wearing heavy insulating clothing. Of course, sweat losses per hour vary greatly from workout to workout.

Even without the adverse effects of dehydration, training in the cold can adversely affect your coordination, fine motor skills, strength, power production, and aerobic power. Dehydration levels of over 2 percent of body weight can also reduce mental concentration and performance in cold weather.

Hypothermia, when your core temperature falls below 98.6°F (37°C), occurs when you lose more heat than is produced. Early warning signs include shivering as well as increased breathing and heart rate, which can progress to fatigue, weakness, disorientation, and even the cessation of shivering. Mild hypothermia can even develop in temperatures of 50°F to 65°F (10°C to 18°C), so be alert for the signs. Events such as triathlon, where you may be wet from the swim, place you at greater risk, as do windy conditions and the second half of long events when your pace can slow and you are generating less heat.

The fact that water solidifies at temperatures below 32°F (0°C) can make optimal hydration a challenge. Endurance athletes who train in cold weather can practice a few warming strategies to keep the fluids flowing.

Sports drinks can be heated before training and placed inside a thermos or a bottle covered with an insulating warmer. Experiment with drinks and flavors that appeal to you when heated. Warm sports drinks are easier to down on a cold winter day than cold ones and can help to maintain your core body temperature.

Tube-fed winter hydration systems are also now available for training in the cold. Hydration systems are handy, as they do not require that you reach for your bottle with cold fingers and thick gloves. There are some newer models that are designed for the cold, but in the coldest temperatures you cannot fight the freeze indefinitely. In order to prevent the drink tube from freezing, buy products with an insulated hose and bite valves covered with insulating caps. In full-on winter weather, make sure that you fill the fluid reservoir with warm or hot fluid. You should also blow back into the drink tube after you have taken a hydrating gulp to prevent fluid from sitting and freezing in the drink tube. And keep the fluid reservoir and hose as close to your body as possible so that your body heat can keep the system warm.

In addition to having fluid strategies that work well in the cold, you should have cold-weather fueling strategies. It is key to start cold-training sessions or events well fueled, as you do burn more calories in colder conditions than in temperate ones. Maintaining blood glucose levels is essential for brain fuel and making good decisions when training in the cold, such as when to turn back and get warm again. During cold-weather training the amounts of both carbohydrate and fat that you burn increase, so you should maintain the same targeted carbohydrate focus in your diet as during the warmer months. Sports drinks provide some needed carbohydrate; however, pre-chopped energy bars or bites, gels, and blocks kept warm inside clothing may also be needed for fueling.

NUTRITION AT HIGH ALTITUDE

Endurance athletes who live, train, or compete at altitude should be aware of how the elevation can affect their body and performance. Breathing at high elevations can be challenging if you are not used to it, and exercising at high elevations places special demands on the respiratory and circulatory systems. The higher the elevation, the less dense the air that you breathe. Altitude hypoxia, or a reduction of oxygen in your body tissues, can result. Fortunately, your body adjusts or "acclimatizes" to altitude, though this process can take up to three weeks. When you travel quickly to altitude, you may experience symptoms such as rapid heart rate, headache, shortness of breath, fatigue, nausea and vomiting, loss of appetite, decreased urine output, and insomnia, often referred to as acute mountain sickness (AMS). This complex of symptoms is most likely to occur in individuals who reside at sea level and ascend rapidly to a high altitude. Symptoms normally develop in 6 to 12 hours, peak at 24 to 48 hours, and subside in 3 to 7 days as your body acclimatizes to the new conditions.

Upon arriving at a high altitude, your body experiences an initial decrease in blood volume designed to concentrate the red blood cells that carry oxygen in your blood. During an adjustment period of 10 to 14 days your body adapts to altitude and makes adjustments that are more permanent. Your blood volume will return to normal or expand, and you will develop more red blood cells if you stay at altitude for several weeks. In addition, your muscles will begin to extract more oxygen from your blood.

Altitude clearly causes metabolic adaptations that affect your nutritional needs. Even relatively moderate elevations of up to 5,000 feet can affect how you should eat and drink. The air at high altitudes is extremely dry, and every breath you take results in fluid loss. "Insensible" fluid losses through your skin also increase. Normally these insensible fluid losses amount to only about ½ a quart (about 1 L) daily; this amount can increase to 2 quarts (about 2 L) daily at high altitudes. This is in addition, of course, to your urinary output and sweat losses during exercise, all of which implies that hydration should be your top concern when you are training or competing at high elevation, especially if you are not yet acclimatized.

Replacing your fluid losses at altitude takes a conscious effort. Always try to keep a source of fluid with you. You may require 4 to 8 quarts (3.8–7.6 L) of fluid daily depending on your training schedule. Light-colored urine indicates that you are matching your fluid losses.

When at altitude, you also have to consider your carbohydrate and calorie intake. Your basal metabolic rate can increase by as much as 40 percent the first few days at altitude; it then gradually drops off to about 15 percent above sea-level values. Overall, your energy needs at altitude may increase by 200 to 300 calories daily. Although this may sound like a simple problem to cure, there is a real decrease in appetite that sets in at altitude, causing you to undereat by several hundred calories daily. Undereating and losing weight at altitude do not result in body fat loss. What is more likely to occur is that your body will utilize valuable protein stores for fuel.

It is best if the extra calories that you take in at altitude come from carbohydrates. High-carbohydrate diets may reduce the effects of acute mountain sickness. They also delay the depletion of muscle glycogen, which will support endurance training at altitude. Another benefit is that carbohydrates are more easily digested and better tolerated than high-fat foods. Keep foods such as energy bars, cereals, crackers, and fresh or dried fruit handy, and have snacks to meet the additional caloric requirements. Small, frequent meals may be better tolerated with the decrease in appetite. "Bonking" can creep up on you more quickly at altitude, making adequate intake of glucose during exercise imperative. Sports drinks clearly provide both needed fluids and carbohydrates.

Although research on vitamin and mineral requirements at altitude is limited, enough is known about iron to suggest that it deserves your attention at higher elevations. Athletes training at altitude should have their iron status monitored regularly. Having adequate iron stores ensures that you will be able to produce needed red blood cells. Besides emphasizing good food sources of iron, you may want to take an iron supplement to boost and maintain your stores of this nutrient. Be careful not to supplement to excess, however, and only take supplements under a physician's supervision. Too much iron causes oxidation and free radical production, which damage cells and are associated with a number of health conditions. Adequate intakes of folate and vitamin B12 from a variety of foods, supplemented with a basic multivitamin if needed, are also essential for red blood cell production.

Focusing on foods high in antioxidants like vitamins C and E may also be beneficial, as exercising at high altitude places "oxidative stress" upon your body. Exercising at altitude may also raise your vitamin E requirements. Food sources of vitamin E include fortified cereals, whole grains, wheat germ, nuts and seeds, green leafy vegetables, and vegetable oils. Recommendations for vitamin E supplementation are currently 100 to 200 IU daily.

EATING WELL ON CAMPUS

College food services usually offer a wide selection of foods for students living in dorms or group home settings such as sororities and fraternities. Campus food courts also provide selections in a variety of locations near classrooms, and of course there is the ever-present vending machine. The college athlete's task is to seek out, from an overwhelming wealth of choices, items that support athletic training, recovery, and good health.

Eating on campus presents several challenges. One is the "all-you-can-eat" setting, with unlimited returns to the table and a wide variety of hot and cold foods that may or may not be prepared with moderate to high amounts of fat and salt. You need to become a savvy consumer in these settings and make wise choices just as you would at any restaurant or fast-food establishment.

Although dining-hall hours of operation are usually fairly generous, student athletes do need to review their class and training schedules and plan when and where they will be eating each day of the week. Late nights of studying may necessitate evening snacking, so keep a stash of healthy choices in your room as well. Remember, in college, you are not on a 9-to-5 schedule. You will need to be flexible with your meal and snack times while giving yourself the consistent mealtime structure required for a healthy diet.

Although it may be tempting to sleep in, make sure that you always start your day with breakfast. Dorm-style breakfast offerings include many choices with wholesome carbohydrates and protein. Consider the standard cold and hot cereals, and gravitate toward whole-grain, low-sugar choices. Skim milk and yogurt add more carbohydrates and high-quality protein to the mix. Be sure to include fruit and whole-grain breads as desired. Peanut butter adds protein, as do eggs. If you do sleep late, try to at least catch the tail end of breakfast time. You can also keep some simple breakfast items in your room, such as cereal, milk, fruit, and yogurt (if you have a mini-fridge), so that skipping breakfast is not necessary even if you do sleep in.

Breakfast choices on campus often go beyond the simple items typically available at home. Food fare that was once limited to weekend brunches, such as omelets, waffles, pancakes, sausage, and bacon, may be available every day. These items can be part of your breakfast choices, but keep portions of high-fat items to reasonable levels.

Most athletes get hungry every 3 to 4 hours, and sometimes even at shorter intervals if a long training session takes place. Although you should sit down to eat lunch and dinner regularly, it is also important to include snacks in your sports diet. Convenient items like yogurt and fruit can be purchased on campus, as can granola bars and sandwiches.

Carry snacks with you as needed, and stake out various campus locations close to your classrooms for healthy choices.

Try not to arrive for your meals famished. You want to have time to look over the hot and cold choices that are available and make healthy selections, rather than rushing to buy the first thing that looks good. If you are overly hungry, you might eat too fast and eat more than you intended. Some food services and group homes post their menus for the week ahead of time, which can be helpful for meal planning. Make your choices based on what looks good and what best fits your nutritional needs. Keep an eye out for whole grains, fruits, and vegetables. Standard items offered usually include a salad bar, a sandwich bar, soups, a baked potato bar, several hot entrées, and a decent variety of desserts.

The salad bar can certainly supplement a healthy meal, but choose wisely if it is your main course. Plenty of fresh vegetables such as carrots, mushrooms, cucumbers, and peppers are great, as are leafy greens such as lettuce and spinach. If the salad is to be a main focus of the meal, be sure to include proteins such as cottage cheese, eggs, tuna, cheese, garbanzo beans, kidney beans, tofu, or turkey. Prepared salads such as pasta salad, potato salad, and marinated vegetable salads also add carbohydrates, but they may contribute some fat as well, so control your portions with these items. Watch out for foods loaded with mayonnaise if you are trying not to overdo your fat intake.

If you like sandwiches at lunchtime, gravitate toward whole-grain breads, but also vary your choices with pita bread and sandwich wraps. Turkey, tuna, peanut butter, and ham all supply good protein. Round out your sandwich with a bowl of soup, some fruit, vegetables, and yogurt or a glass of milk. Higher-calorie items would include a large bagel or submarine sandwich, French fries, and milkshakes. Baked potato bars, like sandwich bars, can provide a good balance of protein and carbohydrates. Spuds can be topped with vegetables, cheese, yogurt, chili, turkey, or various sauces. Monitor portions of items such as sour cream, butter, gravies, and cream soups.

Hot entrées are available at both lunch and dinner in college dining halls and can run the gamut from healthy stir-fries to high-fat fried foods, though recent years have seen a wider variety of healthy entrées offered at the dorm. Ask questions about how the foods have been prepared, and request specific portion sizes. You can also ask for sauces to be served on the side so that you can control your own portion sizes of these items, which are often high in fat. Veggie and turkey burgers make good low-fat choices, as do pasta plates with red sauces, grilled or broiled fish, and other grilled meats. Regularly offered sides that are smart choices include steamed rice, baked potatoes, skim milk and yogurt, fresh fruit, and soups.

Desserts are often in abundant supply at the college cafeteria. A self-serve frozen yogurt machine and side toppings make a good choice. Ice cream, cakes, and pies may also be available on a regular basis, but they are probably the highest in calories. More reasonable options include fruit bars, yogurt bars, and popsicles as well as sorbet and baked or fresh fruit. But set limits on your consumption of desserts. One a day or several per week may be fine, depending on your energy needs.

EATING WELL WHEN TRAVELING

Endurance athletes may frequently be presented with the need to make healthy food choices on the road. It is important to consider how traveling affects your pre-competition nutrition program and plan accordingly. Special meals that reduce fat content or add more fruits and vegetables can be ordered on airlines with advance notice. Or you can pack items that can be consumed when traveling. You might want to purchase low-fat airport food options for consumption on the plane. Be familiar with what is offered at your hometown airport. Many airports have websites that list the restaurants in various terminals so that you can plan your meals for the trip home.

When traveling—by road or plane—try to bring bottled water with you to make sure you maintain good hydration levels. Make healthy choices at airports whenever possible. Aim for turkey sandwiches or wraps for lower-fat choices and plenty of carbohydrates. Choose low-fat frozen yogurt, fruit juices, soft pretzels, low-fat milk, baked potatoes, and/or smoothies. Plan ahead and pack some of your favorite nonperishable items, such as energy bars, granola bars, cereals, packets of instant breakfast mix, dried fruit, whole-grain crackers, powdered sports drinks, meal replacements, instant soups, fruit juices, and any other items that travel safely.

You might also investigate the food options at your destination before you leave. Call ahead to your hotel and find out about food establishments in the area. Internet searches also provide valuable travel information. Table 14.1 provides some suggested meal and snack choices for traveling.

Here is a travel plan checklist:

• Find out what to expect at your travel destination. Some locations may be in small towns with limited grocery options. Athletes who have traveled to this location before are often the best source of information.

TABLE *14.1* MEAL AND SNACK CHOICES WHILE TRAVELING

MEAL	FOOD CHOICES
Breakfast	• Choose dry or cooked cereals, juices, fresh fruits, waffles, French toast, and/or pancakes. • Keep margarine and butter to a minimum. • Order skim milk and low-fat yogurt. • Bagels and muffins with small amounts of peanut butter and jam are good choices as well. • Omelets made with egg whites are fine, but go easy on the cheese. Ask for vegetable fillings instead.
Lunch	• Try to frequent restaurants that have low-fat sandwiches made from poultry or lean meats. Low-fat tuna salads may be available. Go easy on the cheese, and ask for extra vegetable toppings whenever possible. • Choose salads that include lean protein, or choose baked potatoes or chili. • A regular-sized hamburger or cheeseburger is fine, but split a small order of French fries with a teammate.
Dinner	• Choose lean meat, fish, or poultry that is broiled, grilled, baked, or blackened. • Ask for potatoes, rice, pasta, or noodles to be prepared with less than the usual amount of fat. • Order your salad with dressing on the side. • Consume breads and rolls, but go easy on the margarine or butter. • Have fruit for dessert whenever possible.
Snacks	• Try fresh or dried fruit, granola bars, and energy bars. • Buy milk chugs and low-fat yogurt whenever possible. • Snack on low-fat crackers, instant soups, and pretzels. • Drink water and other fluids.

- Plan your accommodations with your ideal meals and length of stay in mind. You may prefer to have full kitchen accommodations before a long race to allow you to carbohydrate-load with your favorite and safest foods.
- If you plan to stay in a hotel, determine if a fridge is available and what type of food storage options you may have.
- Pre-arrange meals for travel on airlines when possible. Pack foods for travel if meals are not served on your flight.
- Take along a supply of portable and nonperishable foods, keeping in mind packing strategies and weight restrictions. Some pre-race foods to pack are canned fruit, dried fruit, energy bars, granola bars, quick-cooking pasta and noodle packs or soups, peanut butter, and jam.
- Watch your eating amounts. Consume just what you need for your nutrition plan and don't let extra sneak in due to airport waiting times and boredom.
- Be aware of fluid losses when traveling, particularly by air.
- When arriving in a new time zone at your destination, try to get on the new meal-time schedule as soon as possible to help your body clock adapt.
- Be aware of water safety and stick with bottled water when necessary, even for brushing your teeth. Ask for beverages without ice. Avoid food from local markets

and stalls and stick with good hotels and well-known restaurants. Make sure that food is well cooked.

- Don't be afraid to ask for what your body needs, such as lean proteins, extra servings of carbohydrates, or less fat in the food preparation.
- Don't fall victim to all-you-can-eat dining; stick to the amounts you need leading up to the race.

APPENDIX A: GLYCEMIC INDEX OF FOODS

As you review the glycemic index (GI) of foods below, this measure of carbohydrate foods may seem to defy common logic. Contrary to popular opinion, most foods high in simple sugars do not raise blood glucose levels any more than do complex starchy foods; in fact, the opposite is often true. Let's look at some test dose results of isolated sugars and some common foods that contain these sugars.

Fruits, though naturally sweet, tend to have a lower GI because they contain mainly fructose, which has a GI of 23. Table or refined sugar, also called sucrose, is composed of one glucose and one fructose molecule and has a GI of 65. Thus, many foods that contain sucrose have a GI of around 60. In contrast, soft white bread such as baguette, which is a complex carbohydrate, has a GI of 95. Honey is another example of a sweet food with a low GI; most varieties have a GI ranging from 35 to 48. Another naturally occurring sugar, lactose, has a GI of 43. Fruited yogurt, which contains both lactose and fructose, has a low GI of 32, despite being perceived as a sugary food.

Glucose and maltodextrin, with GIs of 100 and 105 respectively, are the main ingredients in most sports drinks and quickly raise blood glucose levels, providing fuel for exercise.

Factors other than type of sugar can affect glycemic index, including the physical form of the food, how swollen the starch content is, the type of starch, the fiber content, the sugar content, acidity, and the fat content. This is why it is important to test a food. See www.glycemicindex.com for the full current list of tested foods.

APPENDIX A GLYCEMIC INDEX OF FOODS

FOOD	SERVING SIZE (OZ.)	(G/ML)	CARBOHYDRATES PER SERVING (G)	GLYCEMIC LOAD PER SERVING	GLYCEMIC INDEX (50 G)
HIGH-GLYCEMIC FOODS (GI >70)					
Potato, white without skin, baked	5	150	27	26	98
Potatoes, instant, mashed	5 (1 cup)	150	27	26	97
Baguette	2	60	30	28	95
Rice milk	8.5	250 ml	32	29	92
Rice, instant, white	5	150	42	37	87
Pretzels	1.5	45	30	25	83
Rice Krispies™ cereal	1	30	26	22	82
Rice cakes	1.5	45	38	31	82
Gluten-free bread	2	60	30	24	80
Cornflakes™ cereal	1	30	26	21	80
Vanilla wafers	1.5	45	32	25	77
Waffles	1.1	35	13	10	76
Doughnut	1.6	47	23	17	76
Total™ cereal	1.5	45	33	25	76
Grape-Nuts™ cereal	1	30	22	16	75
Soda crackers	1.6	50	34	25	74
Cheerios™ cereal	1.5	45	30	22	74
Watermelon	5 (1 cup)	130	11	8	72
Bagel, white, frozen	2.3	70	35	25	72
Millet, boiled	5	150	36	26	71
Bread, white	2	60	28	20	71
MODERATE-GLYCEMIC FOODS (GI 55–70)					
Special K™ cereal	1.5	45	32	22	69
Pancakes, from mix	2.5	76	28	19	67
Croissant	1.9	57	26	17	67
Shredded Wheat cereal	1	30	20	13	67
Cream of Wheat™	8.5 (1 cup)	250	26	17	66
Pineapple	8 (1 cup)	240 ml	20	13	66
Rye bread	2	60	18	12	66
Oat kernel bread	1.5	45	29	19	65
Cantaloupe	8	240 ml	12	8	65
Muffin, banana, oat and honey	1.7	50	26	17	65
Beets	2.7	80	7	4	64
Raisins	1 (¼ cup)	36	32	20	64
Rye crispbread	1.5	38	32	20	63
Sweet corn	2.7	80	18	11	62
Couscous, boiled	5	150	35	21	61
Fig, dried	2 (2 whole)	60	26	16	61
Papaya	4	120	29	17	60
Bran muffin	1.9	57	24	14	60

FOOD	SERVING SIZE (OZ.)	(G/ML)	CARBOHYDRATES PER SERVING (G)	GLYCEMIC LOAD PER SERVING	GLYCEMIC INDEX (50 G)
MODERATE-GLYCEMIC FOODS (GI 55–70), *CONTINUED*					
Oat bran, raw	0.8 (½ cup)	23	30	18	59
Basmati, white rice	5	150	38	22	58
Spaghetti, white, durum wheat	6	180	44	26	58
Kiwifruit	4 (1 whole)	120	12	7	58
Ice cream	5 (1 cup)	148	32	18	57
Pita bread, white	1.5	45	25	15	57
Orange juice, from concentrate	8.5	250 ml	26	15	57
Wild rice	5	150	32	18	57
Pumpernickel bread	2	60	24	14	56
Muesli	1.5	45	29	16	55
Popcorn	0.7	20	10	6	55
Frosted Flakes™ cereal	1 (¾ cup)	30	28	15	55
All-Bran™ cereal	1.5	45	31	17	55
LOW-GLYCEMIC FOODS (GI <55)					
Pound cake	1.8	53	28	15	54
Quinoa	5	150	25	13	53
Buckwheat	5	150	30	15	51
Bread, whole-grain	2	60	26	13	51
Jam, strawberry	2 (3 tbsp.)	60	26	13	51
Mango	4 (1 small)	120	15	8	51
Banana, ripe	4 (1 medium)	120	25	13	51
Rice, brown	5	150	33	16	50
Porridge oatmeal	8.5	250 ml	23	11	49
Grapefruit juice	8.5	250 ml	20	9	48
Pudding, chocolate, instant	3.3	100 ml	16	7	47
Bulgur	5	150	26	12	46
Kudos® granola bar	1.7	50	30	14	45
Soy milk, low-fat	8.5	250 ml	10	4	45
Sweet potato	5	150	25	11	44
Honey (52% fructose)	0.8	25	21	9	43
Nectarine	4	120	9	4	43
Lactose	(test portion)	10	10	4	43
Garbanzo beans	5	150	22	9	42
Pear, Bartlett	5.5 (1 medium)	166	25	10	41
Strawberries	5 (1 cup)	144	10	4	40
Apple juice	8.5	250 ml	25	10	39
Pinto beans, dried, boiled	5	150	26	10	39
Apple	4	120	16	5	34
Apricots, dried	2 (2 medium)	60	22	7	32

Continues >

ᴀᴘᴘᴇɴᴅɪx A   **GLYCEMIC INDEX OF FOODS** *continued*

FOOD	SERVING SIZE (OZ.)	(G/ML)	CARBOHYDRATES PER SERVING (G)	GLYCEMIC LOAD PER SERVING	GLYCEMIC INDEX (50 G)
LOW-GLYCEMIC FOODS (GI <55), *CONTINUED*					
Fettucine	6	180	46	15	32
Yogurt, fruited	6.5	195	33	11	32
Milk, skim	8.5	250 ml	13	4	32
Spaghetti, whole-grain, cooked	6 (1 cup)	180	44	14	32
Black beans, cooked	5 (¾ cup)	150	23	7	30
Peach	4 (1 large)	120	13	4	28
Lentils	5 (¾ cup)	150	18	5	28
Grapefruit	4 (½ medium)	120	11	3	25
Barley	5 (1 cup)	150	42	9	22
Cherries	4 (1 cup)	120	12	3	22
Kidney beans		150	25	5	19

SOURCES: WWW.GLYCEMICINDEX.COM AND *THE GLUCOSE REVOLUTION* (MARLOWE & COMPANY). ACCESSED 2011.

Note: Values can vary depending on form of food, how food is prepared, and type of study conducted.

APPENDIX B:
GLOSSARY OF VITAMINS AND MINERALS

APPENDIX *B* GLOSSARY OF VITAMINS AND MINERALS

VITAMINS	DRIS (DAILY REFERENCE INTAKE)	MAJOR SOURCES	MAJOR FUNCTIONS
WATER-SOLUBLE			
Thiamin (vitamin B1)	*Males* 14–70 yrs: 1.2 mg *Females* 14–70 yrs: 1.1 mg	Wheat germ, whole-grain breads and cereals, organ meats, lean meats, legumes	Energy production from carbohydrates; essential for healthy nervous system
Riboflavin (vitamin B2)	*Males* 14–70 yrs: 1.3 mg *Females* 14–18 yrs: 1.0 mg 18–70 yrs: 1.1 mg	Milk and dairy products, green leafy vegetables, lean meats, beans	Energy production from carbohydrates and fats; essential for healthy skin
Niacin (nicotinamide, nicotinic acid)	*Males* 14–70 yrs: 16 mg *Females* 14–70 yrs: 14 mg	Lean meats, fish, poultry, whole grains, peanuts	Energy production from carbohydrates, synthesis of fat, blocks release of FFA
Vitamin B6 (pyridoxine)	*Males* 14–50 yrs: 1.3 mg 51–70+ yrs: 1.7 mg *Females* 14–18 yrs: 1.2 mg 19–50 yrs: 1.3 mg 51–70+ yrs: 1.5 mg	Liver, lean meats, fish, poultry, legumes, bran cereal	Plays role in protein metabolism, necessary for formation of hemoglobin and red blood cells and synthesis of essential fatty acids; required for glycogen breakdown
Vitamin B12 (cobalamin)	*Males* 14–70+ yrs: 2.4 mcg *Females* 14–70+ yrs: 2.4 mcg	Lean meats, poultry, dairy products, eggs	Plays role in formation of red blood cells and metabolism of nervous tissue; involved in folate metabolism, formation of DNA
Folic acid (folate)	*Males* 14–70+ yrs: 400 mcg *Females* 14–70+ yrs: 400 mcg	Green leafy vegetables, legumes	Plays role in red blood cell and DNA formation
Biotin	*Males* 14–18 yrs: 25 mcg 19–70+ yrs: 30 mcg *Females* 14–18 yrs: 25 mcg 19–70+ yrs: 30 mcg	Meats, legumes, milk, egg yolks, whole grains	Plays role in metabolism of carbohydrates, protein, fat
Pantothenic Acid	*Males* 14–70+ yrs: 5 mg *Females* 14–70+ yrs: 5 mg	Liver, lean meats, eggs, salmon, all animal and plant foods	Plays role in metabolism of carbohydrates, protein, fat
Vitamin C	*Males* 14–18 yrs: 75 mg 19–70+ yrs: 90 mg *Females* 14–18 yrs: 65 mg 19–70+ yrs: 75 mg	Citrus fruits, green leafy vegetables, broccoli, peppers, strawberries, potatoes	Essential for connective tissue development, plays role in iron absorption; antioxidant; plays role in wound healing
FAT-SOLUBLE			
Vitamin A (retinol, provitamin carotenoids)	*Males* 14–70+ yrs: 900 mcg *Females* 14–70+ yrs: 700 mcg	Liver, milk, cheese, fortified margarine, carotenoids in plant foods (orange, red, deep green in color)	Maintains healthy tissue in skin and mucous membranes, essential for night vision; plays role in bone development

Continues >

APPENDIX B GLOSSARY OF VITAMINS AND MINERALS *continued*

VITAMINS	DRIS (DAILY REFERENCE INTAKE)	MAJOR SOURCES	MAJOR FUNCTIONS
FAT-SOLUBLE, *CONTINUED*			
Vitamin D (cholecalciferol)	*Males* 14–70 yrs: 600 IU (15 mcg) 70+ yrs: 800 IU (20 mcg) *Females* 14–70 yrs: 600 IU (15 mcg) 70+ yrs: 800 IU (20 mcg)	Vitamin D–fortified milk and margarine, fish oil, metabolized by sunlight on skin	Increases intestinal absorption of calcium, promotes bone and tooth formation, plays role in preventing colon cancer and autoimmune diseases, such as type 1 diabetes and rheumatoid arthritis
Vitamin E (tocopherol)	*Males* 14–70+ yrs: 15 mg *Females* 14–70+ yrs: 15 mg	Vegetable oils, margarine, green leafy vegetables, wheat germ, whole-grain products	Plays role in formation of red blood cells; antioxidant
Vitamin K (phylloquinone)	*Males* 14–18 yrs: 75 mcg 19–70+ yrs: 120 mcg *Females* 14–18 yrs: 75 mcg 19–70+ yrs: 90 mcg	Liver, soybean oil, spinach, cauliflower, green leafy vegetables	Essential for normal blood clotting
MAJOR MINERALS			
Calcium	*Males* 14–18 yrs: 1,300 mg 19–50 yrs: 1,000 mg 51–70+ yrs: 1,000 mg *Females* 14–18 yrs: 1,300 mg 19–50 yrs: 1,000 mg 51–70+ yrs: 1,200 mg	Milk, cheese, yogurt, dried peas and beans, dark green leafy vegetables	Plays role in bone formation, enzyme activation, nerve impulse transmission, muscle contraction
Phosphorus	*Males* 14–18 yrs: 1,250 mg 19–70+ yrs: 700 mg *Females* 14–18 yrs: 1,250 mg 19–70+ yrs: 700 mg	Protein foods such as meat, poultry, fish, eggs, milk, cheese, dried peas and beans, whole grains	Plays role in bone formation, cell membrane structure, B-vitamin activation, component of ATP-CP and other important organic compounds
Magnesium	*Males* 14–18 yrs: 410 mg 19–30 yrs: 400 mg 31–70+ yrs: 420 mg *Females* 14–18 yrs: 360 mg 19–30 yrs: 310 mg 31–70+ yrs: 320 mg	Milk, yogurt, dried beans, nuts, whole grains, tofu, green vegetables, chocolate	Plays role in protein synthesis, glucose metabolism, muscle contraction
TRACE MINERALS			
Iron	*Males* 14–18 yrs: 11 mg 19–70+ yrs: 8 mg *Females* 14–18 yrs: 15 mg 19–50 yrs: 18 mg 51–70+ yrs: 8 mg	Organ meats, lean meats, poultry, shellfish, dried peas and beans, whole-grain products, green leafy vegetables	Plays role in hemoglobin formation, oxygen transport

VITAMINS	DRIS (DAILY REFERENCE INTAKE)	MAJOR SOURCES	MAJOR FUNCTIONS
TRACE MINERALS, *CONTINUED*			
Zinc	*Males* 14–70+ yrs: 11 mg *Females* 14–18 yrs: 9 mg 19–70+ yrs: 8 mg	Organ meats, meat, fish, poultry, shellfish, nuts, whole-grain products	Involved in energy metabolism, immune function
Copper	*Males* 14–18 yrs: 890 mcg 19–70+ yrs: 900 mcg *Females* 14–18 yrs: 890 mcg 19–70+ yrs: 900 mcg	Organ meats, meat, fish, poultry, shellfish, nuts, bran cereal	Plays role in use of iron and hemoglobin by body, involved in connective tissue formation and oxidation
Fluoride	Adequate intake *Males* 14–18 yrs: 3 mg 19–70+ yrs: 4 mg *Females* 14–70+ yrs: 3 mg	Milk, egg yolks, drinking water, seafood	Plays role in tooth and bone formation
Selenium	*Males* 14–70+ yrs: 55 mcg *Females* 14–70+ yrs: 55 mcg	Meat, fish, poultry, organ meats, seafood, whole grains and nuts from selenium-rich soil	Forms part of antioxidant enzyme
Chromium	*Males* 14–50 yrs: 35 mcg 51–70+ yrs: 30 mcg *Females* 14–18 yrs: 24 mcg 19–50 yrs: 25 mcg 51–70+ yrs: 20 mcg	Organ meats, meats, oysters, cheese, whole-grain products, beer	Enhances insulin function as glucose tolerance factor
Iodine	*Males* 14–70+ yrs: 150 mcg *Females* 14–70+ yrs: 150 mcg	Iodized table salt, seafood, water	Forms part of thyroxine, which plays a role in reactions involving cellular energy
Manganese	Adequate intake *Males* 14–18 yrs: 2.2 mg 19–70+ yrs: 2.3 mg *Females* 14–18 yrs: 1.6 mg 19–70+ yrs: 1.8 mg	Beet greens, whole grains, nuts, legumes	Plays role in essential enzyme systems
Molybdenum	*Males* 14–18 yrs: 43 mcg 19–70+ yrs: 45 mcg *Females* 14–18 yrs: 43 mcg 19–70+ yrs: 45 mcg	Legumes, cereal grains, dark green leafy vegetables	Plays role in essential enzymes involved in carbohydrate and fat metabolism

APPENDIX C: COMPARISON OF SPORTS NUTRITION PRODUCTS

APPENDIX C COMPARISON OF SPORTS NUTRITION PRODUCTS

PRODUCT	TYPE OF CARBOHYDRATE	CARBOHYDRATE CONCENTRATION (%)	CALORIES	CARBO-HYDRATES (G)	SODIUM (MG)
COMMERCIAL SPORTS DRINKS (8 OZ. OR 240 ML SERVING)					
Accelerade	Sucrose, fructose, maltodextrin (also contains 4 gm protein per serving)	8	93	17	127
All Sport	Fructose, sucrose	8	70	19	55
Amino Vital	Fructose (also contains 740 mg of amino acids)	3	35	8	10
Body Fuel	Maltodextrin, fructose	7	70	17	70
Cytomax	Fructose, maltodextrin, polylactate, glucose	8	83	19	70
e-Fuel	Maltodextrin, fructose	7	70	18	130
EFS	Complex carbohydrates, sucrose, dextrose (also contains 1.5 g of amino acids)	8	72	18	188
Endura	Glucose polymers, fructose	6	60	15	92
Endurathon	Maltodextrin, trehalose, ribose, fructose, glucose, sucrose (also contains 4 g of protein)	7	90	16	200
Exceed	Glucose polymer, fructose	7	70	17	50
Gatorade	Sucrose, glucose	6	50	14	110
Gatorade Endurance Drink	Sucrose, glucose	6	60	15	200
Gleukos	Glucose	7	70	17	40
Gookinaid	Glucose, fructose	5	43	10	69
GU Electro-lyte Brew	Maltodextrin, Fructose	5	50	13	250
GU20	Maltodextrin, fructose	6	52	13	120
HEED	Maltodextrin	5	48	12	31
Hydra Fuel	Glucose polymer, fructose, glucose	7	66	16	25
Hydro-BOOM	Maltodextrin, sucrose, glucose, fructose	7	70	17	160
Ironman Perform	Glucose, fructose	7	70	17	190
Met-Rx ORS	Rice syrup solids, glucose	8	70	19	125
Perform	Glucose, fructose, maltodextrin	7	60	16	110
Performance	Maltodextrin, fructose	10	100	25	115
Power Ade	Fructose, sucrose	6	55	14	50
PowerBar Endurance Sports Drink	Maltodextrin, dextrose, fructose	7	70	17	160
PR Solution	Maltodextrin, fructose	13	120	30	50

APPENDIX D: CREATING THE OPTIMAL TRAINING DIET

Meal planning need not be a frustrating experience for dedicated endurance athletes—and you don't have to employ a personal chef or learn to make gourmet meals. But like your training program, meal planning does require forethought, organization, and flexibility. With practice, your meal-planning skills will become second nature. Some fundamentals of meal planning follow.

PLANNING YOUR DAILY MEALS

Have a well-organized and well-equipped kitchen. Make sure that you have the basic tools: a microwave, a steamer, a countertop portable grill, a toaster oven, a set of microwave-proof cookware, and a slow cooker. Other handy items include a large skillet or wok, a rice cooker, a lasagna pan, and sharp knives. Always store items in the same places—knowing where everything is located makes putting together meals much easier.

Plan out your week's meals beforehand. Think ahead to what meals you will need to cook, pack, or eat out based on that week's schedule. How many dinners will you cook at home? Account for healthy takeout, eating out, and leftovers. Where will you be for lunch? Do you need to pack a full lunch, or just extras? Will your training schedule require you to have energy bars or carbohydrate drinks on hand? Make a shopping list as you plan; if you can shop only once for the week, plan to consume the fresh vegetables and fruit early on and save frozen or canned items for later.

Develop a meal schedule. For example, you could always have chicken on Monday nights, fish on Thursdays, and stir-fries on Fridays. Vary the types of vegetables and side dishes to obtain a variety of nutrients. Sometimes it is easier to achieve variety when you prepare dinner for an entire family; when cooking for just one or two people, try to obtain variety on a weekly basis, switching the grains, fruits, and vegetables you consume.

Keep nonperishable stock food items amply supplied. A well-stocked cupboard of items such as rice, pasta, whole grains, instant couscous, and other dry items and canned goods can help you in a pinch when fresh food supplies run low or during heavy training weeks. Some quick meals made from these ingredients are black bean burritos (freeze the tortillas); pasta and tomato sauce; stir-fries made from frozen chicken, instant rice, and frozen vegetable mixes; and canned chili with bread or crackers.

Go grocery shopping every week for fresh items. Have a designated grocery-shopping day and time and make it part of your weekly schedule. Don't put off shopping until it is convenient to go—it may never be convenient! In the long run, going shopping once a week is much less time-consuming than having to make several quick trips to the store to grab a few needed items each time. Try to find one supermarket that has all the items you need. Go during off-peak times to avoid crowds, and don't mull over items that are not on your shopping list. If you can't make it to the supermarket some weeks, find a grocery store or online grocery system that accepts phone, fax, or Internet delivery orders.

Keep a running list of items that need to be replenished. Have a pad and pen handy in the kitchen. When you notice that items are running low or are used up, add them to your list. Trying to remember everything you need while shopping at the grocery store may not be the best strategy for a busy athlete.

Batch-cook meals, make extra portions, and freeze single servings. This strategy can be a great time-saver. Set aside a lighter training day to cook items such as soup, chili, and lasagna. When cooking regular meals, make an extra portion for the next day to save on preparation time or to have a nice midday meal. Freeze single-item portions in plastic containers or oven-ready aluminum foil pans for later use on heavy training days.

Pack meals, snacks, and food supplements for the next training day the night before. If your next day's schedule is full, pack your foods and snacks the night before. Having some portioned items and fresh foods in the fridge will make this task as simple as possible. Plan snacks that can be eaten on the run.

Acquire a repertoire of quick and easy-to-prepare meals. Anyone can become a proficient cook, and it does not have to be a time-consuming project. Be on the lookout for quick and simple recipes. Ask friends for some of their quick meal ideas. Focus on recipes like stir-fries, rice dishes, burritos, and pastas.

Take advantage of food shortcuts. Purchase chicken tender strips, beef stir-fry strips, frozen pre-cooked shrimp, and rotisserie chickens. Try frozen vegetable stir-fry mixes, pre-cut fruits, pre-seasoned and cut tofu, ready-to-heat soups, fresh pastas (you can freeze them), and canned beans, chickpeas, and other legumes.

BREAKFAST, LUNCH, AND SNACKS

Breakfast really is the most important meal of the day. It revs up your body's metabolism and refills liver glycogen stores that have become depleted overnight. It can be an important recovery meal after a solid early-morning training session. If you tend to skip breakfast, eat a medium-sized lunch, and feast at dinner, you may be not only compromising your recovery but also cheating your body of important nutrients. Skipping breakfast is also a terrible weight-management strategy because it sets you up for increased hunger and overeating later in the day.

Breakfast should keep you feeling satisfied for three hours or so until you are hungry again. Inserting a mid-morning snack into your eating plan enables you to stretch out the span of time between breakfast and lunch. If your energy needs are high, eat a substantial breakfast. Eat calorically dense cereals such as granola or muesli. A large glass of juice can add a substantial amount of calories and carbohydrates, which is good if you need the carbs to supply energy for your morning workout. Adding some protein to your breakfast can help keep you comfortably full until the next meal.

Depending on your schedule, you may need to consume breakfast on the fly. Bringing breakfast with you as you leave for work or school is better than skipping it altogether. Quick choices include yogurt, bananas, dried fruit, bagels, muffins, and fruit smoothies made with yogurt and granola.

APPENDIX D.1   SIMPLE SUGGESTIONS FOR STOCKING YOUR PANTRY

FOR THE FREEZER	FOR THE REFRIGERATOR	FOR THE CUPBOARD
Chicken tenders	Fresh fruit	Dried pasta
Cooked shrimp	Fresh vegetables (including pre-washed salad greens, mini-carrots)	Rice
Lean ground beef		Couscous
Lean pork fillets	Juices	Quinoa
Cubed meat for stir-fries	Milk (dairy, soy, rice)	Pilaf mixes
Soy and garden burgers	Yogurt	Tabouleh
Textured vegetable proteins	Eggs	Canned beans
Egg substitute	Reduced-fat cheese	Canned tuna
Variety of breads	Butter or margarine	Peanut butter and other nut butters
Waffles	Lean deli meats	Instant stuffing mixes
English muffins	Fresh pasta	Canned soup
Muffins	Sauces and condiments (including salsa, marinades)	Instant soup and grain cups
Tortillas		Seasoning mixes
Pre-cooked pasta and rice		Cold cereal assortment
Frozen vegetables		Oatmeal and farina
Stir-fry mixes		Low-fat crackers
Sorbet		Dried fruit
Frozen fruit		Granola bars
		Nuts and sunflower seeds
		Pretzels
		Fig Newtons®

Your lunch should provide you with quality carbohydrates balanced with a healthy proportion of proteins and fats. Eat lunch when hunger first sets in, as this is a sign that your body needs fuel. Packing a lunch takes more time and planning than purchasing one at a restaurant or fast-food establishment, but it is well worth the effort because you can ensure that you have lean proteins and the right type and amount of fats. Some people enjoy eating leftovers from the previous night's dinner, but sandwiches are also good if last night's leftovers seem too repetitive. Good protein options are lean beef, hummus, turkey, chicken, tuna, and low-fat cottage cheese. Liven up that turkey sandwich with add-ons such as avocado, lettuce leaves, cucumber, tomato, sprouts, and low-fat cheese. High-carbohydrate items that you can include with your lunch are fruits, pretzels, raw vegetables, yogurt, low-fat chips, low-fat crackers, and vegetable and bean soups.

When your energy needs are high, snacks give you a nice calorie boost. They can also provide you with fuel before training sessions and keep hunger at bay until you can sit down for a full meal. Many elite athletes swear by snacking. Plan some serious snacking in your diet. If there is a particular time of day when you experience an energy lull, snacking may make all the difference. The table "Breakfast and Snack Ideas" lists some tasty breakfast and snack ideas.

LABEL-READING TIPS

Food labels help you determine the nutritional breakdown of foods. The ingredients list is a good place to start. Because the ingredients are listed by weight, the one that makes up the largest percentage of a food by weight will be the first item listed; the one that makes up the next largest percentage by weight will be the second listed, and so on. So, for example, if you are trying to incorporate more whole-wheat flours and other whole grains into your diet, this part of the label will help you decide among brands of bread, pasta, and the like. Look for whole-wheat flour to be the first ingredient.

Before going any further, look for the part of the label that lists the serving size, and compare it with the amount that you actually eat. The portions you consume may be double those on the package, and you should adjust the nutrition information accordingly. To evaluate whether a food will significantly impact your carbohydrate intake, check for the total grams of carbohydrates per serving. You can then determine how far that particular food will go toward providing the carbohydrates you need to help you meet your training requirements for the day.

APPENDIX D.2   BREAKFAST AND SNACK IDEAS

BREAKFAST	SNACKS
Cooked oatmeal with raisins, cinnamon, and low-fat milk	Peanut butter-and-jelly sandwich
Open-face English muffin halves broiled with cheese, and fruit on the side	Hard and soft pretzels
	Baked potato with low-fat cheese
Omelet made with egg substitute and vegetables, with toast, juice, and milk	Crackers with peanut butter
	Muffin or bagel with jam and low-fat cream cheese
Yogurt with fresh fruit and a low-fat muffin	Yogurt with fruit
Whole-grain cereal with milk and fruit	Bowl of soup with crackers
Fruit smoothie made with yogurt, fresh or frozen fruit, and granola	Pasta or bean salad
	Fresh fruit, low-fat cheese, and nuts
Whole-grain bread with peanut butter, banana, and honey	Cottage cheese and fruit
	Instant breakfast mix and fruit
Any leftovers that sound appealing	Hummus and crackers or pita bread
	Fruit smoothie
	Milk and fruit

Total fat grams as well as calories from fat are also listed. To determine the percentage of calories from fat, divide the fat calories per serving by the total calories per serving and multiply by 100. Keep high-fat foods in perspective. Your fat intake needs to be considered in the context of an entire day. Your total day's intake should include some foods that contain healthy fats—as long as you don't go overboard with fatty foods or eat the wrong type of fats. Some foods, such as dried pasta, are very low in fat, while others, such as margarine, provide a relatively high amount of fat. As long as the percentage of fat for the day averages out to 20 to 25 percent of your total intake, you are in the ballpark. (See Chapter 2 for information on healthy versus unhealthy fats.)

The Daily Value (DV) for various vitamins and minerals provided on the nutrition label is based on a 2,000-calorie intake. The percentage indicates if a food is high or low in a nutrient such as calcium, fiber, or vitamin C. A food is considered to be a good source of a nutrient if it provides 20 percent of the DV. Besides increasing your intake of foods high in specific nutrients, use the DV to avoid excess fat, saturated fat, and cholesterol.

DIETARY RULES FOR RESTAURANTS

Like many North Americans, you probably eat out several times weekly. Lunch is the meal most frequently eaten away from home, followed by dinner and then breakfast. You may eat out at restaurants, in a cafeteria, at your desk, and even in your car.

Regardless of where you eat your meal out, the basic strategies are the same. Watch for hidden and added fats, and keep a close eye on portions. Despite your high energy requirements for endurance training, not all restaurant meals fit nicely into your nutrition plan. They may be too high in fat to become a frequent indulgence and may not provide the healthy ingredients that you require. It is important to learn what healthy food choices are available at your favorite restaurants. Ask questions about how foods are prepared, and don't hesitate to request modifications. Often you can creatively outsmart the menu and enjoy your meal knowing that it will be good for you.

FAST FOOD

Fast food—especially supersized meals and grease-laden French fries—can provide excessive amounts of fat. But it is possible to make choices that fit into a sports diet at some fast-food establishments. Have a small hamburger that provides only 2 or 3 ounces of meat rather than the large one. Order a baked potato instead of French fries. Choose a broiled chicken sandwich over chicken pieces, which are generally fried. The same goes for fish sandwiches, as they come dripping with plenty of unwanted oil. Order skim milk or juice instead of sugary sodas. Salads and vegetables may be on the menu, but watch out for the dressings. Limit the sauces and toppings.

Many fast-food establishments now provide good sandwich choices. You can choose lean roast beef, ham, turkey, or chicken and limit oils, mayonnaise, and cheese. Go for baked chips and pretzels. Chicken fajitas or tacos can also make good lower-fat choices. Frozen yogurt and low-fat milkshakes are better for you than deep-fried pastries or cookies.

Another fast-food choice that can fit into your sports nutrition plan is a vegetarian thin-crust pizza. Some establishments also have a soup-and-baked-potato bar. Bean burritos and soft tacos may also be available, or possibly chili, bagels, English muffins, waffles, pancakes, and cereals.

ETHNIC CUISINE

If you eat out frequently, you have probably enjoyed many types of ethnic cuisines. These cultural edibles can fit into a healthy training diet if you know what choices to make and can avoid consuming hidden fats. The sampling of ethnic cuisine below includes only a few of the many cultural options available in most large and medium-sized cities. Take a commonsense approach to any ethnic cuisine, whether Indian, Thai, Vietnamese, African, Russian, or Middle Eastern, looking for lean protein options and low-fat alternatives.

Italian Cuisine

Italian food is a popular favorite and can be consumed at a variety of settings—upscale, family-style, or fast-food. With an emphasis on grains and vegetables, Italian eating can be quite healthy. Some relatively light, low-fat choices are starches such as spaghetti, risotto, and polenta; vegetables such as zucchini and even tomato-based sauces; and lean meats such as chicken, veal, shrimp, and grilled fish. Herbs, vinegar, garlic, and crushed red peppers may be available at the table to spice up your food. Fill up on minestrone, and top your pasta with marinara or red clam sauce. Order your salad dressing on the side, and have an Italian ice for dessert. You can also make special requests—for example, you can ask your waiter to remove the olive oil from the table or have the chef remove the skin from your chicken.

There are also plenty of heavier choices at Italian restaurants. Starches such as garlic bread and focaccia are usually loaded with fat, as are fried vegetables and meats like salami, prosciutto, and sausage. Watch out for high-fat cheeses and dishes prepared with cream, butter, and even olive oil, which may be relatively healthy as far as oils go but still contains plenty of fat calories. Go easy on the antipasto plate and the olive oil served with bread. Alfredo sauce, Italian sausage, lasagna, and parmigiana dishes are all high in fat because of the ingredients and methods of preparation.

Mexican Cuisine

Like Italian food, Mexican cuisine contains both light and heavy choices. Many staples of Mexican cuisine can be considered low-fat, including items such as whole beans, refried beans prepared without oil, tortillas, rice cooked without oil, grilled vegetables, and salsa. Grilled proteins, such as shrimp, fish, and chicken, are good choices, as are whole black beans. You can also fill up on gazpacho, marinated vegetables, and burritos (but go easy on the cheese).

Heavier choices at Mexican restaurants include tortilla chips, chimichangas, and taco shells. Avocados (guacamole), olives, sour cream, and cheese are also high in fat. Watch out for chorizo, cheese, sour cream, and oil used in cooking, which may contribute a significant amount of fat, especially saturated fat, to a meal. Avoid items on the menu with descriptions that say "smothered in cheese."

Chinese Cuisine

Chinese cuisine, providing a variety of regional cooking styles, is a frequent favorite at mall eateries and small neighborhood restaurants. Although there are light choices in Chinese cooking, there are also many high-fat pitfalls. To keep your meal on the light side, look for stir-fried vegetables. Almost every Chinese restaurant will have a variety to choose from, such as snowpeas, bamboo shoots, water chestnuts, cabbage, baby corn, and broccoli.

Lean proteins found in Chinese dishes include shrimp, chicken, tofu, and lean cuts of beef and pork, usually mixed with vegetables in some sort of stir-fry combination. Chinese dishes may also contain low-fat fruits, such as pineapple and orange sections. Condiments such as mustard, soy sauce, ginger, duck sauce, and garlic will not increase the fat content of your meals.

Chinese cuisine contains plenty of high-fat choices, however. Everyone is familiar with the fatty breaded and fried sweet-and-sour dishes. Fried rice has twice the calories of steamed rice, with all the additional calories coming from oil. Fried noodles and egg rolls also up your fat intake. Stay away from fried seafood, pork, spare ribs, and duck with skin. Stir-fried dishes that contain nuts and peanuts will also be much higher in fat, as will any choices in which oil is used heavily. Request that your dish be prepared with as little oil as possible, and try to split entrees, as portions are often large.

SALAD BARS

Visits to the salad bar are often well intended but can result in surprisingly high-fat meals. Beside those healthy raw vegetable items like spinach, tomatoes, broccoli, and green peppers are plenty of items mixed with fat or sitting in oil. Some of the less healthy choices are pasta salad, potato salad, marinated vegetables, cheeses, and bean salads made with oil. Go easy on portions of these items. Of course, try to keep salad dressing portions reasonable as well.

Salad bars have plenty of carbohydrates and fiber and can help you keep your protein portions low and reasonable. Obviously, fresh greens and plain raw vegetables are your best bet. Starches on the salad bar may include garbanzo beans, kidney beans, green peas, crackers, and pita bread. Lean-protein salad bar choices include plain tuna, cottage cheese, hard-boiled egg, ham cubes, and feta cheese. Avoid most cheeses and pepperoni. Keep marinated vegetable portions small, and watch out for salads made with mayonnaise, such as tuna or chicken salad, seafood salad, macaroni salad, and potato salad. Peanuts, sesame seeds, and sunflower seeds provide good fats and can be used in small amounts.

MEAL-PLANNING TIPS FOR VEGETARIANS

- Include a protein-rich food at all meals and snacks.
- Add milk, fortified soy or rice milk, or yogurt to every meal or snack.
- Use nuts, butters, hummus, and low-fat cheeses (soy and regular) for toppings on breads, bagels, and crackers.
- Add nuts and seeds to a fruit-and-yogurt snack.
- Make tofu and tempeh stir-fries.
- Experiment with quick and easy bean recipes to make burritos, casseroles, and salads.
- Make thick soups and stews with beans and lentils.
- Experiment with all the meat-replacer soy products on the market, such as tofu dogs and burgers.
- Make casseroles, lasagna, and stuffed pasta shell recipes with tofu.
- Most health-food stores and the health-food sections of many supermarkets provide a wide selection of vegetarian food choices and convenience items.
- The number of textured vegetable protein products has increased significantly in the past several years. You can now buy products that resemble and taste like hot dogs, burgers, or breakfast sausage. Many of these products make quick and easy lunch ideas.
- Tofu can be substituted for chicken in most recipes. Seasoned tofu is available, and you can also season the recipe to spice up tofu's milder taste.
- Substitute vegetable broth when recipes call for beef or chicken stock. Vegetable broth is available in many supermarkets and most health-food stores.
- Canned lentils, garbanzo beans, and other beans are a quick and nutritious vegetarian option. When time allows, soak the dried lentil and bean versions. Bean and lentil recipes can be batch-cooked and frozen for later use.
- If you need assistance, find a vegetarian cookbook that provides meal ideas suited to athletes.
- Include protein-rich foods at every meal. Because vegetarian options are not as concentrated in protein as animal sources, you need to include adequate portions at most meals and snacks.
- Purchase calcium-fortified soy and rice milks if you drink these products instead of dairy milk.
- Purchase iron-fortified cereals and consume them with products high in vitamin C, such as orange juice.

APPENDIX E: SAMPLE MENUS

Nutritional requirements need to be tailored to the unique needs of individual athletes, and they will change even for individual athletes at various phases in their training program. A periodized nutrition plan requires adjustments in total intake of carbohydrates, proteins, and fats through each training cycle as well as for various types of training sessions within a training cycle (see Chapter 4).

The sample menus provided here are therefore not meant to be followed precisely—individual athletes or their sports dietitian must design personalized menus that are appropriate for personal nutrient and energy needs; however, these serve as a guide to how food intake might be balanced for various levels of training. If you know your calorie intake and nutrient needs, you may find that you can choose menus from the list that are a fairly good match for your current training cycle and use them to help you get started in improving your sports nutrition diet, making adjustments for your own tastes and requirements. Experiment with various food items and portion sizes to find out what works best for you.

Because of the timing of training most common among endurance athletes—and the frequency of training, with some athletes training twice daily—most of these menus provide one or two snacks a day. In some of the menus, one of these is a light snack that can be consumed before very early-morning training, a time when a full breakfast may not be tolerated. The timing of food and fluid intake can, and should, be adjusted to accommodate individual tolerances and training schedules. Consult Chapter 5 for more information on making adjustments in meal and snack timing before and after training. Also, many endurance athletes may need additional amounts of water and other fluids for adequate daily hydration. Monitor your weight before and after different types of training sessions so that you will be familiar with your sweat rate, and be sure to drink enough fluids to replace these losses adequately (see the sidebar "Estimating Your Sweat Losses" in Chapter 5).

Sports drinks and gels can also be added to these sample menus. You may choose to use sports nutrition products in place of some of the snacks because of their convenience and easier tolerance around exercise. If so, keep in mind that these products typically replace a grain or fruit serving on the menus in regard to a caloric equivalent.

Consider enlisting the services of a sports dietitian or nutritionist who can provide you with personalized meal plans as you prepare for an event or competition.

APPENDIX E MEAL PLANS

BASE

BASE CYCLE MEAL PLANS

2,200 CALORIES	2,400 CALORIES	2,700 CALORIES
340 g carbohydrates (60%) 99 g protein (18%) 56 g fat (22%)	346 g carbohydrates (58%) 99 g protein (17%) 68 g fat (25%)	380 g carbohydrates (56%) 130 g protein (19%) 75 g fat (25%)
Breakfast Orange juice, 1 c. (240 ml) French toast, 2 slices Syrup, ½ c. (120 ml) Strawberries, 1 c. (240 ml)	**Breakfast** English muffin Cream cheese, 2 tbsp. (30 ml) Jam, 2 tbsp. (30 ml) Grapefruit juice, 12 oz. (360 ml) Egg, 1 medium	**Breakfast** Oatmeal, cooked, 1 ½ c. (360 ml) Skim milk, 8 oz. (240 ml) Wheat germ, 4 tbsp. (60 ml) Bread, 2 slices Jam, 2 tbsp. (30 ml) Orange juice, 8 oz. (240 ml)
Lunch Low-fat cheese, 2 oz. (60 g) Bread, 2 slices Tomato, 1 medium Yogurt with fruit, 1 c. (240 ml) Pear, 1 medium	**Lunch** Pinto beans, ½ c. (120 ml) Rice, cooked, 1 c. (240 ml) Tortilla, 1 medium Salsa, 4 tbsp. (60 ml) Cheese, 1 oz. (30 g) Avocado, ¼ whole	**Lunch** Chicken, 4 oz. (120 g) Bread, whole-grain, 2 slices Mayonnaise, light, 2 tbsp. (30 ml) Rice and bean salad, ½ c. (120 ml) Grapes, 1 c. (240 ml)
Snack Crackers, 8 small Hummus, ½ c. (120 ml) Skim milk, 8 oz. (240 ml)	**Snack** Granola bar Peaches, 2 medium Almonds, 1 tbsp. (15 ml)	**Snack** Energy bar Banana, 1 medium Yogurt with fruit, 8 oz. (240 ml)
Dinner Rice, cooked, 1 ½ c. (360 ml) Shrimp, cooked, 6 oz. (180 g) Red pepper, 1 whole Broccoli, cooked, 1 c. (240 ml) Sesame oil, 1 tbsp. (15 ml)	**Dinner** Pasta, cooked, 2 c. (480 ml) Lean beef, 3 oz. (90 g) Marinara sauce, 1 c. (240 ml) Green salad, 2 c. (480 ml) Salad dressing, 2 tbsp. (30 ml)	**Dinner** Tofu, 6 oz. (180 g) Asian noodles, cooked, 2 c. (480 ml) Vegetables, 2 c. (480 ml) Sesame oil, 2 tbsp. (30 ml)
Snack Frozen yogurt, 1 c. (240 ml) Fruit slices, ½ c. (120 ml)	**Snack** Frozen yogurt, 1 c. (240 ml) Blueberries, ½ c. (120 ml)	

3,000 CALORIES	3,400 CALORIES	3,800 CALORIES
450 g carbohydrates (60%) 115 g protein (15%) 83 g fat (25%)	510 g carbohydrates (60%) 130 g protein (15%) 95 g fat (25%)	570 g carbohydrates (60%) 140 g protein (15%) 105 g fat (25%)
Snack Toast, 1 slice Jam, 1 tbsp. (15 ml) Juice, 8 oz. (240 ml)	**Snack** Energy bar Juice, 8 oz. (240 ml) Banana, 1 medium	**Snack** Toast, 2 slices Jam, 2 tbsp. (30 ml) Peanut butter, 1 tbsp. (15 ml) Juice, 8 oz. (240 ml)
Breakfast Oatmeal, cooked, 1 c. (240 ml) Skim milk, 8 oz. (240 ml) Raisins, 2 tbsp. (30 ml) Banana, 1 large Juice, 8 oz. (240 ml)	**Breakfast** Granola, 1 cup (240 ml) Soy milk, 8 oz. (240 ml) Nuts, 12 Berries, 1 c. (240 ml) Juice, 8 oz. (240 ml)	**Breakfast** Muesli, 1 c. (240 ml) Skim milk, 8 oz. (240 ml) Raisins, 3 tbsp. (45 ml) Juice, 8 oz. (240 ml)
Snack Granola bar, 1 medium	**Snack** Bagel, 3 oz. (90 g) Jam, 2 tbsp. (30 ml) Orange, 1 medium	**Snack** Yogurt with fruit, 6 oz. Nuts, 24 Banana, 1 medium

Continues >

APPENDIX E MEAL PLANS *continued*

BASE CYCLE MEAL PLANS, *CONTINUED*

BASE

3,000 CALORIES	3,400 CALORIES	3,800 CALORIES
Lunch Chicken salad, 3 oz. (100 g) Bread, whole-grain, 2 slices Avocado, 3 slices Potato salad, low-fat, 1 c. (240 ml) Grapes, 15	**Lunch** Roast beef, 4 oz. (120 g) Cheese, low-fat, 1 oz. (30 g) Roll, 2 oz. (60 g) Pasta salad, ½ cup (120 ml) Pear, 1 medium	**Lunch** Tuna salad, 4 oz. (120 g) Bread, whole-grain, 2 slices (60 g) Pretzels, 2 oz. (60 g) Vegetable mix, 1 c. (240 ml) Plums, 2 small
Snack Cottage cheese, ½ cup Pretzels, 1½ oz. (45 g) Apple, 1 medium	**Snack** Yogurt with fruit, 6 oz. (180 ml) Nuts, 24	**Snack** Crackers, 2 oz. (60 g) Cream cheese, 1 tbsp. (15 ml) Dried apricots, 12
Dinner Pork, cooked, 5 oz. (150 g) Stir-fry vegetable mix, 1 cup Canola oil, 1 tbsp. (15 ml) Brown rice, cooked, 1½ c. (360 ml)	**Dinner** Burrito: Beans, 1 c. (240 ml) Rice, cooked, ⅔ c. (160 ml) Chicken, 4 oz. (120 g) Tortilla, 1 large, 2 oz. (60 g) Salsa, ½ c. (120 ml) Vegetable mix, 1 c. (240 ml)	**Dinner** Fish, 5 oz. (150 g) Sweet potato, 1 large Salad mix, 2 c. Salad dressing, 3 tbsp. (45 ml) Vegetables, cooked, 1 c. (240 ml) Bread, 2 slices
Snack Yogurt, 6 oz. Peach, 1 medium	**Snack** Ice cream, low-fat, 1 c. (240 ml) Fruit, ½ cup (120 ml)	**Snack** Frozen yogurt, 8 oz. Berries, 1 c.

BUILD CYCLE MEAL PLANS

BUILD

2,200 CALORIES	2,500 CALORIES	2,800 CALORIES
370 g carbohydrates (67%) 100 g protein (18%) 33 g fat (15%)	410 g carbohydrates (66%) 120 g protein (19%) 42 g fat (15%)	455 g carbohydrates (65%) 125 g protein (18%) 53 g fat (17%)
Breakfast Toast, 2 slices Jam, 2 tbsp. (30 ml) Juice, 8 oz. (240 ml) Egg, 1 medium Banana, 1 medium	**Breakfast** Bagel, 4 oz. (120 g) Jam, 2 tbsp. (30 ml) Peanut butter, 1 tbsp. (15 ml) Juice, 8 oz. (240 ml)	**Breakfast** Cereal, 1½ oz. (45 g) Soy milk, 8 oz. (240 ml) Juice, 8 oz. (240 ml) Berries, 1 c. (240 ml)
Snack Crackers, 1 oz. (30 g) Hummus, 2 tbsp. (30 ml) Apple, 1 medium	**Snack** Yogurt, 8 oz. (240 ml) Granola, ½ cup (120 ml) Raisins, 1 tbsp. (15 ml)	**Snack** Bagel, 4 oz. (120 g) Honey, 2 tbsp. (30 ml) Peanut butter, 1 tbsp. (30 ml) Juice, 8 oz. (240 ml)
Lunch Ham, 3 oz. (100 g) Bread, 2 slices Kidney bean salad, 1 c. (240 ml) Grapes, 30	**Lunch** Burrito: Beans, ½ c. (120 ml) Tortilla, 1 large Chicken, 3 oz. (90 g) Salsa, ½ c. (120 ml) Rice, cooked, ⅔ c. (180 ml) Peppers, ½ c. (120 ml)	**Lunch** Turkey, 3 oz. (90 g) Bread, 2 slices Lentil salad, ½ c. (120 ml) Vegetable mix, 1 c. (240 ml) Juice, 8 oz. (240 ml)
Snack Granola bar Pear, 1 small Nuts, 12	**Snack** Pretzels, 2 oz. (60 g) String cheese, 1 oz. (30 g) Plums, 2 medium	**Snack** Yogurt, 8 oz. (240 ml) Raisins, 3 tbsp. (45 ml) Nuts, 12

BUILD

BUILD CYCLE MEAL PLANS, *CONTINUED*

2,200 CALORIES	2,500 CALORIES	2,800 CALORIES
Dinner Stir-fry: Shrimp, 5 oz. (150 g) Vegetable mix, 1 c. (240 ml) Brown rice, cooked, 1½ c. (360 ml) Sesame oil, 1 tbsp. (15 ml)	**Dinner** Fish, 6 oz. (180 g) Baked potato, 1 medium Bread, 2 slices Vegetable, 1 c. (240 ml)	**Dinner** Pasta, cooked, 2½ cups (600 ml) Marinara sauce, 1 c. (240 ml) Salad, 2 c. Salad dressing, 4 tbsp. (60 ml) Chicken breast, 3 oz. (90 g)

3,000 CALORIES	3,700 CALORIES	4,500 CALORIES
430 g carbohydrates (58%) 176 g protein (23%) 63 g fat (19%)	630 g carbohydrates (68%) 130 g protein (14%) 75 g fat (18%)	775 g carbohydrates (67%) 140 g protein (12%) 105 g fat (21%)
Breakfast Bagel, 4 oz. (120 g) Peanut butter, 2 tbsp. (30 ml) Citrus juice, 12 oz. (360 ml) Banana, 1 medium Yogurt, plain, 1 c. (240 ml)	**Breakfast** Grits, cooked, 1 c. (240 ml) Raisins, 2 tbsp. (30 ml) Yogurt, nonfat, plain, 1 c. (240 ml) Dried cherries, 10 Cashews, 1 tbsp. (15 ml)	**Breakfast** Pancakes, 4 small Maple syrup, ¾ c. (180 ml) Banana, 1 medium Raisins, 2 tbsp. (30 ml) Nuts, 1 tbsp. (15 ml) Soy milk, 12 oz. (360 ml) Sports drink, 40 oz. (1,200 ml)
Lunch Tuna, 4 oz. (120 g) Mayonnaise, 1 tbsp. (15 ml) Pita bread, 1 round Pretzels, 1½ oz. (45 g) Raw vegetable salad, 1 c. (240 ml)	**Lunch** Hummus, ½ c. (120 ml) Pita bread, 2 rounds Celery, pepper, carrots, 2 c. (480 ml) Apple juice, 12 oz. (360 ml)	**During training** Sports drink, 40 oz. (1,200 ml)
Snack Soy or dairy milk, 12 oz. (360 ml) Peach slices, 1 c. (240 ml) Granola, low-fat, ¼ c. (60 ml)	**Snack** Bagel, 2 oz. (60 g) Nut butter, 2 tbsp. (30 ml) Apple, 1 large	**Lunch** Burrito: Chicken, 5 oz. (150 g) Rice, cooked, 2 c. (480 ml) Pinto beans, cooked, 1 c. (240 ml) Avocado, ¼ whole Salsa, ½ c. (120 ml)
Dinner Halibut, 8 oz. (240 g) Buckwheat, cooked, 1½ c. (360 ml) Asparagus, 1 c. (240 ml) Canola oil, 2 tsp. (10 ml)	**Dinner** Pork tenderloin, 8 oz. (240 g) Rice, cooked, 1½ c. (360 ml) Corn, ½ c. (120 ml) Mushrooms, ¼ c. (60 ml) Bread, 2 slices Olive oil, 4 tsp. (20 ml)	**Dinner** Linguine, cooked, 3 c. (720 ml) Mixed vegetables, 1 c. (240 ml) Bread, 2 slices Olive oil, 2 tbsp. (30 ml) Salad, 2 c. (480 ml) Salad dressing, 2 tbsp. (30 ml)
Snack Sorbet, 1 c. (240 ml) Fig cookies, 3 small	**Snack** Sherbet, 1 c. (240 ml) Raspberries, 1 c. (240 ml)	**Snack** Frozen yogurt, 2 c. (480 ml) Cookies, 2 Strawberries, 1 c. (240 ml)

Continues >

TRANSITION

TRANSITION CYCLE MEAL PLANS

2,200 CALORIES	2,500 CALORIES	2,800 CALORIES
290 g carbohydrates (51%) 143 g protein (25%) 60 g fat (24%)	415 g carbohydrates (64%) 110 g protein (17%) 53 g fat (19%)	335 g carbohydrates (51%) 139 g protein (21%) 83 g fat (28%)
Breakfast Cooked grain cereal, 1 c. (240 ml) Banana, 1 medium Cottage cheese, ½ c. or egg, 1 medium Nuts, 1 tbsp. (15 ml)	**Breakfast** Oatmeal, cooked, 1 c. (240 ml) Apple, 1 medium Juice, 8 oz. (240 ml)	**Breakfast** Muesli, ¾ c. (180 ml) Apple, 1 medium Raisins, 2 tbsp. (30 ml) Soy or dairy milk, 1 c. (240 ml) Almonds, 2 tsp. (10 ml)
Snack Recovery smoothie: 12 oz. soy or dairy milk (360 ml) Frozen fruit, 1 c. (240 ml)	**Snack** Yogurt, 6 oz. (180 ml) Strawberries, 1 c. (240 ml)	**Snack** Granola bar Peach, 1 medium
Lunch Low-fat tuna salad, 3 oz. (90 g) Bread, 2 slices Lentil or pasta salad, ½ c. (120 ml)	**Lunch** Chicken, 3 oz. (100 g) Bread, whole-grain, 2 slices Pretzels, ¾ oz. (22 g) Pear, 1 large	**Lunch** Chicken tacos: Chicken, 3 oz. (90 g) Kidney or pinto beans, cooked, ½ c. (120 ml) Rice, cooked, 1 c. (240 ml) Tortillas, corn, 2 Oil, 2 tsp. (10 ml)
Dinner Salmon, 6 oz. (180 g) Buckwheat or rice, cooked, 1 c. (240 ml) Asparagus, 1 c. (240 ml) Salad, 2 c. (480 ml) Olive oil, 2 tsp. (10 ml) Salad dressing, 2 tbsp. (30 ml)	**Dinner** Beef strips, 3 oz. (90 g) Noodles, cooked, 2 c. (480 ml) Bread, 1 slice Olive oil, 2 tsp. (10 ml) Mixed vegetables, 1 c. (240 ml)	**Dinner** Risotto: Beef, 4 oz. (120 g) Broccoli, 1 c. (240 ml) Rice, 1½ c. cooked (360 ml) Bread, 2 slices Oil, 2 tsp. (10 ml)
Snack Sorbet or frozen yogurt, ½ c. (120 ml) Peach, 1 medium	**Snack** Bagel, 3 oz. (90 g) Peanut butter, 1 tsp. (5 ml)	**Snack** Papaya, 1 medium Crackers, 2 oz. (60 g) Cream cheese, 2 tbsp. (30 ml)

2,800 CALORIES	3,800 CALORIES	4,300 CALORIES
405 g carbohydrates (58%) 125 g protein (18%) 90 g fat (24%)	550 g carbohydrates (58%) 160 g protein (17%) 105 g fat (25%)	610 g carbohydrates (56%) 168 g protein (15%) 137 g fat (29%)
Breakfast Waffles, 4 squares Syrup, ½ c. (120 ml) Berries, 1 c. (240 ml) Hard-boiled egg, 1 Soy or dairy milk, 12 oz. (360 ml)	**Breakfast** Raisin bran, 1½ c. (360 ml) Milk, 8 oz. (240 ml) Grapefruit, 1 medium Bagel, 3 oz. (90 g) Cheese, low-fat, 2 oz. (60 g)	**Breakfast** Bran flakes, 1 c. (240 ml) Milk, 1 c. (240 ml) English muffins, 2 Cheese, low-fat, 2 oz. (60 g) Smoothie: Soy or dairy milk, 12 oz. (360 ml) Banana, 1 medium Wheat germ, 1 tbsp. (15 ml) Sports drink, 40 oz. (1,200 ml)

TRANSITION CYCLE MEAL PLANS, *CONTINUED*

2,800 CALORIES	3,800 CALORIES	4,300 CALORIES
Lunch Roast turkey, 3 oz. (90 g) Avocado or hummus, 2 tbsp. (30 ml) Toasted pita, 1 round Plums, 3 medium Soy or dairy milk, 8 oz. (240 ml) Yogurt, nonfat, 6 oz. (180 g)	**Snack** Recovery smoothie: Skim milk, 16 oz. (480 ml) Juice, 4 oz. (120 ml) Granola, ½ c. (120 ml) Banana, 1 medium	**Lunch** Beef and bean burritos: Beef, 8 oz. (240 g) Rice, cooked, ½ c. (120 ml) Beans, 1 c. (240 ml) Tortillas, 2 large Salsa, 1 c. (240 ml) Canola oil, 4 tsp. (35 ml)
Snack Pear, 1 large Crackers, 12	**Lunch** Peanut butter, 1 tbsp. (15 ml) Jam, 2 tbsp. (30 ml) Bread, 2 slices Pear, 1 medium	**Snack** Gingersnaps, 6 Juice, 8 oz. (240 ml)
Dinner Pasta, 3 c. (720 ml) cooked Marinara sauce, 1½ c. (360 ml) Lean beef, 3 oz. (90 g) Bread, 2 slices Salad, 2 c. (480 ml) Olive oil, 1 tbsp. (15 ml) Salad dressing, 2 tbsp. (30 ml)	**Snack** Orange, 1 medium Yogurt with fruit, 8 oz. (240 ml) Granola bar, 1 medium Nuts, 24	**Dinner** Tofu stir-fry: Tofu, 4 oz. (120 g) Brown rice, 1½ c. cooked (360 ml) Sweet peppers and broccoli, cooked, 1 c. (240 ml) Sesame oil, 1 tbsp. (15 ml)
	Dinner Grilled chicken, 6 oz. (180 g) Sweet potatoes, 10 oz. (300 g) Peas, cooked, 1 c. (240 ml) Bread, 2 slices Olive oil, 5 tsp. (50 ml) Fruit salad, 1 c. (240 ml)	**Snack** Granola bar Ice cream, 1 c. (240 ml) Chocolate syrup, 2 tbsp. (30 ml) Nuts, 2 tsp. (10 ml)
	Snack Sorbet, 1 c. (240 ml) Strawberries, 1 c. (240 ml)	**Snack** Granola bar Ice cream, 1 c. (240 ml) Chocolate syrup, 2 tbsp. (30 ml) Nuts, 2 tsp. (10 ml)

VEGETARIAN MEAL PLANS

2,200 CALORIES	2,400 CALORIES	3,000 CALORIES
348 g carbohydrates (62%) 95 g protein (17%) 53 g fat (21%)	390 g carbohydrates (63%) 105 g protein (17%) 56 g fat (20%)	475 g carbohydrates (67%) 102 g protein (14%) 60 g fat (19%)
Breakfast Farina, cooked, 1 c. (240 ml) Skim milk, 8 oz. (240 ml) Nuts, 1 tbsp. (15 ml) Apple, 1 medium Orange juice, 12 oz. (360 ml)	**Breakfast** Muesli, ¾ c. (180 ml) Soy or dairy yogurt, 8 oz. (240 ml) Blueberries, 1 c. (240 ml)	**Breakfast** Waffles, 2 small Maple syrup, 4 oz. (120 ml) Raspberries, 1 c. (240 ml) Skim milk, 1 c. (240 ml)
Lunch Soy burger, 1 patty Bun, 1 whole Cheese, low-fat, 1 oz. (30 g) Lentil or bean salad, ½ c. (120 ml) Vegetables, raw, 1 c. (240 ml) Avocado, ¼ whole	**Lunch** Garbanzo beans, ⅓ c. (80 ml) Salad greens/vegetables, 3 c. (720 ml) Pita, 1 large Cheese, low-fat, 2 oz. (60 g) Grapefruit juice, 8 oz. (240 ml)	**Lunch** Hummus, ½ c. (120 ml) Rice, cooked, ½ c. (120 ml) Lentil salad, ½ c. (120 ml) Pita bread, 1 round Carrots and celery, 2 c. (480 ml)

TRANSITION

VEGETARIAN

Continues >

APPENDIX *E* **MEAL PLANS** *continued*

VEGETARIAN MEAL PLANS, *CONTINUED*

2,200 CALORIES	2,400 CALORIES	3,000 CALORIES
Dinner Kidney beans, 1 c. (240 ml) Rice, cooked, 1 c. (240 ml) Tortilla, 1 medium Green salad, 1 c. (240 ml) Salad dressing, 2 tbsp. (30 ml)	**Snack** Energy bar, 1 medium Apple, 1 medium	**Snack** Bagel, 4 oz. (120 g) Cheese, low-fat, 2 oz. (60 g) Apple, 1 medium
Snack Granola bar Peach, 1 medium Yogurt with fruit, 8 oz. (240 ml)	**Dinner** Tempeh, ¾ c. (180 ml) Rice, cooked, 1½ c. (360 ml) Broccoli, cooked, 1 c. (240 ml) Sesame seed oil, 1 tbsp. (15 ml)	**Dinner** Tofu, 4 oz. (120 g) Soba noodles, cooked, 2 c. (480 ml) Greens, cooked, 1 c. (240 ml) Sesame oil, 1 tbsp. (15 ml)
	Snack Orange, 1 medium Almonds, 2 tsp. (10 ml)	**Snack** Pear, 1 large

2,900 CALORIES	3,400 CALORIES	3,700 CALORIES
470 g carbohydrates (62%) 113 g protein (15%) 78 g fat (23%)	550 g carbohydrates (65%) 120 g protein (14%) 77 g fat (21%)	610 g carbohydrates (66%) 134 g protein (14%) 83 g fat (20%)
Breakfast Pancakes, 4 small Syrup, 6 tbsp. (90 g) Raisins, 2 tbsp. (30 ml) Apple juice, 8 oz. (240 ml) Eggs, 2 medium	**Breakfast** Oatmeal, cooked, 1½ c. (360 ml) Skim milk, 1 c. (240 ml) Wheat germ, 2 tbsp. (30 ml) Orange juice, 12 oz. (360 ml) Yogurt, 1 c. (240 ml) Apple, 1 large Sports drink, 40 oz. (1,200 ml)	**Breakfast** Bran flakes, 1½ c. (360 ml) Wheat germ, 2 tbsp. (30 ml) Soy or dairy milk, 8 oz. (240 ml) Peach, 1 medium Nuts, 12
Snack Soy or dairy yogurt with fruit, 8 oz. (240 ml) Almonds, 2 tbsp. (30 ml)	**Snack** Pretzels, 2 oz. (60 g) Hummus, ½ c. (120 ml) Raw vegetables, 1 c. (240 ml)	**Snack** Recovery Drink Juice, 12 oz. (360 ml) Yogurt, 1 c. (240 ml) Banana, 1 medium
Lunch Bean soup, 1½ c. (360 ml) Rye crackers, 4 Vegetable salad, 1 c. (240 ml) Soy milk, 12 oz. (360 ml)	**Lunch** Thin-crust pizza, cheese, 3 slices Green salad, 2 c. (480 ml) Salad dressing, 2 tbsp. (30 ml) Soy milk, 8 oz. (240 ml)	**Lunch** Nut butter, 2 tbsp. (30 ml) Bread, 2 slices Bean soup, 1 c. (240 ml) Raw vegetables, 1 c. (240 ml)
Dinner Potato, 1 large Kidney beans, 1 c. (240 ml) Cheese, low-fat, 1 oz. (30 g) Green salad, 2 c. (480 ml) Salad dressing, 3 tbsp. (45 g)	**Dinner** Spaghetti, cooked, 3 c. (720 ml) Marinara sauce, 2 c. (480 ml) Parmesan cheese, 3 tbsp. (45 ml) Italian bread, 2 slices Olive oil, 1 tbsp. (15 ml)	**Dinner** Tofu, 8 oz. (240 g) Peas, 1 c. (240 ml) Noodles, cooked, 2 c. (480 ml) Rolls, 2 Vegetable oil, 2 tbsp. (30 ml) Green salad, 2 c. (480 ml) Salad dressing, 2 tbsp. (30 ml) Sports drink, 40 oz. (1,200 ml)
Snack Frozen yogurt, 1 c. (240 ml) Banana, 1 medium	**Snack** Sorbet, 1½ c. (360 ml) Fig bars, 2	**Snack** Yogurt, 8 oz (240 ml) Mango, 1 large Crackers, 12

VEGETARIAN

APPENDIX F:
ESTIMATING SWEAT LOSS—WORKSHEET

SWEAT LOSS **CALCULATOR**

1 CHECK WEIGHT* BEFORE AND AFTER TRAINING TO CALCULATE WEIGHT LOSS.

WEIGHT BEFORE		WEIGHT AFTER		AMOUNT OF WEIGHT LOST		OZ. (ML)

*Check weight without clothing, if possible.

TIME PERIOD (1 HOUR IS PREFERABLE)

2 CONVERT AMOUNT OF WEIGHT LOSS TO OZ. (ML) OF FLUID.

E.g., a 2-lb. weight loss = 30 oz. of fluid / E.g., a l-kg weight loss = 1,000 ml of fluid

OZ. (ML) OF FLUID LOST

3 RECORD AMOUNT OF FLUID CONSUMED DURING TRAINING SESSION.

E.g., Squeeze bottles are 20–24 ounces/600–720 ml

OZ. (ML) OF FLUID CONSUMED

4 ADD AMOUNT OF FLUID LOST AND FLUID CONSUMED.

FLUID LOST + FLUID CONSUMED =   OZ. (ML)

5 DIVIDE TOTAL OZ. (ML) OF WEIGHT LOSS BY NUMBER OF HOURS OF TRAINING TO DETERMINE AMOUNT OF OZ. LOST IN SWEAT PER HOUR.

TOTAL FLUID LOST ÷ HOURS OF TRAINING =   FLUID LOSSES IN OZ. (ML) PER HOUR

EXAMPLE:

1. Weight before training: 165 lb. (75 kg)
   Weight after training: 164 lb. (74 kg)

2. **Total weight loss: 1 lb. (0.5 kg) = 15 oz. (500 ml) fluid**

3. Consumed 30 oz. (960 ml) fluid during 1-hour bike ride.
   30 oz. (960 ml) fluid

4. Add fluid lost and fluid consumed.
   15 oz. (500 ml) + 30 oz. (960 ml) = 45 oz. (1,460 ml)

5. Divide total sum of weight loss by hours of training.
   45 oz. (1,060 ml) / 1 hour of training = 45 oz. per hour for sweat losses

Armstrong, L. E. 2000. *Performing in Extreme Environments.* Champaign, IL: Human Kinetics.

Armstrong, L. E. 2002. Caffeine, body fluid–electrolyte balance, and exercise performance. *International Journal of Sport Nutrition and Exercise Metabolism* 12(2): 189–206.

Armstrong, L. E. 2005. Fluid, electrolyte, and renal indices of hydration during 11 days of controlled caffeine consumption. *International Journal of Sport Nutrition and Exercise Metabolism* 15(3): 252–265.

Ball, T., et al. 1995. Periodic carbohydrate replacement during 50 minutes of high-intensity cycling improves subsequent sprint performance. *International Journal of Sport Nutrition and Exercise Metabolism* 5(2): 151–158.

Beals, K. 2004. *Disordered Eating Among Athletes.* Champaign, IL: Human Kinetics.

Beals, K., and M. Manore. 1994. The prevalence and consequences of subclinical eating disorders in female athletes. *International Journal of Sport Nutrition and Exercise Metabolism* 4(2): 175–195.

Beelen, M., et al. 2010. Nutritional strategies to promote exercise recovery. *International Journal of Sport Nutrition and Exercise Metabolism* 20(6): 515–532.

Below, P., et al. 1995. Fluid and carbohydrate ingestion independently improve performance during 1 hour intense exercise. *Medicine and Science in Sports and Exercise* 27: 200–210.

Benson, J., et al. 1996. Nutritional aspects of amenorrhea in the female athlete triad. *International Journal of Sport Nutrition and Exercise Metabolism* 6(2): 134–145.

Berning, J. 1996. The role of medium chain triglycerides in exercise. *International Journal of Sport Nutrition and Exercise Metabolism* 6(2): 121–133.

Betts, J. A., and C. Williams. 2010. Short-term recovery from prolonged exercise: Exploring the potential for protein ingestion to accentuate the benefits of carbohydrate supplements. *Sports Medicine* 40(11): 941–959.

Betts, J. A., et al. 2008. Increased carbohydrate oxidation after ingesting carbohydrate with added protein. *Medicine and Science in Sports and Exercise* 40(5): 903–912.

Blom, T., et al. 1987. The effects of different post-exercise sugar diets on the rate of muscle glycogen resynthesis. *Medicine and Science in Sports and Exercise* 19: 491–496.

Brand-Miller, Jennie, et al. 2003. *The New Glucose Revolution Complete Guide to Glycemic Index Values.* New York: Marlowe.

Brooks, G., et al. 1991. Increased dependence on blood glucose after acclimatization to 4,300 meters. *Journal of Applied Physiology* 70(2): 919–927.

Brown, G., et al. 2000. Effect of anabolic precursors on serum testosterone concentrations and adaptations to resistance training in young men. *International Journal of Sport Nutrition and Exercise Metabolism* 10(3): 340–359.

Bruce, C. R., et al. 2000. Enhancement of 2000-m rowing performance after caffeine ingestion. *Medicine and Science in Sports and Exercise* 32(11): 1958–1963.

Burke, L. M. 2010. Fueling strategies to optimize performance: Training high or training low? *Scandinavian Journal of Medicine and Science in Sports* 20 (supplement 2): 48–58.

Burke, L. M., and J. A. Hawley. 2002. Effects of short-term fat adaptation on metabolism and performance for prolonged exercise. *Medicine and Science in Sports and Exercise* 34(9): 1492–1498.

Burke, L. M., et al. 1993. Muscle glycogen storage after prolonged exercise: Effect of the glycemic index of carbohydrate feedings. *Journal of Applied Physiology* 75(2): 1019–1023.

Burke, L. M., et al. 1996. Muscle glycogen storage after prolonged exercise: Effect of the frequency of carbohydrate feedings. *American Journal of Clinical Nutrition* 64: 115–119.

Burke, L. M., et al. 2000. Effect of fat adaptation and carbohydrate restoration on metabolism and performance during prolonged cycling. *Journal of Applied Physiology* 89(6): 2413–2421.

Burke, L. M., et al. 2002. Adaptations to short-term high-fat diet persist during exercise despite high carbohydrate availability. *Medicine and Science in Sports and Exercise* 34(1): 83–91.

Burke, L. M., et al. 2004. Carbohydrate and fat for training and recovery. *Journal of Sports Sciences* 22(8): 15–30.

Burke, L. M., et al. 2005. Effect of carbohydrate intake on half-marathon performance of well-trained runners. *International Journal of Sport Nutrition and Exercise Metabolism* 15(6): 573–589.

Butterfield, G., et al. 1992. Increased energy intake minimizes weight loss in men at high altitude. *Journal of Applied Physiology* 72(5): 1741–1748.

Campbell, W., et al. 1997. Effects of chromium picolinate and resistance training on body composition in older men. *Medicine and Science in Sports and Exercise* 29(5): S277.

Carey, A., et al. 2001. Effects of fat adaptation and carbohydrate restoration on prolonged endurance exercise. *Journal of Applied Physiology* 91(1): 115–122.

Catlin, D., et al. 2000. Trace contamination of over-the-counter androstenedione and positive urine test results for a nandrolone metabolite. *Journal of the American Medical Association* 284(20): 2618–2621.

Chryssanthopoulos, C., et al. 2002. The effect of a high carbohydrate meal on endurance running capacity. *International Journal of Sport Nutrition and Exercise Metabolism* 12(2): 157–171.

Clancy, S., et al. 1994. Effects of chromium picolinate supplementation on body composition, strength, and urinary chromium loss in football players. *International Journal of Sport Nutrition and Exercise Metabolism* 4: 142–153.

Clarkson, P. 1991. Nutritional ergogenic aids: Chromium, exercise, and muscle mass. *International Journal of Sport Nutrition and Exercise Metabolism* 1: 289–293.

Clarkson, P. 1992. Nutritional ergogenic aids: Carnitine. *International Journal of Sport Nutrition and Exercise Metabolism* 2: 185–190.

Conley, M., and M. Stone. 1996. Carbohydrate ingestion/supplementation for resistance exercise and training. *Sports Medicine* 21(1): 7–17.

Cox, G. R., et al. 2002. Effect of different exercise protocols of caffeine intake on metabolism and endurance performance. *Journal of Applied Physiology* 93(3): 900–909.

Cox, G. R., et al. 2010. Daily training with high carbohydrate availability increases exogenous carbohydrate oxidation during endurance cycling. *Journal of Applied Physiology* 109(1): 126–134.

Cox, G. R., et al. 2010. Race-day carbohydrate intakes of elite triathlete contesting Olympic-distance triathlon events. *International Journal of Sport Nutrition and Exercise Metabolism* 20(4): 299–306.

Coyle, E. 2004. Fluid and fuel intake during exercise. *Journal of Sports Sciences* 22(8): 39–55.

Coyle, E., et al. 2001. Low-fat diet alters intramuscular substrates and reduces lipolysis and fat oxidation during exercise. *American Journal of Endocrinology and Metabolism* 280(3): E391–E398.

Crowe, M. J., et al. 2003. The effects of B-hydroxy-B-methylbutarate (HMB) and HMB/creatine supplementation on indices of health in highly trained athletes. *International Journal of Sport Nutrition and Exercise Metabolism* 13(2): 184–197.

Currell, K., and A. E. Jeukendrup. 2008. Superior endurance performance with ingestion of multiple transportable carbohydrates. *Medicine and Science in Sports and Exercise* 40(2): 275–281.

Davis, J. 1996. Carbohydrates, branched chain amino acids, and endurance: The central fatigue hypothesis. *Gatorade Sports Science Exchange* 9(2).

Decombaz, J., et al. 1993. Effect of l-carnitine on submaximal exercise metabolism after depletion of muscle glycogen. *Medicine and Science in Sports and Exercise* 25: 733–740.

Decombaz, J., et al. 2011. Fructose and galactose enhance post-exercise human liver glycogen synthesis. *Medicine and Science in Sports and Exercise,* March 10 (Epub).

DeSouza, M. J., et al. 2010. High prevalence of subtle and severe menstrual disturbances in exercising women: Confirmation using daily hormone measures. *Human Reproduction* 25(2): 491–503.

Dunford, Marie. 2006. *Sports Nutrition: A Practice Manual for Professionals.* Chicago: American Dietetic Association.

Fallowfield, J., et al. 1995. The influence of ingesting a carbohydrate-electrolyte beverage during 4 hours of recovery on subsequent endurance capacity. *International Journal of Sport Nutrition and Exercise Metabolism* 5: 285–299.

Febbraio, M. A., et al. 1996. Carbohydrate feedings before prolonged exercise: Effect of glycemic index on muscle glycogenolysis and exercise performance. *Journal of Applied Physiology* 81(3): 1115–1120.

Fiala, K. A. 2004. Rehydration with a caffeinated beverage during the nonexercise periods of 3 consecutive days of 2-a-day practices. *International Journal of Sport Nutrition and Exercise Metabolism* 14(4): 419–429.

Foster-Powell, K., and J. Brand-Miller. 1995. International tables of glycemic index. *American Journal of Clinical Nutrition* 62 (supplement): 871–893.

Gleeson, M., et al. 2004. Exercise, nutrition, and immune function. *Journal of Sports Sciences* 22(8): 115–125.

Graham, T., and L. Spriet. 1996. Caffeine and exercise performance. *Gatorade Sports Science Exchange* 9(1).

Grandjean, A. C., et al. 2000. The effect of caffeinated, non-caffeinated, caloric, and non-caloric beverages on hydration. *Journal of the American College of Nutrition* 19(5): 591–600.

Green, H., et al. 1992. Altitude acclimatization and energy metabolic adaptation in skeletal muscle during exercise. *Journal of Applied Physiology* 73 (6): 2701–2708.

Haff, G. G., et al. 2000. Carbohydrate supplementation attenuates muscle glycogen loss during acute bouts of resistance exercise. *International Journal of Sport Nutrition and Exercise Metabolism* 10(3): 326–339.

Havemann, L., et al. 2006. Fat adaptation followed by carbohydrate-loading compromises high-intensity sprint performance. *Journal of Applied Physiology* 100(1): 194–202.

Hellsetn-Westing, Y., et al. 1993. The effect of high-intensity training on purine metabolism in man. *Acta Physiologica Scandinavica* 149: 405–412.

Hulston, C. J., and A. E. Jeukendrup. 2008. Substrate metabolism and exercise performance with caffeine and carbohydrate intake. *Medicine and Science in Sports and Exercise* 40(12): 2096–2104.

Hulston, C. J., and A. E. Jeukendrup. 2009. No placebo effect from carbohydrate intake during prolonged exercise. *International Journal of Sport Nutrition and Exercise Metabolism* 19(3): 275–284.

Hulston, C. J., et al. 2009. Exogenous carbohydrate with glucose plus fructose intake during exercise. *Medicine and Science in Sport and Exercise* 41(2): 357–363.

Ivy, J. L., et al. 1988. Muscle glycogen storage after different amounts of carbohydrate ingestion. *Journal of Applied Physiology* 64(5): 2018–2023.

Ivy, J. L., et al. 1988. Muscle glycogen synthesis after exercise: Effect of time of carbohydrate ingestion. *Journal of Applied Physiology* 64(4): 1480–1485.

James, A. P., et al. 1999. Muscle glycogen supercompensation: Absence of gender-related differences. *European Journal of Applied Physiology* 85(6): 533–538.

Jentjens, R. L. P., et al. 2004. High oxidation rates from combined carbohydrates ingested during exercise. *Medicine and Science in Sports and Exercise* 36(9): 1551–1558.

Jentjens, R. L. P., et al. 2004. Oxidation of combined ingestion of glucose and fructose during exercise. *Journal of Applied Physiology* 96(4): 1277–1284.

Jeukendrup, A., et al. 1997. Carbohydrate-electrolyte feedings improve 1 hour time trial cycling performance. *International Journal of Sports Medicine* 18(2): 125–129.

Jeukendrup, A. E. 2010. Carbohydrates and exercise performance: The role of multiple transportable carbohydrates. *Current Opinion in Clinical Nutrition and Metabolic Care* 13(4): 452–457.

Jeukendrup, A. E., and E. S. Chambers. 2010. Oral carbohydrate sensing and exercise performance. *Current Opinions in Clinical Nutrition and Metabolic Care* 13(4): 447–451.

Jeukendrup, A. E., and M. J. Gibala. 2009. Protein plus carbohydrate does not enhance 60-km time-trial performance. *International Journal of Sport Nutrition and Exercise Metabolism* 19(4): 335–337.

Jeukendrup, A. E., and L. Moseley. 2010. Multiple transportable carbohydrates enhance gastric emptying and fluid delivery. *Scandinavian Journal of Medicine Science in Sports* 20(1): 112–121.

Kang, J., et al. 1995. Effect of carbohydrate ingestion subsequent to carbohydrate supercompensation on endurance performance. *International Journal of Sport Nutrition and Exercise Metabolism* 5: 329–343.

Kenney, W. L. 2004. Dietary water and sodium requirements for active adults. *Gatorade Sports Science Exchange* 17(1): 1–6.

Kimber, N. E., et al. 2002. Energy balance during an Ironman triathlon in male and female triathletes. *International Journal of Sport Nutrition and Exercise Metabolism* 12: 47–62.

King, D., et al. 1999. Effect of oral androstenedione on serum testosterone and adaptation to resistance training in young men. *Journal of the American Medical Association* 281(21): 2020–2028.

Kirwan, J. P., et al. 1988. Carbohydrate balance in competitive runners during successive days of intense training. *Journal of Applied Physiology* 65(6): 2601–2606.

Kovacs, E. M. R., et al. 2002. Effect of high and low fluid intake on post-exercise rehydration. *International Journal of Sport Nutrition and Exercise Metabolism* 12: 14–23.

Kreider, R., et al. 1998. Creatine supplement: Analysis of ergogenic value, medical safety, and concerns. *Journal of Exercise Physiology* 1(1): 1–11.

Lambert, E., et al. 2001. High-fat diet versus habitual diet prior to carbohydrate loading: Effects on exercise metabolism and cycling performance. *International Journal of Sport Nutrition and Exercise Metabolism* 11: 209–225.

Lemon, P., et al. 1992. Protein requirements and muscle mass/strength changes during intensive training in novice bodybuilders. *Journal of Applied Physiology* 73(2): 767–775.

Lemon, P., et al. 1995. Do athletes need more dietary protein and amino acids? *International Journal of Sport Nutrition and Exercise Metabolism* 5: S39–S61.

Loucks, A. B., and J. R. Thuma. 2003. Luteinizing hormone pulsatility is disrupted at a threshold of energy availability in regularly menstruating women. *Journal of Clinical Endocrinology and Metabolism* 88(1): 297–311.

Macdermid, P. W., and S. R. Stannard. 2006. A whey-supplemented high-protein diet versus a high-carbohydrate diet: Effects on endurance cycling performance. *International Journal of Sport Nutrition and Exercise Metabolism* 16(1): 65–77.

Madsen, K., et al. 1996. Effects of glucose, glucose plus branched-chain amino acids, or placebo on bike performance over 100 km. *Journal of Applied Physiology* 81(6): 2644–2650.

Manore, M. M. 2002. Dietary recommendations and athletic menstrual dysfunction. *Sports Medicine* 32(14): 887–901.

Mason, W., et al. 1993. Carbohydrate ingestion during exercise: Liquid versus solid feedings. *Medicine and Science in Sport and Exercise* 25: 966–969.

McConnell, G., et al. 1996. Effect of timing of carbohydrate ingestion during exercise performance. *Medicine and Science in Sports and Exercise* 28: 1300–1304.

Millard-Stafford, M., et al. 1992. Carbohydrate-electrolyte replacement improves distance running performance in the heat. *Medicine and Science in Sports and Exercise* 24: 940–943.

Millard-Stafford, M., et al. 2005. Recovery from run training: Efficacy of a carbohydrate-protein beverage? *International Journal of Sport Nutrition and Exercise Metabolism* 15(6): 610–624.

Miller, S. L., et al. 2003. Independent and combined effects of amino acids and glucose after resistance training. *Medicine and Science in Sports and Exercise* 35(3): 449–455.

Nicholas, C. W., et al. 1997. Carbohydrate intake and recovery of intermittent running capacity. *International Journal of Sport Nutrition and Exercise Metabolism* 7(4): 251–260.

Nissen, S., et al. 1996. Effect of leucine metabolite B-hydroxy-B-methylbutarate on muscle metabolism during resistance training exercise. *Journal of Applied Physiology* 81(5): 2095–2104.

Parkin, J., et al. 1997. Muscle glycogen storage following prolonged exercise: Effect of timing of ingestion of high glycemic index food. *Medicine and Science in Sports and Exercise* 29(2): 220–224.

Pascoe, D., and L. Gladden. 1996. Muscle glycogen resynthesis after short-term, high-intensity exercise and resistance exercise. *Sports Medicine* 21(2): 98–118.

Paul, D. R., et al. 2001. Carbohydrate-loading during the follicular phase of the menstrual cycle: Effect on muscle glycogen and exercise performance. *International Journal of Sport Nutrition and Exercise Metabolism* 11(4): 430–441.

Pedersen, D. J., et al. 2008. High rates of muscle glycogen resynthesis after exhaustive exercise when carbohydrate is co-ingested with caffeine. *Journal of Applied Physiology* 105(1): 7–13.

Peters, E., et al. 1993. Vitamin C supplementation reduces the incidence of post-race symptoms of upper-respiratory-tract infection in ultramarathon runners. *American Journal of Clinical Nutrition* 57(2): 170–174.

Pfeiffer, B., et al. 2009. The effect of carbohydrate gels on gastrointestinal tolerance during a 16-km run. *International Journal of Sport Nutrition and Exercise Metabolism* 19(5): 485–503.

Pfeiffer, B., et al. 2010. Carbohydrate oxidation from a carbohydrate gel compared with a drink during exercise. *Medicine and Science in Sports and Exercise* 42(11): 2038–2045.

Pfeiffer B., et al. 2010. Oxidation of solid versus liquid carbohydrate sources during exercise. *Medicine and Science in Sports and Exercise* 42(11): 2030–2037.

Pfeiffer, B., et al. 2011. Carbohydrate oxidation from a drink during running compared with cycling exercise. *Medicine and Science in Sports and Exercise* 43(2): 327–334.

Pizza, F., et al. 1995. A carbohydrate loading regimen improves high intensity, short duration exercise performance. *International Journal of Sport Nutrition and Exercise Metabolism* 5: 110–116.

Reed, M. J., et al. 1989. Muscle glycogen storage post-exercise: Effect of mode of carbohydrate administration. *Journal of Applied Physiology* 66(2): 720–726.

Roy, B., and M. Tarnopolsky, et al. 1998. Influence of differing macronutrient intakes on muscle glycogen resynthesis after resistance exercise. *Journal of Applied Physiology* 84(3): 890–896.

Roy, R., et al. 1997. Effect of glucose supplement timing on protein metabolism after resistance training. *Journal of Applied Physiology* 82(6): 1882–1888.

Sawka, M. N., et al. 2005. Human water needs. *Nutrition Reviews* 63(6): S30–S39.

Sherman, W. M., et al. 1989. Effects of 4-hour pre-exercise carbohydrate feedings on cycling performance. *Medicine and Science in Sports and Exercise* 21(5): 598–604.

Sherman, W. M., et al. 1991. Carbohydrate feedings 1 hour before exercise improves cycling performance. *American Journal of Clinical Nutrition* 54(5): 866–870.

Shirreffs, S., et al. 1996. Post-exercise rehydration in man: Effect of volume consumed and drink sodium content. *Medicine and Science in Sports and Exercise* 28(10): 1260–1271.

Simonsen, J. C., et al. 1991. Dietary carbohydrate, muscle glycogen, and power output during rowing training. *Journal of Applied Physiology* 70(4): 1500–1505.

Slater, G., et al. 2001. B-hydroxy-B-methylbutarate (HMB) supplementation does not affect changes in strength and body composition during resistance training in trained men. *International Journal of Sport Nutrition and Exercise Metabolism* 11(3): 384–396.

Slater, G. J., et al. 2006. Preparation of former heavyweight oarsmen to compete as lightweight rowers over 16 weeks: Three case studies. *International Journal of Sport Nutrition and Exercise Metabolism* 16(1): 108–121.

Smith, J. S., et al. 2002. The effect of pre-exercise glucose ingestion on performance during prolonged swimming. *International Journal of Sport Nutrition and Exercise Metabolism* 12(2): 136–144.

Stanko, R., et al. 1990. Enhanced leg exercise endurance with a high-carbohydrate diet and dihydroxyacetone and pyruvate. *Journal of Applied Physiology* 68(5): 1651–1656.

Stanko, R., et al. 1990. Enhancement of arm exercise endurance capacity with dihydroxyacetone and pyruvate. *Journal of Applied Physiology* 68(1): 119–124.

Stellingwerff, T., et al. 2006. Decreased PDH activation and glycogenolysis during exercise following fat adaptation with carbohydrate restoration. *American Journal of Physiology, Endocrinology, and Metabolism* 290(2): E380–E388.

Tarnopolsky, M. A. 1997. Post-exercise protein-carbohydrate and carbohydrate supplements increase muscle glycogen in men and women. *Journal of Applied Physiology* 83(6): 1877.

Tarnopolsky, M. A., et al. 2001. Gender differences in carbohydrate loading are related to energy intake. *Journal of Applied Physiology* 91(1): 225–230.

Tarnopolsky, Mark, ed. 1999. *Gender Differences in Metabolism.* Boca Raton, FL: CRC Press.

Thompson, D., et al. 2001. Prolonged vitamin C supplementation and recovery from demanding exercise. *International Journal of Sport Nutrition and Exercise Metabolism* 11: 466–481.

Thompson, J., et al. 1996. Effects of diet and diet-plus-exercise programs on resting metabolic rate: A meta-analysis. *International Journal of Sport Nutrition and Exercise Metabolism* 6: 41–61.

Tipton, K. D., and R. R. Wolfe. 2004. Protein and amino acids for athletes. *Journal of Sports Science* 22(1): 65–79.

Volek, J., and W. Kramer. 1996. Creatine supplementation: Its effect on human and muscular performance and body composition. *Journal of Strength and Conditioning Research* 10(3): 200–210.

Walker, L., et al. 1997. Effect of chromium picolinate on body composition and muscular performance in collegiate wrestlers. *Medicine and Science in Sports and Exercise* 29(5): S278.

Wallis, G. A., et al. 2007. Dose-response effects of ingested carbohydrate on exercise metabolism in women. *Medicine and Science in Sports and Exercise* 39(1): 131–138.

Wojcik, J. R., et al. 2001. Comparison of carbohydrate and milk-based beverages on muscle damage and glycogen following exercise. *International Journal of Sport Nutrition and Exercise Metabolism* 11(4): 406–419.

Yaspelkis, B., et al. 1993. Carbohydrate supplementation spares muscle glycogen during variable-intensity exercise. *Journal of Applied Physiology* 75(4): 1477–1485.

Yeo, W. K., et al. 2008. Fat adaptation followed by carbohydrate restoration increases AMPK activity in skeletal muscle from trained humans. *Journal of Applied Physiology* 105(5): 1519–1526.

INDEX

Absorption, 132, 144–145, 146, 255, 291, 292
Acclimatization, 139, 141, 151, 152, 154, 252, 255, 366, 370
Acute mountain sickness (AMS), 370, 371
Adenosine triphosphate (ATP), 80–82, 84–85, 86, 181, 208, 222
Adequate Intake (AI), 5, 6, 52
Aerobic capacity, 78, 83, 86, 87, 101, 105, 108, 247, 265, 287, 305
  anaerobic capacity versus, 79–80
Aging, 324, 326
  muscle mass and, 175, 325
Alcohol, 64, 160, 197, 324, 330, 333
  bone mass and, 351
  calories from, 8, 9 (table)
  fat and, 194
  as nonnutritive nutrient, 8–12, 14
Allergies, food, 68, 315, 331, 335–340
Alternatives, whole-grain, 26, 26 (table)
Amenorrhea, female athletes and, 348–349
Amino acids, 35, 36, 182, 203, 211, 212–213, 223
Anaerobic capacity, 78, 79–80, 83, 86, 101, 304
Anaerobic threshold, 176, 234, 264, 307
Anemia, 55, 291, 321, 329
  iron and, 65, 191, 292
Anorexia, 343, 344, 345, 346, 347
Antibodies, 35, 336, 339
Antioxidants, 8, 25, 27, 28, 33, 51, 56, 57, 69, 70, 71, 72, 318, 359, 360, 371
Artificial sweeteners, 12, 299, 330

Bacteria, 31, 34, 330, 332, 335
Base cycle, described, 104
Beta-carotene, 28, 30, 58, 69, 70, 361
Bicarbonate, 224, 225–226
Binge eating, 344, 345, 346, 347
Bioelectrical Impedance Analysis (BIA), 189
Bladder hydration systems, 253, 258, 269, 274, 278
Blocks, 149, 154, 164, 174, 277, 300, 369
Blood, 159, 367
  clotting, 60, 72
  flow, 220, 265, 299
Blood glucose, 20, 80, 81, 82, 88, 147, 154, 156, 218, 236, 239, 242, 245, 252, 273, 287, 307, 308, 312, 313, 327, 377

decrease in, 134, 136, 142
exercise and, 130
glycemic index and, 21, 23, 25
low, 128, 255, 340, 355
maintaining, 34, 132, 135, 136, 138, 145, 265, 269, 272, 273, 275, 281, 287, 297, 329, 340, 341, 342, 369
Blood pressure, 9, 31, 151, 152, 222, 323
Blood sodium, 250, 297, 367
  low, 70, 128, 150, 151, 295, 357
Blood sugar, 20, 21, 255, 270
Body composition, 76, 175, 200, 290–291
  changes in, 92, 176, 186, 187, 188, 190–195, 198, 237–238, 323
  ergogenic aids and, 208, 210–218
  goals for, 92, 100, 101, 128, 176, 192, 195, 236, 291, 344
Body fat, 80, 82, 103, 184, 192, 208, 275, 287, 306, 346, 358, 368
  checking, 177, 187–190, 193, 283
  decrease in, 106, 175, 291, 302, 324, 344, 371
  gain in, 186, 191, 284, 312, 359
  goals for, 191, 192, 268, 343
  health/endurance sports and, 187 (table)
  levels of, 238, 268, 308, 309
  low, 187, 268, 271
  performance and, 185, 186
  weight and, 186, 188
Body mass, 94, 192, 323, 349
  lean, 106, 185, 188, 193, 194, 196, 216, 268, 319, 325
Body temperature, 139, 365, 366, 368
Body weight, 81, 99, 139, 190, 322, 345
  carbohydrates and, 161, 171, 249
Bone building, 60, 350–352
Bone density, 320, 326, 348, 350, 351, 352
Bone health, 60, 191, 267, 347–352, 363
  vitamin D and, 63–64, 352
Bone mass, 60–61, 357
  increase in, 351–352
  low, 317, 324, 348, 349, 351, 352
Brain, 191, 369
  boosting, 138, 260
  carbohydrates and, 142, 150
  glucose and, 142
Branched chain amino acids (BCAAs), 182
Breakfast, 163, 310, 372, 374, 388–390
  carbohydrate-based, 280, 297, 322

eating, 197, 297, 314, 322–323
ideas for, 288–289, 391
Build cycle, 105–107, 266–268
Bulimia nervosa, 343, 345, 346

Caffeine, 10, 64, 218, 219–221, 229, 279, 337
  consuming, 7, 349
  dehydration and, 6–8
  limiting, 6, 11, 299, 330
  performance and, 8, 220
  rehydration and, 160
Calcium, 13, 39, 68, 69, 71, 123, 150, 318, 321, 332, 356
  absorption of, 63, 64, 67, 349
  bone density and, 320, 326
  consuming, 60–61, 63–64, 267, 308, 326, 329, 330, 347, 348, 349, 350, 351, 357, 358
  loss, 64, 117, 351, 352
  pregnancy and, 329–330
  required, 61 (table), 332, 352
  sources of, 61, 62 (table), 64, 308, 320, 329–330, 348
Calories, 18, 31, 51, 36, 75, 122 (table), 167, 183, 213, 237, 252, 283, 306, 314
  activity level and, 92–93
  alcohol, 9 (table), 194
  balance of, 274, 328
  burning, 191, 248, 359
  carbohydrates and, 98, 124
  consuming, 82, 85, 91, 95, 102, 107, 108, 117, 121, 122, 196, 197, 250, 252, 265, 300, 301, 312, 318, 327, 328, 329, 349, 352, 359, 361, 363, 364, 371, 396
  covert, 11–12, 14
  decrease in, 108, 191, 195, 266, 325, 359
  endurance sports and, 92 (table)
  fat and, 100, 122–123
  inadequate, 361, 363, 371
  muscle building and, 178–179
  required, 90–93, 108, 248, 265, 270–271, 305, 307, 310, 325, 360, 371
  restricting, 98, 191, 193, 266, 276, 291, 309, 346
  sources of, 38, 124, 321
  training and, 91, 92 (table), 93, 94, 95, 114, 192
  weight loss and, 103, 194–195

413

Cancer, 9, 26, 31, 39, 52, 55, 58, 70, 72, 318
Carbohydrate loading, 107, 164, 245, 246, 248, 249, 261, 270, 275, 277, 278, 293, 296–297, 298, 302, 311–312, 312, 375
  plan for, 294, 362
  pre-competition, 164–168
Carbohydrates, 2, 4, 8, 56, 72, 74, 75, 81, 83, 121, 128, 141, 246, 257, 260, 268, 274, 300, 319, 320, 329, 353, 358, 369, 373, 374, 377
  adjustments in, 106, 129, 342
  balance of, 18, 240, 241
  body weight and, 161, 171, 249
  boost from, 277, 279, 280, 289
  calories and, 97–98, 124, 183, 266, 283
  carrying, 170, 277, 308
  classification of, 18, 21
  complex, 19–20, 21, 38, 147, 148, 377
  concentrated, 18, 23, 145, 167, 313
  consuming, 11, 17, 18, 20, 36, 51, 76, 82, 85, 97, 98, 99, 106, 108, 109, 113, 114–115, 116, 119, 122, 126, 130, 132, 133, 134, 135, 136, 146, 138, 142, 148, 149, 153–154, 156, 158, 161, 162, 164–165, 168–170, 177, 180, 181, 196, 240, 243, 244, 245, 250, 252, 254, 255, 261, 266, 269, 270, 271, 268, 272, 277, 279, 281, 282, 288, 289, 290, 294, 297, 298, 306, 311, 312, 325, 342–343, 354, 355–356, 357, 361, 362, 363, 364, 366, 371, 396
  content of, 110–113 (table)
  decrease in, 104, 194, 196, 253
  easily digested, 163, 165, 271, 275, 279, 280, 282, 294
  FODMAPs, 332, 334, 335
  liquid, 133, 148–149, 156, 242, 269, 271
  low-fiber, 114, 167, 249, 294
  low-glycemic, 21, 136, 199
  muscle building and, 178–179
  optimal, 18, 146, 161
  performance and, 20, 135, 145
  planning, 109, 114–116
  pre-event, 169–170, 269
  protein and, 157, 180, 184, 265
  quality, 20–21, 100
  recovery and, 96–99, 156–157, 193, 200, 343
  replacing, 149, 261, 300, 302, 361
  required, 95, 99, 100, 101, 109, 116, 117, 128, 157, 248, 265, 300, 307, 309, 325, 371
  simple, 18–19, 19–20, 21, 32, 146
  solid, 148–149, 156, 242

sources of, 1, 90, 114, 146–147, 148–149, 154, 247, 257, 272
  sports drinks and, 148, 242, 257, 278, 294
  stored, 35, 36, 79, 88, 98, 132, 164, 171, 270, 320
  training and, 90, 96–98, 102, 106, 108, 114–115, 126, 132–133, 193, 239, 314, 333, 342, 356
  wholesome, 21, 109, 163, 320, 372
Cardiovascular system, 55, 130, 139, 222, 326
Carotenoids, 28, 30, 58–59, 59 (table), 70, 72
Celiac disease, 315, 317, 331, 336, 338–339
Chloride, 60, 68, 71, 150
Cholesterol, 9, 34, 41, 44, 72, 74, 117, 123, 216–217, 323
Chromium, 59, 214–215
Collagen, 64, 359, 360
Constipation, 67, 331, 334, 335, 339, 345
Continuous Glucose Monitoring (CGM), 342
Copper, 59, 67, 292
Core temperature, 141, 368, 369
Cramping, 70, 287, 313, 315
Creatine, 201, 207, 208, 210, 223
Creatine-phosphate (CP), 79, 83, 84, 178, 181
Cross-training, 233, 264, 275, 304, 305, 351, 352, 368

Dairy, 33, 37, 39, 116, 180, 332
Dehydration, 3, 15, 136, 137, 145, 152, 158, 167, 189, 221, 247, 253, 268, 293, 345, 356, 368
  caffeine and, 6–8
  dealing with, 129, 138–139, 140, 295, 299, 300, 321, 366
  GI problems and, 139, 154
  minimizing, 32, 131, 138, 139, 140–141, 243, 298, 299
  risk of, 9, 138–139, 140, 270, 297
  signs of, 139–140, 154, 321, 326
  stomach emptying and, 255
  sweat loss and, 278
  weight loss and, 11
Designer waters, 4, 11–12, 14, 12 (table)
Diabetes, 31, 32, 39, 222, 315, 317, 318, 323, 325, 340–343
Diarrhea, 287, 299, 331, 339, 345
Diet, 2, 81, 329, 331–332, 344, 361
  balanced, 33, 53, 63, 75, 178, 265, 308, 317, 318, 319, 361
  carbohydrates and, 18, 19–20, 25, 354, 363
  elimination, 336–337
  gluten-free, 339–340

health and, 17, 20, 33, 53, 124, 324, 372
  high-carbohydrate, 165, 166, 311, 312, 363, 371
  high-fat, 100, 354
  inadequacies in, 50, 51, 191–192
  modification of, 47, 197, 284, 318, 353
  muscle-building, 183 (table)
  optimal, 109, 335, 387–394
  performance, 50, 129, 203
  periodizing, 101–102, 354–356
  planning, 2, 34, 99, 113–117, 164, 387–394
  rigid, 191, 268, 290, 309
  training, 17, 75, 77, 129, 202, 235, 248, 276, 304, 317, 331, 340
  vegetarian, 39, 51, 65, 124, 317, 318, 319
Digestion, 20, 132, 144–145, 238, 231, 261, 277, 278, 336
  exercise and, 239
  fiber and, 34
  time for, 131, 133
  water and, 5
Disordered eating, 324, 343–344, 346–347
Docosahexaenoic acid (DHA), 42, 45, 46, 330
Drinking, 147, 155, 159, 252, 254, 267, 296, 307
  body weight and, 322
  GI upset and, 153
  intensity and, 272, 273
  opportunities for, 141
  performance and, 254
  regular, 278, 322
  timing, 151, 152, 153, 272, 298
  training and, 136, 158, 160–161, 257

Eating, 268, 376
  boredom/stress and, 122
  disordered, 324, 343–344, 346–347
  healthy, 47, 305
  patterns, 122, 196, 198, 358
  planning, 198, 375
  pre-exercise, 132–133, 135, 197, 244, 288
  quality, 2, 291
  restrictive, 191, 195
  schedules and, 133–134, 239
  social, 196, 199, 310, 311
  timing of, 238, 299
  training and, 109, 133–134, 239, 257–258, 349
  travel and, 374–376
Eating Disorder Not Otherwise Specified (EDNOS), 343, 346, 347
Eating disorders, 324, 343–347, 348, 349

Electrolytes, 59, 68, 71, 76, 141, 236, 240, 243, 257, 287, 322, 345, 357, 366
  consuming, 138, 261, 342
  loss of, 11, 130, 138, 150–151, 246, 261, 346–347
  replacing, 152–155, 223, 267, 295, 300, 302
  tablets, 155, 252, 254, 258, 300
Elimination diet, 336–337
Endurance, 228, 245, 256, 260, 263, 264, 354, 362, 365
  aerobic, 286
  training, 1–2, 77, 90, 104, 127, 141, 149, 178, 184, 185, 255, 257, 371
Energy, 50, 145, 147, 176, 194, 218, 252, 269, 299, 307, 320, 359, 361
  aerobic/anaerobic, 84, 85
  boosts, 289, 301
  consuming, 47, 77, 178, 196, 319, 321, 323, 348, 349
  drop in, 185, 196, 240
  low, 126, 176, 196, 240
  needs, 90, 91, 92–96, 98, 149, 236–237, 314, 371
  production of, 84–86, 90, 126, 203, 304, 319
  required, 90–96, 126, 200, 309, 325, 328
  systems, 78, 79–80, 83, 83 (table), 84
  training and, 28, 38, 79, 96, 101, 106, 196, 265, 276, 307
Energy bars, 135, 149, 154, 184, 201, 202, 223, 238, 252, 257, 260, 271, 272, 275, 279, 281, 299, 300, 306, 312, 329
  calcium in, 351
  carrying, 269, 277, 313
  consuming, 114, 162, 164–165, 168
Environmental conditions, 254, 159, 236, 255, 266, 270, 287, 290, 298, 302, 313, 315, 321, 365
Enzymes, 31, 35, 36, 64, 158, 201, 203–204, 333, 359
Ergogenic aids, 76, 202, 209 (table), 229
  body composition and, 208, 210–218
  checklist for, 225–226
  common, 207–208, 207–222, 224–228
  performance and, 218–222, 224–228
  safety with, 204–207
Essential fatty acids, 38, 40, 99, 100, 117, 121, 320, 334
  omega-3, 42, 45, 121, 194
  omega-6, 42, 194
  sources of, 43–44 (table), 76
Estimated Average Requirement (EAR), 52
Estrogen, 61, 216, 349

Fat, 2, 4, 8, 56, 86, 88, 116, 117, 118 (table), 121, 126, 129, 135, 171, 179, 191, 219, 248, 266, 274
  alcohol and, 194
  balancing, 18, 241
  burning, 37, 89, 130, 162, 193, 201, 203, 218, 261, 266, 283, 353, 354, 355, 359
  calories from, 100, 122–123, 283
  consuming, 17, 36, 38, 41, 47, 51, 98, 100, 102, 106, 108, 123, 180, 197, 237, 240, 250, 277, 294, 308, 310, 325, 334, 354, 372, 373
  dietary, 41, 41 (table), 193, 334, 359
  facts/figures about, 38, 40–41
  healthy, 25, 40, 76, 109, 117, 126, 163, 308, 320, 334
  hidden, 115, 121, 197
  hydrogenated, 308
  loading, 353–354
  losing, 36, 40, 122, 185–199, 211, 219, 374
  monounsaturated, 41, 42, 117, 194
  polyunsaturated, 42
  required, 95, 99–100, 101, 102, 128, 169
  saturated, 37, 38, 39, 40–41, 123, 308, 317
  sources of, 1, 41 (table), 90, 120 (table)
  storing, 35, 37, 100, 130, 353
  training and, 90, 102, 106, 108
  trans, 40–41, 44
  unsaturated, 41,
Fatigue, 15, 65, 126, 140, 148, 149, 196, 220, 268, 270, 282, 292, 311, 314, 321, 329, 339
  anaerobic system and, 79
  described, 127–128
  mental, 128, 301
  nutrition and, 128
Fiber, 2, 21, 23, 25, 30, 84, 123, 161, 299, 327, 334
  fitting in, 31, 34, 197, 299, 318
Fluid loss, 3, 4, 5, 128, 139, 140, 160, 252, 268, 281, 307, 321, 363, 368, 375
  monitoring, 306
  recovery and, 159
  replacing, 6, 265, 366, 367, 370
Fluids, 3, 47, 130, 155, 253, 254, 257, 268, 300, 320
  accessibility of, 153
  adequate, 161, 289
  balance, 155, 246, 287, 297
  caffeine and, 7, 7 (table)
  carbohydrates and, 144, 253, 254
  carrying, 170, 267, 282, 308
  consuming, 1, 4–7, 10, 11, 12, 119, 121, 136, 137, 138, 140, 141, 143,

152, 153, 154, 155, 158–159, 244, 249, 253, 254, 256, 269, 270, 274, 277, 279, 289, 290, 293, 296, 298, 300, 301, 307
  obtaining, 140, 152, 268
  recovery, 121, 158–159, 296
  replacing, 152–155, 267, 300, 302, 307, 367
  required, 100, 159, 267, 290, 306–307, 326, 329, 371
Folate, 55, 327, 328, 338, 371
Folic acid, 51, 54–55, 327, 328
Food and Drug Administration (FDA), 14, 203, 204, 217, 336
Food intolerances, 317, 336, 337
Food journals, 119–122, 126, 196, 198, 200, 337
Foods, 113–117, 119
  animal, 40, 44, 318
  carbohydrate contents of, 110–113 (table), 115, 119, 293, 310
  choosing, 106, 109, 196, 242, 311
  consuming, 17, 198, 314, 322, 342
  convenience, 47, 308, 392
  easily digested, 244, 250
  ethnic, 392–394
  fatty, 40, 123, 167, 197, 308
  fiber-rich, 34, 170
  folate-rich, 55, 55 (table)
  healthy, 31, 318, 372, 374
  high-carbohydrate, 162, 168 (table), 294, 296
  iron-rich, 74, 329
  low-fiber, 132, 168 (table), 171
  nutrient-dense, 20, 50, 51, 156, 265, 325, 326
  plant, 37, 38, 39, 54, 74, 319
  pre-race, 246, 293, 375, 387
  preparing, 169, 258, 310, 376, 388
  processed, 2, 258, 335
  protein content of, 37 (table)
  recovery, 121, 162, 241, 296
  sensitivities to, 331, 335–340
  training and, 239–240, 300
Fructose, 19, 23, 32, 33, 146, 148, 299, 332, 333, 377
Fruits, 26, 33, 56, 58, 71, 72, 115–116, 117, 168, 184, 197, 238, 253, 290, 299, 308, 311, 312, 314
  choosing, 29 (table)
  consuming, 28–30, 39, 318, 351, 374
  fiber from, 31
  nutrition from, 29, 360
Fuel, 86, 149, 178, 181, 198, 236, 272, 284, 319, 323
  adequate, 89, 275
  calories from, 81 (table)
  consuming, 129, 152
  depletion of, 78, 128, 129, 242, 311
  exercise and, 86 (fig.), 130, 141–142

heart rate and, 87–88
high-quality, 17
intensity and, 77, 83 (fig.), 89
performance and, 132
recovery and, 28, 102
replacing, 129, 131, 141, 152–155
training and, 89, 98, 102, 128, 134,
    257, 261, 287–288
using, 82–84, 178
Fueling, 149, 169, 236, 241, 244, 247,
    271, 272, 281, 287, 293, 298, 302,
    309, 340, 342
on bike, 268–269
cold and, 368–369
leanness and, 283
long run, 288–289
plans for, 153, 174, 258–259, 293,
    341, 343

Gastric emptying, 145, 146, 154, 161,
    271
Gastrointestinal (GI) distress, 31, 34,
    65, 128, 140, 167, 170, 220, 229,
    272, 296, 317, 331, 335
amino acids and, 212
iron and, 67
Gastrointestinal (GI) system, 19, 132,
    135, 140, 146, 153, 247, 248, 249,
    253, 254, 255, 299
adaptation by, 238, 287
blood glucose and, 239
dehydration and, 139, 154
endurance sports and, 268
fiber and, 31
gels and, 154
Gels, 20, 154, 168, 201, 202, 238, 242,
    243, 247, 252, 253, 257, 258, 272,
    279, 281, 298, 299, 312, 329, 342,
    369, 396
caffeine-containing, 229, 260
carbohydrate, 15, 135, 149, 174, 278,
    280, 300
carrying, 269, 277, 313
choosing, 278, 294
consuming, 163, 164, 254, 255, 261,
    273, 288, 298
GI problems and, 154
gluten-free, 340
sodium-containing, 294, 367
water and, 246
Glucose, 4, 23, 32, 55, 81, 89, 146, 221,
    222, 340–341, 371, 377
adequate, 255
boost from, 301
brain and, 142
carbohydrates and, 320
fiber and, 31
fructose and, 148
maintaining, 214, 364, 366
metabolism of, 71, 214

muscle fibers and, 141
polymers, 19, 148
sucrose and, 148
Gluten, 338–340
Glycemic index (GI), 22 (table), 24,
    135–136, 147, 377–380
blood glucose and, 21, 23, 25
low, 25, 161, 199, 341
Glycemic load (GL), 22 (table), 24
Glycogen, 5, 36, 53, 82, 153, 156, 167,
    218, 248, 254, 269, 294, 311, 320
depletion of, 80, 96–97, 129, 131,
    194, 220, 242, 272, 297, 346–347,
    355
loading, 107, 166, 362, 364
muscle, 54, 89
protein and, 55
replenishing, 81, 98–99, 106, 157,
    265, 272, 275, 294
stores, 81, 82, 89, 166, 179, 239, 249,
    281, 294, 354, 355, 361
Glycolysis, 79, 83, 85, 86, 181, 224
Good Manufacturing Processes
    (GMPs), 204–205, 207
Grains, 2, 72, 114–115, 117, 319, 340
whole, 25–26, 27, 33, 39, 47

Headaches, 222, 321, 339, 370
Health, 18, 47, 130, 317, 372
dehydration and, 140
diet and, 17, 20, 323
management of, 185, 197, 325
optimal, 25, 35, 52, 286
problems, 117, 323, 324
Heart disease, 26, 39, 40, 52, 55, 70, 71,
    226, 318
fiber and, 31
risk of, 8, 9, 38, 41, 117
Heart rate, 94, 220, 221, 247, 369, 370
exercise and, 89
fuel and, 87–88
increased, 139
Heart rate monitors, 87, 88, 94
Heat, 193, 368, 369
dealing with, 141, 151, 252, 255,
    326, 366
dehydration and, 138
nutrition and, 367
sweating and, 138
Heat illness, 140, 356, 365–366
Hemoglobin, 35, 65, 67, 74, 291, 292,
    360
High-density lipoprotein (HDL), 8–9,
    40
High-fructose corn syrup (HFCS), 19,
    32–33, 333
Hormones, 4, 35, 36, 56, 60, 61, 158,
    203, 216, 305, 348, 349
calories and, 351
growth, 212, 214

imbalance in, 191, 238
replacing, 349
sex, 352
stress, 361
synthesis of, 359
thyroid, 217
Hunger, 80, 131, 197, 241, 248, 270, 287,
    293, 372
preventing, 143, 196, 198, 297
training and, 132, 136, 241
Hydration, 3, 121, 137, 145, 153, 163,
    169, 170, 181, 189, 236, 244, 246,
    247, 273, 275, 277, 281, 287, 290,
    296, 297, 298, 301, 322, 370
adequate, 89, 100, 167, 289, 312
caffeine and, 6, 8
cold and, 368–369
environmental conditions and,
    139, 313
focusing on, 242, 282, 314
guidelines for, 100, 258, 267, 272,
    289
improving, 10, 11, 148, 174, 321, 329
indicators of, 249, 282
maintaining, 6, 10–11, 152, 159, 170,
    181, 254–255, 258, 259, 277, 281,
    308, 357, 374
optimal, 4, 236, 273, 280, 369
plans for, 174, 258–259, 280, 293
pre-race, 171, 293
sports drinks and, 171, 282, 300
strategies for, 11, 15, 140, 322 (table)
systems, 154, 244, 246, 258, 277, 369
training and, 11, 136–138, 138–142,
    257
Hyperglycemia, 340
Hyperhydration, 221, 297
Hypertension, 39, 318, 325
Hypoglycemia, 134, 143, 266, 282, 287,
    329, 340, 341
developing, 131, 135, 154, 255, 270
preventing, 269, 270, 342
Hyponatremia, 70, 150, 250, 295, 296,
    297, 298
developing, 151–152, 367, 300
Hypothermia, 255, 369

Immune system, 1, 17, 35, 42, 49, 63, 72,
    76, 213, 271, 315, 336, 356
boosting, 155, 360–361
carbohydrates and, 18
suppressing, 361
Insulin, 23, 132, 134, 333, 335, 340, 341,
    342, 343
Intensity, 78, 104–105, 181, 255, 256,
    257, 258, 264, 300, 366
dehydration and, 139
high, 105, 276, 280, 282, 305, 327
nutrition and, 77, 89, 266, 272,
    273, 288

training, 84, 92, 96, 107, 113, 130, 149, 153–154, 155, 159, 161, 166, 229, 242, 243, 252, 267, 274, 281, 282, 304, 308, 309, 341, 358

Intervals, 96, 129, 141, 142, 227, 263, 264, 306, 307, 355

Iron, 37, 59, 60, 68, 123, 291–292, 318, 326, 329, 330, 338, 361, 371
 absorption of, 56, 65, 66, 291
 anemia and, 65, 191, 292
 consuming, 64–67, 74, 267, 271, 292, 321, 329
 menstruation and, 65, 308
 recovery and, 360
 required, 74, 308
 sources of, 66 (table), 67, 74, 267, 291, 321
 vitamin C and, 66, 291

Iron deficiency, 65, 74, 291, 292, 321

Ironman, 146, 152, 165, 233, 234, 236, 249, 255
 calories for, 248, 252
 nutrition for, 247, 250, 252

Irritable bowel syndrome (IBS), 315, 317, 331–335

Juices, 14, 32, 33, 115–116, 117, 145, 168, 183, 184, 197, 242

Labels, checking, 33, 40, 121, 122–123, 161, 184, 333, 351, 390–391

Lactate threshold, 87, 88, 89, 105

Lactic acid, 5, 79, 83, 85, 87, 89, 106, 224, 305, 330, 366

Lactose, 19, 32, 63, 182, 299, 332–333, 338, 377

Lactose intolerance, 61, 117, 332, 336, 339

Laxatives, 344, 345, 346, 347

Lipids, 31, 40, 58, 325, 327

Liver glycogen, 80–81, 134, 170, 174
 depleting, 60, 138, 239, 297
 replenishing, 130, 131, 132, 136, 170, 282, 287, 323
 stores, 247, 259, 269, 288, 292, 309

Low-density lipoprotein (LDL), 40, 41, 72

Magnesium, 60, 64, 68, 69, 71, 356, 358

Marathons, 285, 287, 295
 nutrition for, 294, 296–298, 302

Meals, 2, 126, 199, 238, 258, 287
 balanced, 197, 240
 healthy, 168, 373, 375
 high-carbohydrate, 169 (table), 239, 266, 302, 309
 liquid, 133, 288, 300
 planning, 35, 47, 109, 113, 136, 164, 165, 171, 183, 194, 200, 241, 241 (table), 283, 293–294, 308, 373,

387, 387–388, 389, 390, 395, 396, 396–402
 pre-exercise, 131, 133, 135, 137 (table), 165, 169 (table), 170, 172 (table), 173, 184, 288, 312, 340
 pre-race, 167, 170, 244, 245, 246, 250, 270, 273, 275, 277, 281, 292–294, 297, 299, 313
 recovery, 241, 322
 sample, 396–402
 timing, 171, 172 (table), 238–240, 293, 299, 314, 375
 travel, 375 (table)
 vegetarian, 395

Meat, 67, 158, 197, 310, 319

Medium chain triglycerides (MCTs), 221

Menopause, 61, 326, 348

Menstruation, 65, 308, 321, 331, 345, 346, 347, 348, 349, 363

Metabolism, 49, 53, 60, 68, 131, 191, 217, 221, 321, 347, 363, 370, 371
 aerobic/anaerobic, 84, 86, 90, 305
 carbohydrate, 55
 energy, 59, 360
 estrogen, 72
 fat, 56, 354
 folic acid, 54
 glucose, 71, 214
 protein, 117
 resting, 92

Minerals, 13, 21, 25, 28, 29, 30, 32, 33, 39, 49–50, 72, 117, 164, 185, 203, 223, 318, 319, 320, 330, 358
 consuming, 1, 52, 59–61, 63–68, 69–70, 327, 329, 361
 deficiency in, 338, 356
 list of, 381–383
 low-dose, 326
 required, 371

Morning noshes, ideas for, 288–289

Multivitamins, 11, 63, 67, 68, 215, 291, 326, 328, 330, 352, 361, 371
 choosing, 69–70, 327

Muscle cramps, 155, 246, 356–358

Muscle damage, 155, 157, 165, 211, 280

Muscle dysmorphia, 344, 346

Muscle glycogen, 75, 81–82, 85, 88, 89, 97, 102, 136, 156, 157, 165, 166, 170, 179, 181, 214, 219, 221, 239, 252, 265, 275, 288, 292, 294, 302, 311, 312, 362, 366
 breakdown/synthesis of, 60, 98, 99, 178, 289, 306
 depletion of, 106, 128, 129–130, 138, 142, 147, 184, 276, 280, 306, 371
 replenishing, 98, 131, 155, 166, 180, 282, 323
 storing, 131, 156, 268, 270
 training and, 97 (fig.)

women and, 362

Muscles, 176, 190, 192, 193, 201, 214, 216, 268, 325
 building, 78, 175, 177–181, 183, 183 (table), 185, 196, 203, 212, 219, 229, 265, 304, 305, 308, 320, 344
 ergogenic aids and, 208
 loss of, 191, 238, 270
 repairing/maintaining, 35, 36, 37, 359
 superloading, 107
 supplements and, 223

Nausea, 139, 140, 222, 336, 339, 370

Nutrients, 3, 4, 12, 18, 25, 30, 31, 34, 50, 64, 67, 68, 69, 115, 119, 123, 207, 318, 330
 balance of, 122, 349
 bone-building, 352
 consuming, 17, 47, 161, 323, 332, 396
 deficiencies in, 52, 206, 346, 356
 essential, 28, 39, 63, 116, 320
 required, 90, 96 (table), 236–237, 329
 specific, 325–327
 vegetarians and, 318, 319

Nutrition, 20, 33, 35, 47, 52, 69, 115, 116, 129, 156, 174, 205, 206, 236, 252, 318, 319, 324
 adequate, 1, 75, 106, 286, 373
 attention for, 278, 282, 314
 breakdown of, 122–123
 competition, 150, 258–259, 271–272, 275, 277–278, 286, 292–294, 296–298, 300–301, 304, 309, 311–313
 considerations about, 231, 235, 244, 246, 271, 286, 315
 fatigue and, 128
 guidelines for, 78, 197, 240, 244, 276, 315, 325
 information on, 92, 122, 200, 203
 intensity and, 266, 272
 issues/by specific groups, 307–309
 long-distance, 251 (table)
 muscle building and, 178–181
 optimal, 18, 247, 361
 performance and, 2, 304, 364
 post-exercise, 76, 160, 256
 pre-race, 249, 259
 problem solving with, 356–364
 recovery, 12, 76, 155, 165, 197, 240, 256, 257, 260, 265, 266, 267, 272, 274, 276, 282, 287, 289–290, 305–307, 309, 323, 358–360, 361, 362, 364
 required, 78, 90, 101, 109, 264, 309, 311, 325, 396
 timing, 162–163, 179–181

training, 130–138, 235–242,
    240, 252–254, 256, 264–269,
    270–271, 274–275, 276–277,
    286–292, 304–309, 363–364
triathlon, 245 (table)
women and, 361–364, 362
Nutrition plans, 44, 170, 196, 231, 243,
    244, 260, 283, 284, 293, 325, 357,
    358, 379, 396
competition, 173, 231
diabetes and, 341
high-energy, 165
personalized, 324
travel and, 375
vegetarians and, 39
Nutrition products, 20, 164–165, 201,
    202, 207
compared, 384–386
Nutritional periodization, 101 (table)

Oils
cod liver, 46
fish, 45–46
liquid, 40, 41
monounsaturated, 41, 42, 121
partially hydrogenated, 40, 44
polyunsaturated, 41, 57, 121
soy/canola, 44
Osteopenia, 345, 348, 350
Osteoporosis, 9, 52, 61, 71, 267, 325,
    326, 338, 345, 348
men and, 349–350
Overhydration, 154, 246, 250, 279, 293,
    295, 296, 307
problems with, 278, 297
Oxygen, 4, 12, 79, 85, 86, 94, 370
transport, 59, 60

Pantothenic acid, 51, 55–56
Performance, 3, 23, 28, 187, 193, 200,
    216, 275, 305, 308, 324, 343
absorption and, 146
aerobic, 265
athletic, 201, 202, 205
body fat and, 185, 186
caffeine and, 8, 219
carbohydrates and, 20, 135, 146
ergogenic aids and, 218–222,
    224–228
impairing, 8, 54, 134, 221, 309,
    321, 368
improving, 54, 134, 135, 146, 148,
    175, 176, 185, 202, 206, 218, 219,
    220, 229, 270, 276, 286, 290, 324,
    344, 353–356
nutrition and, 2, 50, 129, 270, 304,
    364
optimal, 6, 25, 35, 176, 320
sports drinks and, 145, 147
training and, 134, 192, 291

vitamins and, 50, 56, 59, 64
women and, 362, 363
Physiological issues, 50, 60, 127, 171,
    234, 324, 325
Phytochemicals, 25, 29, 50, 72, 360
Phytonutrients, 28, 30, 33, 72, 185, 318
Portions, 18, 102, 198, 238, 277, 281,
    294, 314, 319, 388
calories and, 122 (table)
checking, 199
size of, 122, 311
Potassium, 28, 60, 68, 71, 150, 357
Power, 77, 78–79, 263, 368
developing, 34, 99, 127, 276
loss of, 191, 238, 268
Prebiotics/probiotics, 335, 361
Pregnant athletes, 327–330
Prohormones, 215–217
Protein, 2, 8, 56, 76, 86, 118 (table), 126,
    128, 129, 135, 155, 158, 163, 248,
    260, 266, 274, 306, 312, 318, 320,
    338, 358, 373
animal, 39, 124, 319
balance in, 18, 179, 213, 241
breakdown of, 162, 191
building, 180, 182, 197, 214
calories from, 116, 183, 283
carbohydrates and, 157, 180, 184, 265
consuming, 17, 35, 36, 38, 39, 47,
    51, 64, 85, 99, 102, 106, 108, 117,
    121, 157, 177, 178, 179, 180, 181,
    196, 240, 250, 265, 279, 290, 325,
    326, 349, 363
easily digested, 165, 250
function of, 35–36
high-quality, 47, 158, 182, 184, 212,
    265, 307, 308, 319
lean, 47, 117, 121, 126, 163, 197, 242,
    271, 277, 320, 376
muscle building, 179, 320
plant, 37, 39, 54, 116, 319
portions of, 161, 162, 277, 294
power from, 34–38
recovery and, 82, 99, 157–158, 200,
    359
required, 36, 38, 95, 99, 100, 101,
    108, 124, 128, 158, 169, 265,
    307, 360
resistance training and, 180, 184
sources of, 1, 37–38, 37 (table), 90,
    179, 184
storage of, 35, 82, 371
synthesis of, 36, 179, 180, 182, 214
training and, 35, 37, 90, 102, 117,
    149–150, 150, 161
vegetarians and, 124–125
weight training and, 181, 185

Recovery, 15, 71, 90, 92, 93, 100, 106,
    121, 155, 166, 176, 178, 181, 184,

236, 239, 241, 242, 264, 270, 278,
    284, 302, 308, 312, 336, 340,
    360, 361, 372
agents, 212
amino acids and, 213
carbohydrates and, 96–99, 156–157,
    193, 200, 343
energy for, 28, 102
foods/fluids for, 121, 158–159, 296
immediate, 98, 156–159
improving, 76, 161, 222, 311, 314,
    319, 358–360
nutrition for, 1, 12, 47, 76, 77, 78,
    90, 155, 155–161, 161 (table),
    165, 197, 240, 256, 257, 260, 265,
    266, 267, 272, 274, 276, 282, 287,
    289–290, 305–307, 309, 323,
    361, 362, 364
optimal, 6, 109, 157
poor, 65, 266, 276, 283, 304, 310
post-exercise, 160–161, 162
protein and, 82, 99, 157–158, 200
sodium and, 159–160, 162
sports drinks and, 261
timing, 238, 240
training and, 240, 315
Recovery drinks, 20, 30, 161, 164, 202,
    249, 290, 351
Refueling, 149, 157, 239, 242, 243, 248,
    268, 269, 277, 279
opportunities for, 258, 278
planning, 293–294
Rehydration, 7, 15, 76, 141, 155, 159, 163,
    186, 222, 240, 242, 243, 247, 260,
    274, 277, 278
techniques for, 160, 290, 367
Resistance training, 99, 106, 130, 178,
    181, 192, 227, 257, 325
carbohydrates and, 180
glutamine and, 214
protein and, 180, 184
Rest, 85, 93, 108, 167, 271, 273
Restaurants, dietary rules for, 391–394
Resting metabolic rate (RMR), 91, 93,
    94, 95, 191
lowering, 185, 192, 193, 194, 196
Running, 244, 285–286, 293
fluid/sodium balance for, 295–296
gastrointestinal distress and, 299
iron and, 291
nutrition and, 254–255

Salt, consuming, 152, 252, 254, 255, 297,
    300, 357, 367, 374
Snacks, 2, 115, 121, 126, 197, 238, 311,
    391 (table)
carbohydrate, 157, 277
consuming, 171, 287, 297, 308, 314,
    322–323
healthy, 323, 372, 373

high-carbohydrate, 169, 239, 266, 309

nutrition, 47, 164

planning, 241, 312, 388–390

protein, 180

recovery, 165, 179, 240, 242

timing, 173, 238–240, 273, 314

training and, 135, 160, 277, 288, 332, 340

travel and, 375 (table)

Sodium, 6, 60, 68, 76, 163, 249, 256, 257, 260, 278, 368

blood pressure and, 151, 152

consuming, 70–71, 150–151, 152, 155, 161, 246, 259, 267, 279, 300, 349

depletion of, 15, 71, 246, 367

fluids and, 295–296

gels and, 294, 367

loss, 138, 150, 159, 160, 240, 252, 255, 357, 358, 366

overhydration and, 250

recovery and, 159–160, 162

sports drinks and, 137, 151–152, 155, 252, 254, 278–279, 357

sweating and, 70, 151, 152, 295, 367

Sodium bicarbonate, 224–226

Speed, 78, 127, 201, 306

training, 129, 141, 142

Sports drinks, 4, 11, 20, 47, 71, 119, 133, 135, 149, 157, 174, 202, 241, 243, 275, 277, 281, 287, 293, 311, 312, 313, 329, 396

carbohydrates and, 148, 242, 253, 257, 278, 294

consuming, 141, 142, 147–148, 153–154, 160, 162, 164, 181, 183, 244, 245, 246, 254, 265, 268, 269, 271, 274, 278, 296, 308, 314, 322, 323, 342

experimenting with, 257, 293

hydration and, 171, 282, 300

performance and, 145, 147

sodium in, 137, 151–152, 155, 246, 252, 254, 278, 278–279, 296, 357, 367

training and, 147, 154, 155

Steroids, 215, 216, 219, 346

Stomach emptying, 140, 253, 254, 255, 268, 272, 277, 279, 299, 300

Strength, 99, 127, 191, 201, 255, 263, 325

building, 34, 175, 184, 195, 229

Strength-to-weight ratio, 283, 325

Strength training, 99, 102, 116, 176, 179, 181, 183, 201, 257, 263, 264

Sucrose, 19, 32, 146, 377

Sugar, 18, 23, 148

complex/simple, 377

risks of, 32–33

Supplements, 50, 51, 58, 59, 63, 68, 76, 109, 121, 133, 136, 164, 168, 204, 208, 215, 249, 348, 350–351

banning of, 203, 204, 207

choosing, 69–70, 206

consuming, 52, 55, 67, 182, 225, 229, 292, 331

cross-contamination and, 202, 207

evaluating, 225–226, 300

high-carbohydrate, 149, 202, 300, 306, 312

legal/effective/safe, 202–203, 205, 207, 267

nutritional, 206, 207, 223

protein, 181, 182, 184, 307

sports nutrition, 10, 164, 168, 169, 173, 201, 249, 258, 259, 266, 271

testing, 202, 205, 208

weight-loss, 201, 217–218

Sweat loss, 139, 149, 158, 174, 240, 243, 253, 261, 265, 267, 268, 290, 297, 307

environmental conditions and, 154

estimating, 141, 143–144, 144 (fig.), 295, 306, 403

fluids and, 136, 141

minimizing, 153, 298

replacing, 145, 153, 366

sodium consumption and, 152

training and, 136, 143

weight monitoring and, 153

Sweat rate, 138, 141, 152, 242, 243, 252, 260, 267, 282, 302, 306, 307, 313, 363, 367

acclimatization and, 154

determining, 144, 174, 296, 357

minimizing, 298

training and, 5

weight and, 295

Sweating, 3, 71, 138, 159, 167, 293, 321, 329, 363

body weight and, 139

calcium and, 60, 352

fluid loss and, 4, 5, 6

iron and, 65, 74

sodium and, 70, 151, 295, 367

Swimming, 242–243, 303, 305, 306

nutrition and, 307–308, 312–313

Synthesis, protein, 36, 177, 179, 180, 182, 360

Tapering, 105, 152, 164, 165, 231, 237, 246, 247, 261, 311, 312, 362

carbohydrates and, 166–167

drinking and, 151

eating for, 248–249

pre-race, 294, 296, 297

Tolerances, 132, 133, 145, 254, 258, 271, 289, 298, 302

determining, 288, 396

fluid, 293

gastrointestinal, 131, 363

gut, 149, 247

Train low, compete high, using, 354–356

Training, 100, 109, 119, 121, 158, 162, 170, 194, 205, 268–269, 311, 319, 349, 364, 372

aerobic/anaerobic, 81, 263, 265, 303, 304

base, 86, 90, 193, 229

blood glucose and, 130

calories and, 91, 92 (table), 93, 94, 95, 192

carbohydrates and, 90, 96, 97–98, 102, 106, 108, 114–115, 126, 132–133, 193, 239, 266, 314, 333, 342, 356

cycles, 75, 90, 101, 102, 104–105, 106, 108, 109, 126, 165, 238, 240, 318, 396

diet for, 17, 75, 77, 129, 202, 235, 248, 304

duration of, 84, 96, 109, 146

early, 133, 134, 239, 323, 355

eating and, 109, 131–133, 133–134, 257–258, 265

endurance, 90, 95, 99, 104, 157, 178, 193, 304

energy for, 28, 38, 79, 96, 101, 107, 118, 196, 265, 307

fluids and, 139, 153, 268, 366

food and, 129, 239–240, 300

fuel for, 86 (fig.), 89, 98, 102, 128, 130, 134, 141–142, 257, 261, 287–288

heavy, 77, 94, 114–115, 126, 138, 214, 240, 289–290, 304, 318, 361

hot-weather, 138–139, 365–366

hunger and, 132, 136, 241

hydration and, 11, 136–138, 138–142, 147, 154, 155, 158, 160–161, 257

intensity of, 80–87, 92, 96, 105, 106, 109, 149, 153–154, 155, 159, 161, 166, 229, 242, 243, 267, 274, 282, 304, 308, 309, 327, 353, 358, 368

muscle glycogen and, 97 (fig.)

nutrition for, 96 (table), 130–138, 235–242, 240, 256, 270–271, 274–275, 276–277, 286–292, 287, 304–309, 337, 363–364

programs, 1, 78, 88, 89, 97, 113, 174, 203, 236, 243, 256, 264, 285, 286, 305, 310, 315, 327, 353, 396

protein and, 35, 37, 90, 102, 106, 108, 117, 149–150, 161

quality, 1, 93, 127, 129, 176, 240, 271, 291, 314

schedules, 98, 126, 133, 235–236, 238, 239, 240, 261, 280, 302, 370, 396
    sweat loss and, 136, 143
    volume of, 105, 276, 290, 358
    weight loss and, 193–194, 307
    women and, 362, 363
Transition, 105, 108, 250, 256, 264–265
    nutrition in, 252–254, 254–255
    refueling/rehydrating in, 278
Travel, eating and, 374–376, 375 (table)
Triathlons, 231, 233, 234, 243, 261
    energy intake for, 236, 237
    nutrition for, 245 (table)

Ultradistance events, 152, 285, 295, 298
Ultraendurance events, 86, 149, 354, 357
Ultrarunning, 298, 300–301
Urine, 159, 254, 255, 293, 341, 366
    light-colored, 249, 267, 277, 282, 289, 296, 297, 312, 357, 370
    production of, 7, 159, 160, 167, 210, 370

Vegans, 39, 61, 68, 124, 318
Vegetables, 26, 28–30, 33, 47, 56, 58, 71, 72, 114, 119, 197, 319, 360, 373
    choosing, 29 (table), 30
    consuming, 28, 30–31, 39, 318, 351
Vegetarians, 39, 51, 63, 65, 67, 68, 116
    nutrition for, 317–319
    planning for, 125, 395
    protein and, 124–125
    types of, 39, 318
Vitamin A, 28, 38, 50, 51, 69, 321, 338, 361

consuming, 58–59, 330
Vitamin B, 25, 39, 51, 53–56, 68, 69, 318, 326, 338, 360, 361
    consuming, 53, 54, 55, 371
Vitamin C, 14, 28, 30, 51, 64, 69, 70, 74, 123, 125, 292, 359
    consuming, 56–57, 360, 371
    food sources of, 56 (table), 67
    iron and, 66, 291
Vitamin D, 38, 39, 50, 51, 68, 69, 318, 320, 321, 338, 347, 361
    bone health and, 63–64, 352
    consuming, 59, 349, 351
    required, 61 (table), 326, 332
Vitamin E, 38, 50, 51, 57–58, 69, 70, 338, 361, 371
    food sources of, 56 (table)
Vitamin K, 38, 50, 51, 59, 64, 338
Vitamins, 21, 25, 28, 30, 32, 49–50, 53–59, 68, 70, 72, 164, 185, 203, 223, 318–320, 358, 371
    consuming, 1, 11, 49, 51, 52, 69, 326, 329, 361
    deficiency in, 50, 51, 338
    fat-soluble, 50, 51, 320, 338
    list of, 381–383
    recovery and, 360
    water-soluble, 51, 56
VO$_2$ max, 82, 87, 88, 105, 142, 176, 228, 234, 325, 362, 363, 366

Water, 3, 4–6, 246, 253, 282, 322, 426
    balance, 35
    bottled, 13–14, 375
    drinking, 12, 31, 142, 159, 254, 269, 355, 367

Weight, 176, 309
    body fat and, 186, 188
    goal for, 100, 192–193, 236, 343
    sweat loss and, 153
    sweat rates and, 295
    training cycles and, 103
Weight gain, 91, 100, 195, 222, 248, 249, 298, 327, 344, 345
    pattern of, 328
    preventing, 359
    unwanted, 284, 347
Weight loss, 11, 51, 91, 143, 186, 237, 240, 266, 271, 302, 310, 344, 347, 371
    calories and, 103, 194–195
    goals for, 191, 193, 194, 195, 200, 291, 302
    guidelines for, 195–199, 268, 309
    performance and, 158
    rapid, 185, 291
    strategies for, 291, 306
    training and, 193–194, 307
Weight management, 10, 13, 82, 129, 143, 154, 186–187, 197, 198, 261, 290, 296, 308, 344
Weight training, 102, 106, 178, 179, 180, 184, 263, 265, 270, 290, 325, 351, 352
    diet for, 181, 183
    protein and, 185
    supplements and, 211

Zinc, 37, 59, 67, 68, 292, 318, 360, 361

Monique Ryan, MS, RD, CSSD, LDN, is a nationally recognized nutritionist with over twenty-five years of professional experience. She is founder of Personal Nutrition Designs, LLC, a nutrition consulting company based in the Chicago area. Monique has developed thousands of nutrition plans for clients in the areas of sports nutrition, weight management, women's health, eating disorder recovery, various medical and health concerns, and disease prevention and wellness.

Monique is currently the sports dietitian for the professional cycling team Team Type 1 and has extensive experience working with elite athletes. She was a member of the Performance Enhancement Team for USA Triathlon, USA Cycling (Women's Road Team), and Synchro Swimming USA up to the 2004 Athens Olympic Games. She has consulted for multiple seasons with the Timex Multisport Team and the Chicago Fire Soccer Team, and was the nutritionist for the Saturn Cycling Team for the 1994 to 2000 racing seasons. Monique has also consulted with professional football, baseball, and basketball players, and team sport athletes competing at the high school and collegiate levels. She has also consulted with many professional endurance triathletes, the Volvo-Cannondale Mountain Bike, Rollerblade Racing, and the Trek-Volkswagen and Gary Fisher Mountain Bike teams. Monique lectures extensively on sports nutrition to coaches, athletic trainers, and amateur athletes. She has presented across the United States and in Canada, Brazil, Australia, and Thailand. Monique is quoted frequently for sports nutrition articles, and her comments have appeared in the *Chicago Tribune, New York Times, Chicago Sun-Times, Runner's World, Fitness, Men's Journal, Men's Health, Outside, Oxygen, Her Sports,* and *Traithlete,* among other publications.

Monique is the author of *Performance Nutrition for Winter Sports, Performance Nutrition for Team Sports,* and *Complete Guide to Sports Nutrition,* as well as over 175 published magazine articles. She was a regular contributor to *VeloNews—The Journal of Competitive Cycling* and to *Inside Triathlon.* She has appeared on CLTV, FOX-TV, and WGN, ABC, and CBS news.

Monique is a member of the Sports, Cardiovascular, and Wellness Nutritionists (SCAN) practice group and is a Certified Specialist in Sports Dietetics (CSSD). She has a Bachelor of Science degree in Nutrition and Dietetics and a Master of Science degree in Nutrition. She is a registered dietitian (RD) licensed in the state of Illinois (LDN), a member of the American College of Sports Medicine (ACSM), and an ACSM Health Fitness Instructor (HFI). Monique regularly participates in the sports of swimming, cycling, running, and snowshoeing and has competed as a licensed cyclist in the sports of road cycling and mountain biking.